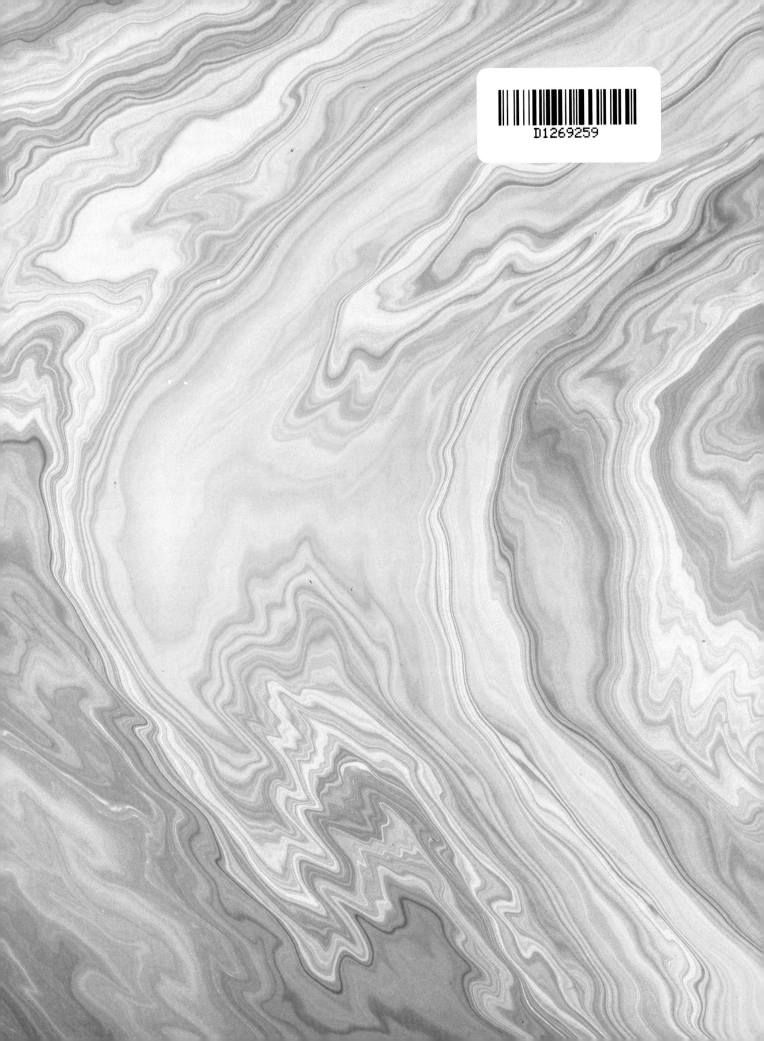

The Art Of Fashion Accessories

A Twentieth Century Retrospective

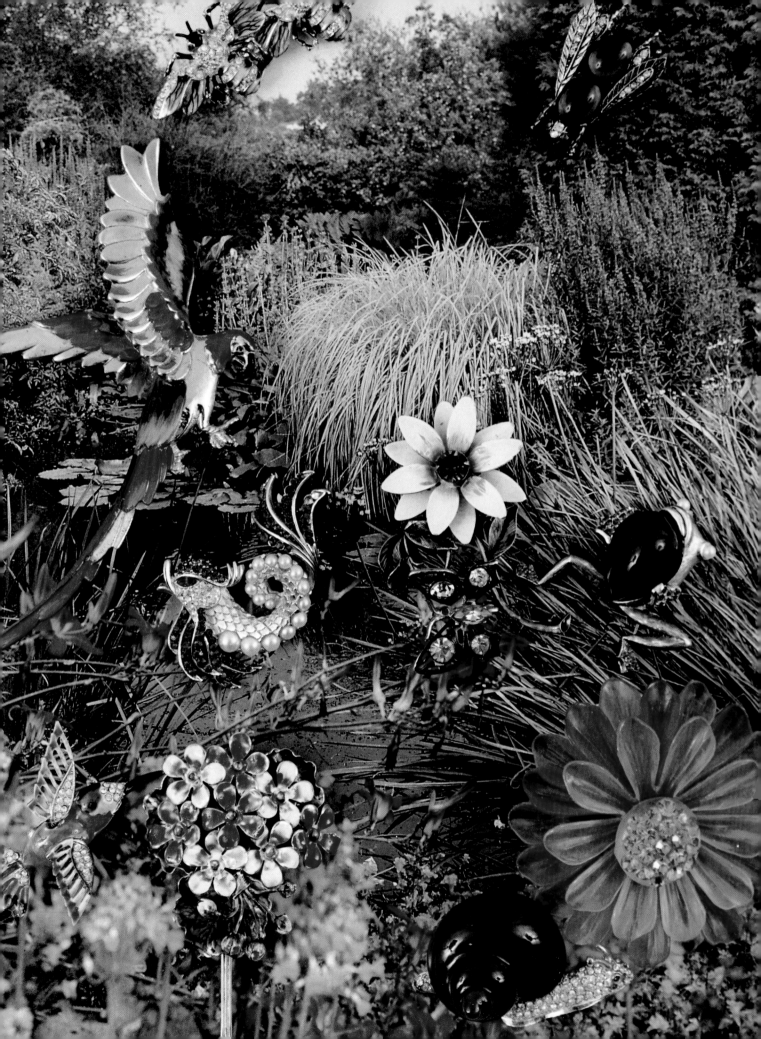

The Art Of Fashion Accessories

A Twentieth Century Retrospective

Joanne Dubbs Ball
Dorothy Hehl Torem

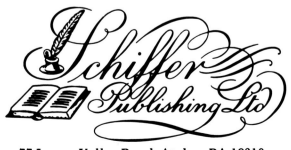

Schiffer Publishing Ltd

77 Lower Valley Road, Atglen, PA 19310

Dedication:

To my parents, Dot and Joe, who are alive in my heart

To my children Chris, Ali and Jake. I will live on through their eyes. They are wonderful, as are Jeffrey, Barbara, Steven, Michael, Neil Alan French, and my very special Aunt Jean, with love to Betty, Gary and Gloria Muroff. To my Milton, who rescued me from the Sixties and spoiled me rotten with riches. I told you I'd love you forever...what better way than to say it in print.

Dorothy Hehl Torem

To my children, Cynthia Ellis Clarke and Brett Hamilton Clarke, who will, I pray, march confidently into the challenges of the 21st Century. May the path be unswerving...and their shoes comfortable!

And to Bob...who makes all things possible.

Joanne Dubbs Ball

ACKNOWLEDGMENTS

We wish to thank the following people for all their help and cooperation in the production of this book: Mel Baker and Brenda Bedrick, *Mel and Me*; Rosalind Becker, *Roz and Sherm*; Clara Braithwaite, Clar-Mar, Warwick, R.I.; Isabel Canovas; Caroline de St. Andre, *Isabel Canovas*; Shirley Clements; Jewel Cook; Michelle Courtois; Barbara Corvino, *Tiffany & Co.*; Jill Speranza, *Tiffany & Co.*; Bridget Devine, *Harry Winston*; Jean Louis Dumas, *Hermes*; Pamela Eldridge, *Barry Kieselstein-Cord*; Frank Fialkoff, *Miriam Haskell*; Roberta Finestone; Elizabeth Gage; Emma Kerr-Smiley, *Elizabeth Gage*; Gai Gherardi, Barbara McReynolds, Ruth Handel, and Beth Herzhaft, *l.a. Eyeworks*; Alan M. Goffman, *The Fine Art of Illustration*; Golden Heart Antiques; Greg Gorman; Leslie Gray; Irma; Joan Castle Joseff; Karl Lagerfeld; Terri Cohen, *Karl Lagerfeld*; E.J. Landrigan; Laurie Fusco, *E.J. Landrigan, Inc./Verdura*; Fred Leighton; Lois Lewis; James Marsh, *Hamilton Watch Co.*; Cathy Bromer, *Hamilton Watch Co.*; Guy McLain, Connecticut Valley Historical Museum; Nicole Miller; Lori Oscher, *Nicole Miller*; Gloria C. Molloy; Barbara Music, *Barbara Music Design*; Newport Historical Society; Elida Olsen, *Elida Olsen et Cie*; Joan Orlen; Peggy Ann Osborne; Rocki Pedersen; Paco Rabanne; Chantal Delinot-Lagraviere, *Paco Rabanne*; Carole Satmary; Jan Schiavino, *Ragtime*; Stephen Sherman, *The Icing*; Michael Castellano, *The Icing!*; Stanley Silberstein,*David Webb, Inc.*; Catherine Stein; Michelle Stoneman; Tim Street-Porter; Veronica Trainer; Vera; James Stocker, *Vera*; Mark Walsh; Jan Walker, *Lord & Taylor*; Vivienne Westwood; Karl Plewka, *Vivienne Westwood*; Simon Barker, *Vivienne Westwood*; Juliet Weber Reid; and Fiona Wong, *Robert Lee Morris*.

With special thanks to Barry Kieselstein-Cord and Robert Lee Morris for their efforts on our behalf; to Rea Lubar for her perseverance...and graciousness; and to Roberta Tepper of *Harper's Bazaar* for her kindness and enthusiasm.

Thanks also to Ralph and June Mogavero, *Directions Plus*; Bob Simas, *East Greenwich Photo Lab*, East Greenwich, R.I.; Karen McLain, *Abar Color Lab*, Providence, R.I.; Magi Motola, international expert on Deco and Fitfties' style, magical friend, and antiques huntress extraordinaire; Hank and Rena Stern, *Renclif* and *Fancy Goods*; Renata McGriff, *D.H.T. Ltd.*; Jack Hehl, *Jack Hehl Antiques*, West Ossipee, N.H.; Susan Clausen, artist, sculptress, toymaker, friend; Kerry Cerio, who helped beyond measure; our persevering husbands, Bob Ball and Milton Torem; and extra special kudos to those masters of persistence, Jake Torem and Alyson Torem-French, who gave "above and beyond." We will be forever grateful to you all.

Published by Schiffer Publishing, Ltd.
77 Lower Valley Road
Atglen, PA 19310
Please write for a free catalog.
This book may be purchased from the publisher.
Please include $2.95 postage.
Try your bookstore first.

We are interested in hearing from authors
with book ideas on related subjects.

Contents

Foreword 7

Part One: The Past Is Prologue 9

Part Two: The Twentieth Century

    Turn of the Century 29

    The Teens 47

    The Twenties 67

    The Thirties 87

    The Forties 111

    The Fifties 137

    The Sixties 163

    The Seventies 175

    The Eighties 187

    The Nineties 203

Epilogue 234

Bibliography 236

Index 237

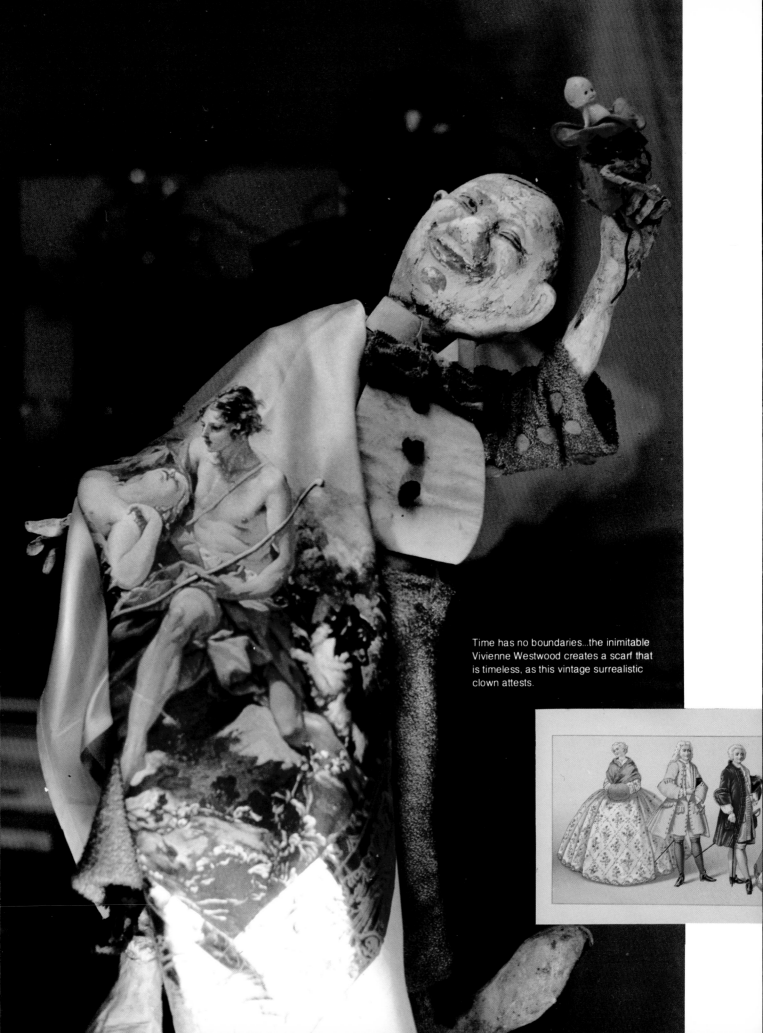

Time has no boundaries...the inimitable Vivienne Westwood creates a scarf that is timeless, as this vintage surrealistic clown attests.

Foreword

IF FASHION IS PUBLIC OPINION EXPRESSED IN DRESS, SHE IS ALSO A PRECIOUS GUIDE TO THE PAST.

Marcel Vertes

If, as the adage goes, "clothes make the man," then it is safe to add that "accessories do indeed make the woman." Although, as we will see, man has accessorized, with sometimes startling results, beyond woman's wildest imaginings. But unlike men, who in overblown splendor frequently became mere mirror images of each other, women, most especially in the 20th century, have had exciting opportunities to set themselves apart from their sisters. For they can change the ambiance of their appearance with the addition of fanciful accessories—and a modicum of imagination.

For example, a dynamic scarf artfully draped at the neck of a dress adds an entirely new dimension to its design. A perky hat worn with a simple sheath imparts an aura of sophistication to an otherwise understated garment. An eye-catching brooch on the lapel of a jacket can also deliver an extra touch of *je ne sais quoi* that separates the imaginative from the mundane. And an elegant handbag can make the difference between simply ordinary and truly "smashing." Even small items like shoe buckles and interesting buttons can become the focal point of a transformation. Many of the world's best-dressed women—as well as the unsung we see everyday on our bustling sidewalks, in busy offices, and the neighborhood grocery stores, who inevitably garner second and third glances from admirers of both sexes—have inherently understood one simple but powerful fact: accessories, both large and small, are imbued with restorative powers. A change of buttons, the addition of a lace collar, or a glittering bib of false jewels can rejuvenate a staple of one's everyday wardrobe into a fashion statement.

There continue to be individuals who, with unabashed verve, grasp that opportunity and thereby add new dimensions to the art of fashion. On the one hand, a glorious, even simple, accessory can proudly stand alone—and the addition of anything else to one's costume only diminishes its impact. On the other, past fashion mavens like Elsa Schiaparelli and Coco Chanel give clear testimony that *more* isn't automatically a hallmark of bad taste and *less* of good. Without question, however, there exists an ineffable quality that enables one individual to carry off a look that would be totally inappropriate for another. Vive le difference!

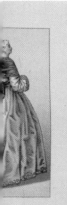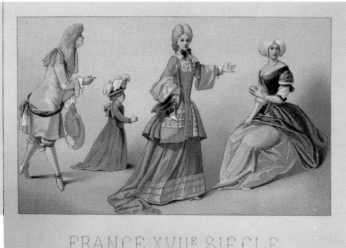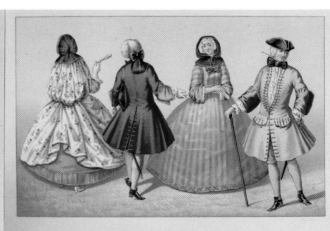

FRANCE XVIIᵉ SIECLE

FRANCE XVIIIᵉ SIECLE

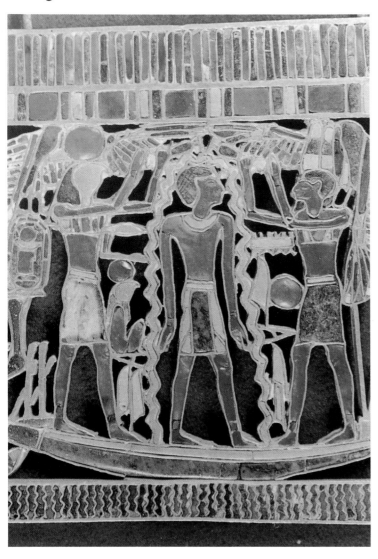

Egyptian pictorial detail.

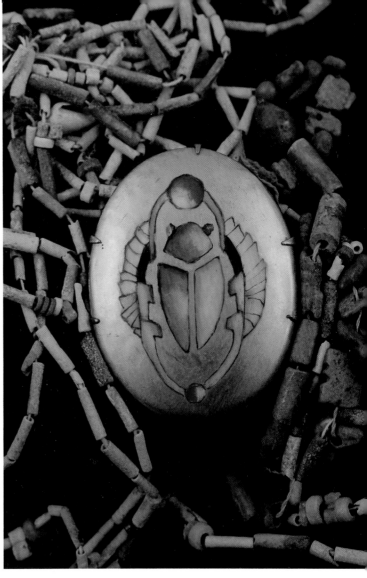

Ancient mummy beads form a suitable
backdrop for an Egyptian Revival
Victorian porcelain brooch.

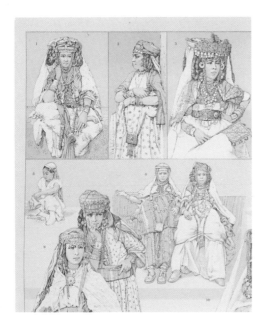

Africa, 1800s.

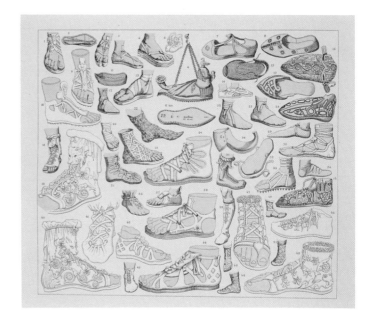

A plethora of Greek shoes from the Pan Hellenic period.

Part One: The Past Is Prologue

FASHION HAS HER OWN LOGIC AND OFTEN WHEN SHE SEEMS AT HER MOST GROTESQUE IT IS FOR REASONS THAT ARE PROFOUNDLY HUMAN.

Marcel Vertes

The Classical Fashions

A detailed history of fashion could fill volumes. It would also *speak* volumes about each century of recorded history, since what is worn reflects not only personal tastes and eccentricities but also the social and political mores of the time. In both subtle and obvious ways, costuming choices are more than just historically significant—they provide insight into the mass psychology that motivated inhabitants of various countries and cultures in all areas of their lives. Intentional or not, there have also been periods when the popular taste was but an updated interpretation of earlier days. By taking a look at those times and places, we can better understand the periods of renewal as they ebb and flow through the world of fashion.   The profound changes in fashion during the 20th century are the culmination of these earlier influences. The basic items of a wardrobe—the dresses, gowns, suits, and coats—are in evolution along with the accessories, and the latter can't be discussed without understanding the social climate that brought about the former. To bring us current, we will briefly hopscotch through centuries past, take a quick look around or linger here and there, and then move on. It would appear, in fact, that there is little in the realm of "modern" apparel that is *really* new. Chances are that someone before us—with some variation—has already tried it.

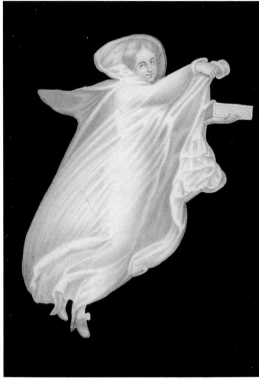

Without question, accessorizing has been an integral part of fashion, and man's nature, since the earliest of times. Why else would Adam have bothered with a fig leaf or Eve draped a flower seductively over one shell-like ear? As Marcel Vertes, 20th century illustrator and fashion aficionado, so succinctly wrote, "Even before the urge to cover one's nakedness, even before modesty came Fashion."[1] And he continued, "At her birth, Fashion was accessible to everybody. Seashells lay scattered just outside the door: one had only to bend down to collect them and string them into necklaces and bracelets."[2]

Vertes was not alone in his assessment, for in his 1907 book *The Heritage of Dress*, Wilfred Mark Webb, then curator of the Eton College Museum, had arrived at much the same conclusion. He wrote:

"Perhaps it will help us if we pause for a moment to consider why clothes are worn at the present day. There is no doubt but that in the case of many garments their ornamental character, real or supposed, is the first consideration. Others are chosen chiefly for protection and warmth, while, as already indicated, the rest suffice to satisfy the claims of modesty. Although the three reasons are now intimately combined, it is practically certain that any one of them is sufficient to have led to the adoption of clothes in the first place, and as if these were not enough there may be other contributing, if not actual causes.

"We may now consider these matters in detail. It would seem from the study of modern peoples, who are still in a very simple state of civilization, as well as from one of the earliest drawings scratched by the cave-men who were contemporary with the mammoth in France, that ornaments are the most primitive part of dress.... The cave-man's sketch shows a woman who is devoid of clothing, but who wears bracelets, while it is said that in the original a necklace can be traced . . .."

Throughout history, the Earth's inhabitants recognized that even the most "utilitarian" of garb could serve multiple purposes. In the beginning the most basic of these were devised out of the simple need for protection. Shoes were to protect the feet—but, oh, what lovely accessories they made. Headgear offered protection from the elements, or one's enemies, and helped to keep one warm. But they, as well as many other items of apparel, became social, economic and political symbols. And thus, consciously or unconsciously, fashion—and the accessories it spawned—told a story that contributed, in no small measure, to the legacy those peoples left behind. And it remains so to this day.

Egyptian Sensuality

Our "fashion journey" begins about 3,000 B.C. in the mysterious Egyptian empire. In the span of the next 3,000 years, the garb of this glorious realm changed but little, and its peoples maintained standards of cleanliness that placed them not only far in advance of other civilizations of the day and prior, but also of the majority that followed. Concern with the perfection of their bodies provided the inspiration for sensual, starkly beautiful garments highlighted by sumptuous accessories. There were embroidered belts, capes, elaborate headpieces, and awesome baubles, including jewelled collars and massive

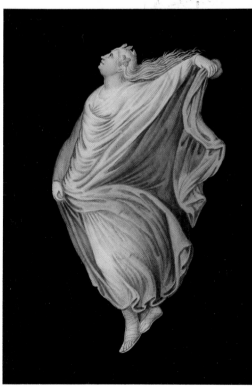

From the Pompeiian era.

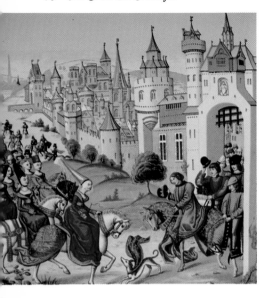

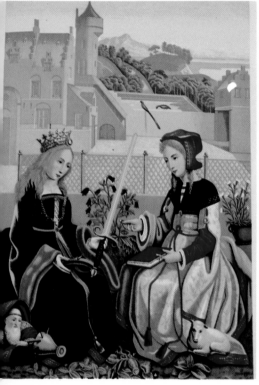

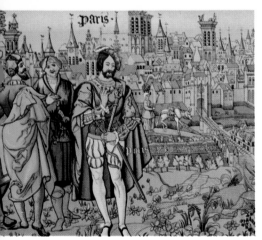

earrings, necklaces, and bracelets. Like the Cretans of the same era, female breasts were often exposed and, especially for ceremonial occasions, the heads of both men and women were covered by wigs.

Cretan Restraint

Cretan men and women of 1600-1450 B.C. must have inherently understood the 20th century's fitness slogan "no pain, no gain," for Cretans of both sexes took pride in displaying their extremely tiny waists, which historians now believe were the result of demonically constructed girdles strapped to them since childhood. Negative health factors resulting from such a painful practice were either unknown or of no concern to them. Fashion dictated . . . and the consequences be damned!

To accentuate these minuscule waistlines, Cretan women wore belts of chased metal in elaborate designs, above which breasts remained bare. Their bell-shaped skirts were intricately decorated, flounced and aproned. This full-skirted look was to be reflected in French fashions many centuries later and even in the hoop skirts of the 19th century antebellum South. They also affected elaborate headdresses, and their hair was ". . . arranged in a variety of ways and surmounted by what may perhaps be regarded as the first 'smart hats' in the history of costume."[3] Coiffures were often intertwined with ribbons and pearls and further accentuated by the many necklaces draped around their necks. The wearing of certain accessories was even mandated: "An Assyrian law of about 1200 B.C. compelled married women to wear veils in public, the earliest record of a custom which has prevailed in these districts until modern times."[4] The headgear worn by Assyrian men during this same period was in the shape of an inverted flower pot, strengthening the argument that not only women have shown cause to be labeled as "slaves to fashion."

Greek Innovation

Like their Cretan "sisters," Greek women of the fifth century B.C. also tied their hair with ribbons. These, however, were fashioned in a cone-shape and looked like projectiles exiting the back of the head. Innovation of another kind was not lost on Greek women engaged in the "world's oldest profession." They gave shoes an intriguing purpose far removed from man's original need to simply protect the soles of his feet, for their gilded footgear was studded with strategically placed nails in the sole, and with each step taken a footprint was left behind that spelled out, "Follow me." Historians believe this same provocative marketing technique was used by courtesans in Lower Egypt, which probably means that *certain* news travels fast and far.

Greek courtesans of the day were given "geisha-like" status, and used many beauty and fashion aids, including masses of jewelry to "ply their trade." Diametrically opposed was the prevailing Greek view of dress, for here was a purity of form allowing for little or no adornments to intefere with the aura of stark simplicity. Women had few opportunities for individuality in matters of dress, but by the fourth century B.C. Greek women were enjoying greater freedom of dress and appearance. They painted their faces with hapless abandon, using white lead for powdering and rouge made from red sulphide and mercury—or mulberries, which were certainly safer. Even then, the medical community knew the dangers to be found in lead and mercury, but their warnings went unheeded. Once again, beauty would not be sacrificed on the alter of good health.

In ancient Greece, the manner in which garments were draped and handled indicated breeding and education. "According to Plato, it was absolutely necessary that a man should know 'how to throw his cloak from left to right as a gentleman should,'"[6] for, like birds preening their feathers, casual movements have often sent out messages far removed from the act itself. Although their garments appeared simple, proper draping consumed much time and was a complex procedure. In contrast, their ankles and thighs were frequently beribboned, and they affected the use of silver and gold-handled walking sticks.

Etruscan Gold Work

This period saw the art of gold-smithing catapulted to its highest levels by the Etruscans, whose culture and dress reflected the influence of both Greece and Asia Minor. In fact, Etruscan gold-smithing encompassed techniques of granulation brought from Asia Minor. This finite art, in which gold is melted and soldered so as not to distort the tiny globules, was of such intricacy it was later lost, not to be recovered until the 19th century.

These people had a deep appreciation of luxury and beauty, and the gold they revered did much to enhance the accoutrements of everyday life, from the objects in their homes to the baubles that they wore. Highly-placed Etruscan women wore intricately repoussé breastplates to signify rank. Shoes were luxurious and important. In fact, this obsession with footwear included an innovative, and surely more glamorous, forerunner to rubberized overshoes of later years, for their version was of hammered bronze! Even

Priceless treasures from the mid-19th century. Venetian earrings with leaf motif of seed pearls, diamonds, and gold, they were crafted in three separate sections, enabling the wearer to adjust lengths at will. Courtesy of Catherine Stein, from her personal collection.

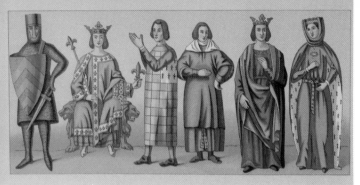

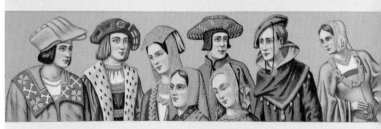

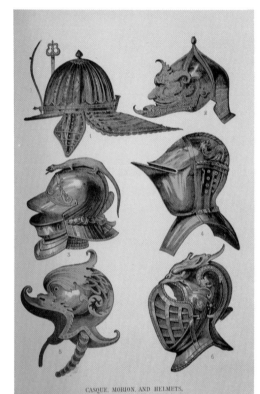

CASQUE, MORION, AND HELMETS,
With and without visors, from the Armeria Real at Madrid.

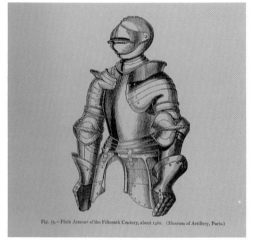

Fig. 53.—Plain Armour of the Fifteenth Century, about 1460. (Museum of Artillery, Paris.)

false teeth, understandably of gold, became a *toothsome* accessory. Etruscan men wore elaborately detailed armor, which served as an accessorizing tool under certain conditions . . . and an absolute necessity under others.

Roman Variety

The various decrees of the Romans, the Etruscans' neighbors to the south, mirrored the rise and fall of the Empire. They ran the gamut from rejection of gold in all forms but that necessary for dental work—which was still in effect as late as 215 B.C.—to a period of supreme excess. During the interim, as restrictions were relaxed, a half-ounce of gold was the limit a women could own, and females were also limited as to how many different colors they could use in their dress. Although the Emperor Claudius had instituted a continuing period of austerity during the first century A.D., by the second century Roman women wore flowing silks of beautiful colors, carried scarves and fans, and were slaves to immaculately coiffed hairdos, compelling Ovid to remark that "A woman should not be a slave to fashion but should choose a hairdo to suit her face."[7]

Roman Excess and the Byzantine Influence

Following the fall of the Western Empire in 476 A.D., the Romans came more and more under the influence of the sensual Orient, just as their Carthaginian neighbors had, and it was then that the beauty of Byzantium permeated the culture of Italy. Many Romans had acquired huge fortunes in the Orient, and this newfound wealth gradually changed the social order for "Never before in history had private individuals commanded so much personal influence or such vast fortunes."[8] As might be expected, what followed was excess—from overeating to extravagant dress. "Moreover the thirst for ostentation extended even to those living on a modest income. In Rome, mused the threadbare Juvenal, 'Everyone dresses above his means.'"[9]

Although men were admonished to wear only signet rings, jewelry and gemstones became an acceptable form of ornamentation for all, and these pieces—including the stones themselves—were replete with intricately painted designs. Engraved stones, cameos, and intaglios enjoyed popularity, along with pearls, which were used both in necklaces and earrings and to embellish the hair and sandals. Jewels were liberally applied to all manner of dress, and gems were even embedded in slippers fashionable Roman women wore indoors. It was even rumored that one Roman matron fastened glittering jewels to the fish in her aquarium! However, this obsession with precious jewels may have reached its apex when Caligula had them plaited into the manes of his horses.

Headbands progressed to tiaras of silver and gold, many covered with jewels and cameos, and to showcase these works of art, wigs became a necessity for fashionable women. Roman women of this later period used beauty spots as a facial "accessory," but not before they'd suffered through the night wearing noxious facial masques, one an odorous concoction of "...sheep fat mixed with bread crumbs soaked in milk,"[10] or, hopefully less popular, another that contained crocodile excrement!

The Byzantine—Justinian and Theodora

The Byzantine Empire must be counted as one of the most influential in culture, fashion and history. The Emperor Justinian, who came to power in the 6th century A.D., and his empress Theodora both played a major role in all three. Justinian spotted Theodora when she appeared as a beauty contestant at one of the Empire's many hippodromes. As Justinian's wife, the Empress Theodora became not only a "fashion plate" but must be classified as one of an elite group of women throughout history who recognized that clothes serve not only to set the wearer apart but to enhance their power by the strength of their style.

Theodora's contribution was not as "just another pretty face," for along with Justinian she was a social reformer, possibly resulting from her own lowly beginnings. Above all else, however, she played a major, if unwitting, role in changing the course of European trade, for she is credited with commissioning a trip to the Orient from which two monks returned with the secret of the origin of silk. Prior to that time, precious silk passed—like state secrets from courier to courier—through the hands of various middlemen on its long journey from East to West. The carefully guarded mystery embedded in the tiny

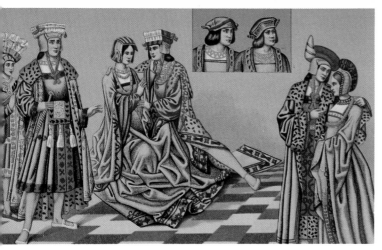

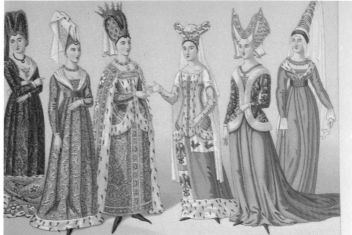

silkworm had given enormous power and wealth to the Orient and created vast fortunes for those middlemen. But with the startling revelation of those monks, that power was swiftly diffused. There is little doubt that the unexpected outcome of Theodora's mission transformed world economics as well as the history of Europe.

One can only marvel at the beauty of Theodora and the splendor of Byzantium as it is captured in the awesome mosaics of San Vitale, where she is resplendently garbed for eternity. As James Laver describes:

> "She wore a long white tunic adorned with...embroideries. Another band, called a *maniakis* embroidered with gold thread and set with precious stones and pearls was draped over her shoulders. . . . she wore a short sleeved robe, with a jewelled belt and fringes at the hem, and a purple cloak embroidered with figures of the Magi. On her head she had an even more splendid diadem than the Emperor's. This was a *stephanos* set with precious stones and with long strings of pearls hanging down on either side. On her feet were closed shoes of soft leather, coloured red and enriched with embroideries."[12]

The Murky Middle Ages and Merovingian Dynasty

In sharp contrast to the regality of Theodora, it was an altogether different "picture" during the 5th century A.D. when Northern Gaul suffered under a Frankish invasion. The Franks accessorized in a comic, yet frightening, manner by today's standards, draping their bodies with seaweed, dying their hair red, and topping the whole glorious mess with a headdress of bison horns (picture that rising out of the sea in a modern-day cult horror movie). Their strength—with more than a little help from the sheer terror instilled by their frightening appearance—established the Merovingian dynasty in 481 A.D., which would continue for the next 300 years. Eventually, seaweed was replaced by more acceptable forms of accessorizing. The once-barbarous Franks also discovered the pleasure of wallowing in excess, developing a penchant for shoes of scarlet leather and hairpins in the shape of ornately jewelled birds and animals.

By the seventh century A.D., even Charlemagne, the Frankish emperor of the Holy Roman Empire, had adopted much of the Byzantine in his dress. The general Frankish attire, however, was simpler, but did involve some interesting accessories, like cross-gartering with studded leather strips extending to the knee. Women of the day draped their gowns with beautiful scarves, and "The hair was dressed in nets of woven beads and precious stones with veils worn on top. Both sexes wore decorative and functional jewelry made in gold, silver, bronze and iron . . . Beads of amber, garnets and other stones were often worn."[13]

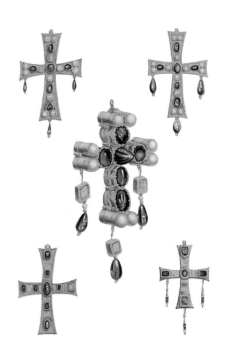

Medieval Modes

From the 9th to the 13th centuries, the Byzantines continued to display brilliant colors like reds and purples, with luxurious silks employed for all manner of dress and, as before, encrusted with pearls and brilliant jewels. Panels on gowns were embroidered with jewels and gold with the ends flowing loosely, after being carefully draped around the body. "Trousers were generally worn by both sexes . . . and . . . often decorated by a jewelled embroidered band running vertically down the line at back and front. The trousers were tucked into high boots or worn over shoes."[14]

Headgear of the Medieval European period ran the gamut from hoods—sometimes covered by wide-brimmed hats—berets, and, for women, veils and *barbettes,* a linen band that was placed under the chin and then drawn tightly over the wearer's temple. Eventually, the peak of the medieval hood expanded into an elongated, five or six foot "tail," thereby allowing the wearer to drape it over the arm or around one's body. This served no utilitarian purpose, but merely flaunted one's social station—inadvertently giving credence to the nursery rhyme "...and dragging their tails behind them."

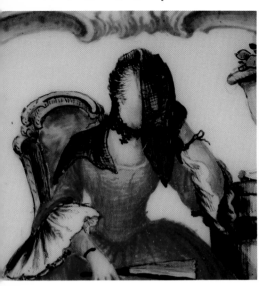

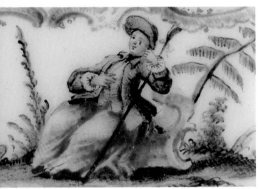

Handpainted 1850's fan with original embroidery and ribbon. Collection of Gloria C. Molloy.

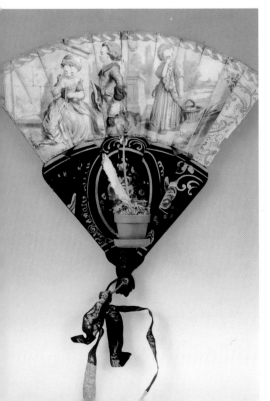

The Renaissance Man . . . and Woman

During the 14th and 15th centuries, the dress of women was not as detailed or elaborate as that of men, and the 15th century spawned a plethora of male hat styles from the elaborate fez to bowler-types to simple flat caps with jewelled ornaments on their upturned brims. One adventuresome soul decided to put his entire head through the simple hood opening that had previously been reserved for his face, and then proceeded to wind the fabric around his head like a turban, giving birth to one of history's most innovative fashions. Over the years it "grew and grew," and assumed various shapes and sizes to eventually play a totally different accessorizing role when someone got the notion to bypass the head and wear it on his shoulder! Even this penchant for the absurd was not original, however, for in the 5th century B.C. Greek women also wore their hats on their shoulders. Defying all reason, the idea became the "rage" of the day, and through the ensuing years it continued to change its purpose, eventually becoming a badge of livery and finally, in the 19th century, the cockade on a coachman's hat.

The history of that venerable fashion mainstay, the shoulder pad, is a similar one. As explained by Wilfred Mark Webb in 1907, "When speaking of padding one might recall the fact that the most usual place in which it is found—in civilian clothes at least—is on the shoulder. The protuberance thus formed . . . was originally intended to prevent weapons from slipping off when they were carried over the shoulder."[15] Men had an understandable need for contrivances to tote not only their weapons but even musical instruments. Over the centuries many styles gained favor, some practical, others purely decorative. One of these, which had its beginnings in medieval times and continued in one form or another into the 18th century, was the baldric, a sash or belt that was slung around one shoulder and then to the opposite hip. These baldrics were highly decorated, mainly of leather or silk, and some even had bells attached—hardly a wise choice when carrying a weapon that might be needed to surprise one's enemy!

The 14th century took men's shoes to heights (or more appropriately, lengths) that it would never see again, and in the process must have caused their wearer more pain than modern women endured at the altar of footwear fashion seven centuries later. Called *crackowes* after Cracow, Poland, where they possibly had their origin, they were pointed to an extent that would make the heartiest woman wince. The church was opposed to this display and ". . . King Edward III even enacted a sumptuary law which laid down that 'no Knight under the estate of a lord, esquire or gentleman, nor any other person, shall wear any shoes or boots having spikes or points exceeding the length of two inches, under the forfeiture of forty pence.'"[16] As might be expected, scofflaws paid no heed, and in ensuing years these footwear atrocities sometimes reached lengths of eighteen inches or more!

Further proof that Edward III was determined to control what his subjects wore can be found in another decree that stipulated: "All esquires and every gentleman under the estate of knighthood, and not possessed of lands or tenements to the yearly amount of 200 marks, shall use in their dress such cloth as does not exceed the value of 4 marks and a half the whole cloth; they shall not wear any cloth of gold, of silk, or of silver, nor any sort of embroidered garment, nor any ring, buckle, nouche, riband nor girdle; nor any ornaments of precious stones, nor furs of any kind; their wives and children shall be subject to the same regulation."[17] This surely put a crimp in the accessorizing proclivities of the British masses but, as in time past, they undoubtedly found a way around it.

What one wore was not only of importance into the grave but well beyond, for in England and Flanders an unusual record remained. Attached to tombstones were memorial tablets with brass figurals and engraved descriptions of the costumes worn by the deceased. Rubbings taken from these stones provide an interesting picture of fashion of the Middle Ages. Animals and birds played a role in headdress of the period. In the animal category, a veil was draped over a wire reconstruction of cows' horns, carrying veiling to "bovine" heights! Somewhat more attractive, although certainly an encumbrance, a later fashion favorite was the butterfly headdress, which recreated the shape of butterfly wings and rose in diaphanous splendor above the wearer's head.

The Middle Ages saw girdles—belts worn around the waist and hips—made of silk, leather, decorative fabrics, and even metals, draped or double-draped over the garment, thereby becoming an ingenious method of displaying other objects like jewels, scented pomanders, keys, and even purses. Styles for men were usually in the form of wide, rigid belts that rested on the hips, with some forming a cage-like, openwork contrivance that was frequently decorated with dangling bells—just another flagrant attention-getter.

A strange Germanic aberration spread from country to country in the early 16th century. Appropriately called *slashing,* it involved the bizarre practice of cutting slits in garments, through which the lining could be pulled. German hose carried this slashing to colorful extremes whereby one leg would be profusely "slashed" in one color and the other leg in yet another. This cutting of one's garments to ribbons was a predominantly male ritual, which once agin illustrates that somehow man was determined to preen. Surprisingly, this fetish continued into the 17th century. For, in 1634, in what was probably a vain attempt to bring certain Puritan mavericks "into line," the governing body of the Massachusetts Colony decreed that "...No man or woman should make or buy slashed clothes 'under penalty of forfeiture of such clothes.'"[18] Possibly to offset the excesses of "slashing," the 16th century ushered in the popularity of a broad shoe of leather, silk, or velvet, frequently ablaze with brilliant jewels.

By the time of the infamous Henry VIII—whose garments were usually so laden with gems that the fabric underneath was totally obscured—fashions seemed to reflect the influence of another art form—architecture, presenting an interesting correlation between fashion and architectural design. For when pointed shoes were abandoned for the broad-toed models, it was ". . . as if to echo the new style of architecture with its flattened arch. Ladies' headdresses ceased to be replicas of Gothic pinnacles and began to resemble Tudor windows."[19]

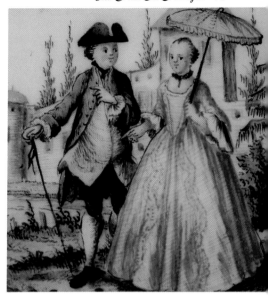

However, while no longer subjecting themselves to footwear designed to maim or at least trip all those they came in contact with, men—and women—decided to transfer this somewhat pleasurable discomfort to the opposite end of their bodies. This restrictive compulsion culminated in a strange allegiance to the ruff. By weaving a drawstring through the upper edge of a shirt and then pulling it very tightly around the neck, this new form of "enduring anything in the name of fashion" made its entry into the world of unusual fashion lore. With the unbending ruff sitting atop high doublet collars, the head was forced to remain erect, supposedly giving its wearer a mantle of aristocracy. Obviously, men could not exert themselves while wearing such a "device"—ergo anyone thus entrapped could never be mistaken for a member of the "working" class.

Not content to "leave ill enough alone," these ruffs became larger and even more uncomfortable as the century progressed—never mind that even the simple act of eating could no longer be accomplished with any ease. In fact, it was reported that one member of royalty was forced to eat her soup with a spoon having a two-foot handle! "The French King Henri III wore a ruff rather more than one foot deep, which contained over 18 yards of linen, all neatly pleated and folded in place with an ironing stick heated on the fire."[20] Women eventually decided to open the ruff and expose their bosoms—with the back of the ruff then fanning out like a wing-like aperture behind their heads.

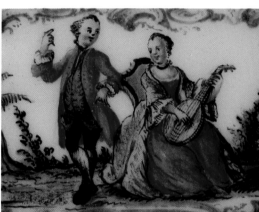

How women coiffed their hair again *rose*—both literally and figuratively—to new heights. This spawned an interesting accessory called a "palisadoe," a wire support over which the hair was raised after it had been fluffed and turned back from the forehead over a pad. Understandably, such a bouffant style made the use of false hair a necessity for all but the most *thick-headed.* To further accentuate this swept-back look, women carried matters to greater extremes by painstakingly (with emphasis on the *pain*) plucking their hairlines to give the illusion of an even higher forehead.

As if all this discomfort wasn't enough for milady, she added to the misery of ruffs, palisadoes, and plucked foreheads by wearing an underskirt called a Spanish farthingale. These consisted of hoops of wire or wood, another forerunner of the crinolines of the nineteenth century. Obviously, only women who "laboured naught" could enjoy the *privilege* of this detriment to sitting, standing, or carefree movement of any kind. The French farthingale compounded the problem, for the wearer then had to stand inside a wheel-like contraption with her skirt attached to the rim. "In the well-known painting *Queen Elizabeth at Blackfriars,* the Queen and all her ladies are seen wearing this singularly unbecoming garment, which made women look as if they were hobby-horses."[21]

The Italians went a step farther by tilting the farthingale with a cushion that gave the garment a bustle-like appearance, with said bustle sometimes widening to an astronomical 48 inches. Another variation of the farthingale was the "bum roll" (a *double entendre* of Elizabethan bawdiness?). This torturous, sausage-shaped device, with the ends joined at the front of the body, caused considerable difficulty in raising or lowering one's arms—somewhat like being permanently attached to an inflatable life-preserver on dry land.

By the mid-16th century, Spain overtook Germany in influencing European fashion, and the bright colors worn by the upper classes succumbed to a trend toward dark, tight, somber clothes. Artwork from the period captures the aura of this elegant, yet brooding, Spanish influence, which replaced at least some of the excessive posturings that went before. Unintentionally, the Spaniards were not without their comedic side, for they were also responsible for the introduction of *bombast*, in which the huge ballooning sleeves both men and women affected during this time were plumped up with whatever "fillings" were at hand, like rags, hair, ". . .or even bran (the least desirable since it had an embarrassing tendency to leak)."[22]

This period also saw the lowly stocking gain a purpose that went beyond the simple act of keeping one's feet warm. Stockings appeared predominantly in the male wardrobe, however, since the leg exposed by wearing breeches demanded delicate hose. Thus, *silk* stockings were initially popular due to the needs of *men* and not women. Far from simple leg adornments, they glistened with gold threads and jewels and were decorated by that old standby, cross gartering—this time with the encircling ribbons tied in a flamboyant bow above the knee. This period also introduced the "clock," the intent of which was to hide unsightly side seams before stockings were constructed in one piece.

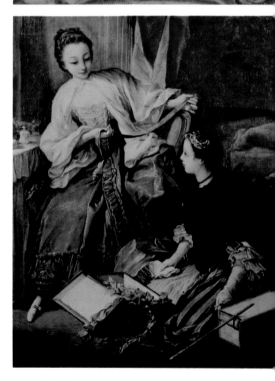

Fashions from the French Empire period are hand-painted in extraordinary detail on porcelain tiles.

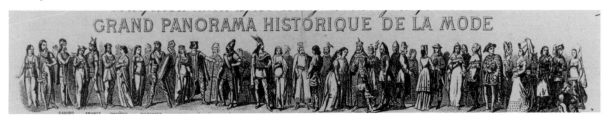

This decorative "clocking" remained even after the "all-in-one-piece" models appeared, and even today are seen as the embroidered or perforated patterns on socks for both sexes.

Prior to the 16th century, and continuing for many years and even centuries thereafter, gloves were more than simply utilitarian, for they were imbued with a ritualistic, ecclesiastical, and superstitious purpose well beyond those of simply warming the hands. In tournaments, they were carried as favors in the headgear of knights. To throw one's gloves in the path of an offender was a deliberate challenge, and gloves have even been used as a provocative means of slapping another's face. It wasn't until 16th century England, however, that fine leather gloves were first manufactured. Many were replete with fringe and gold embroidery, doused with perfume, and carefully tucked into a belt. Again, these were mainly a gentleman's accessory, as were linen and lace handkerchiefs. All in all, the 16th century produced some remarkable fashions, and as James Laver observed in *Costume & Fashion,* "The clothes and accessories of the upper classes in Europe had indeed reached an astonishing degree of elaboration and refinement . . ."[23]

By the 17th century, that wearable "torture chamber," the ruff, had been replaced, at least in England, by the more civilized "falling collar." (The proverbial stubborn Dutchmen, however, persisted in wearing ruffs like cartwheels around their necks for some years to come.) Gentlemen of the 1600s, including the Dutch and Danish, also wore a boot that was tight around the ankles but bulged out at mid-calf into a decorative, wide "bucket" top. This formed a large open circle just under the knee, giving foot attire the look of modern-day wine coolers.

Concealed by their skirts, women's shoes were understandably plain, but one type that piqued female imaginations was a platform style, with some soles rising to such awesome proportions that they looked more like stilts than shoes. These were called *chopines* and dated from an earlier time in Venice, as noted by Hamlet's remark, "'Your ladyship is nearer heaven than when I saw you last, by the altitude of a chopine.'"[24] Not to be outdone, men embellished their boots with lace and perched gigantic rosettes on the vamps of their shoes. Women's headgear of the period remained simple, and rather than wearing hats they pulled small black taffeta hoods over their heads or placed delicate fichus of lace on top.

Female accessorizing wasn't limited to the embellishment of clothing, for although most footwear and headcoverings were a bit dull, women compensated with the beauty marks and startling patches that appeared on their faces—a fad that lasted for fifty years, reemerging many times since. This too can be classified as a form of accessorizing and took all manner of shapes and sizes, from glittering stars and moon-like crescents to horse-drawn coaches.

The Restoration

The restoration of Charles II to England's throne in 1660 brought about another French-inspired fashion, with ribbons everywhere. They covered breeches and waistbands, and were bunched in massive clumps on shoulders and any other available space the wearer fancied. As one observer noted, "We hear of a suit and cloak of satin trimmed with thirty-six yards of ribbon in bunches used on one pair of petticoat breeches."[25] To compound the offense, these breeches—called Rhinegraves—were so large that Samuel Pepys wrote in his 1661 diary that one could easily put both legs into a single "compartment." English women fared far better with this look of contrived dishevelment, probably relieved to finally wear looser clothing and attractively tousled hairdos. However, "The general effect of men's clothes at this period was of fantastic negligence, well suited to the moral climate of the Restoration Court."[26]

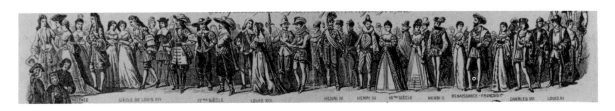

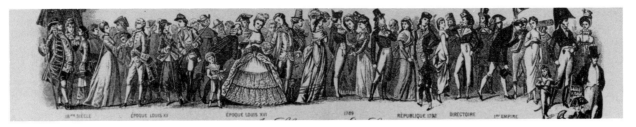

Instigated by Charles II in the mid-1660s, another *restoration* took place, this one in fashion, and deviating, at least temporarily, from the French influence. These included buckled shoes—again with jewelled adornments—and, of lasting importance, Persian-inspired vests and waistcoats. The vest, and its longer version, the waistcoat, permanently influenced men's fashions, and were forerunners of many variations, for women as well as men. The necktie also had its beginning in this era, although these early cravats were merely the hanging fronts of turned-down collars without the common knot of later years.

The French were not about to be upstaged by the English, and in the late 17th century, Louis XIV of France—who ascended to the throne in 1661 and was responsible for the triumph of Versailles—established himself as the high arbiter of fashion. Indeed "the enormous prestige of the court of Versailles resulted all over Europe in a readiness to accept the superiority of France in matters of fashion."[27] Included in this "superiority" was a male head-covering called a periwig. Those worn by fashionable men were heavy and cumbersome, but soldiers and other active persons couldn't don them and effectively perform their duties, making two versions necessary—the "campaign" wig and the "traveling" wig. At no time was appearing sans wig a consideration among the elite, and this accessory remained in favor among the Western European upper classes for nearly a hundred years.

Although French women were enamored of these elaborate wigs, English ladies chose to tie their hair with a ribboned bow in the front, a trend that had also belatedly made its way from France to England. As with most fillips of fashion, simple beginnings harvested questionable "improvements," which built one upon another until the English woman was no better off than her wigged counterpart across the Channel. First, lace was added, and later a cap with a wire frame to support this ever-growing headpiece, which was then appropriately called a *commode* or *tower.* Its reign lasted only a decade, however, until this towering affront also made its way into the murky annals of fashion has-beens.

18th Century Revolutionaries

In the 18th century, hats for men took on an air of singular importance, and their "ups and downs" eventually became what was referred to as a *cocked* hat; that is, the brim on one side or the other, or front or back, turned up, eventually giving birth to the popularity of the three-cornered hat. As in other fashions, "cocking" was reserved for the aristocracy and men never went bareheaded except in the presence of royalty.

A small version of the tricorne hat was paramount to a fashion picture that speaks a thousand words! They were worn by the Macaronis of the 1760s, a group of idle rich young Englishmen, who, following a grand tour of Italy, formed the infamous Macaroni Club, which was devoted to exaggerations of fashion deliberately intended to provoke. With tiny tricorne hats perched atop gigantic foot-high wigs, the Macaronis presented a comical sight—and probably gave staid matrons the vapors—when these hats were doffed in greeting with the tips of their canes or swords! Adding to this "dandy" outfit ". . . fobs, two in number, were attached to his waistcoat and he always carried a jeweled snuff box, a gold-knobbed walking cane with a tassel and a diamond-hilted sword. He wore striped stockings and red-heeled shoes and often, to complete the picture, an artificial nosegay."[28] The Macaronis were not the first to attempt to bring foppery to its ultimate, for in the 1400s, Venetian youth had done the same, with clubs called "Companies of the Hose" striving to outdo one another in outrageous behavior and adornments. Their excessive "dandyism" included such affectations as carrying perfumed balls to mask the noxious fumes emanating from the canals.

Women of the time made their own outlandish fashion statements. Indeed, from the Middle Ages to the dawn of the 20th century, women's skirts continued to expand and take on all manner of idiosyncracies. As Vertes, who graphically referred to them as "mobile prisons," later observed, "All that time women from the waist to the ground were

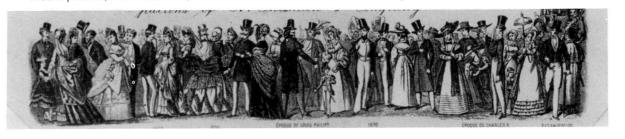

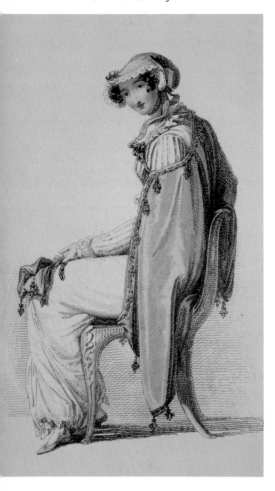

Terminally exhausted! A charming illustration from 1831.

The quintessential solid gold pocketwatch. Courtesy of June Whitlaw Nogavero and Margaret Robinson Propes.

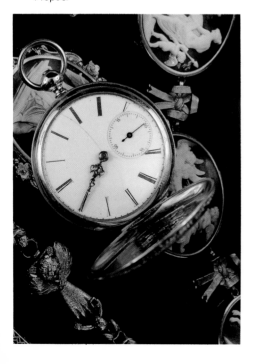

more than a mystery—one might say they did not exist."[29] France did its part to keep this record intact by instigating the highly questionable restoration of the farthingale. These *paniers* or *baskets* marked the return to dome-shaped hoops, once again designed to emphasize tiny waists. The dome later took on oval dimensions, and then progressed to an oblong shape. Sometimes as wide as six feet, these skirts were obviously unmanageable, but the navigational problems that ensued were eased by the invention of collapsible side panels. In the French court, an elaborate robe was worn over this contraption, which had a V-shaped opening through which the top of an embellished petticoat could peek. In contrast, hairdos were shaped to the head, which only exaggerated the voluminous skirts beneath.

But not for long! This trend was reversed with the influence of Marie Antoinette when elaborate coiffures and wigs became the focus, rapidly progressing beyond the boundaries of reason—or good taste. In fact, "Hairstyles were loaded with flowers . . . a kitchen garden, a plate of fruit, or even a ship in full sail. These structures were so elaborate that once dressed, a lady's coiffure was expected to last at least a month, and often two months, no doubt with unsavoury results, since the hair would be mingled with lard and whiting to keep it in place."[30] These tonsorial nightmares prompted the need for another accessory—the "head scratcher," a decorative long-handled contrivance frequently made of ivory or wood, with which the scalp could scratched.

Two names from the French court of this period remain permanently ensconced in the fashion history of the period . . . Madame de Pompadour, who became the arbiter of elegant fashion prior to the Revolution, and the aforementioned Marie Antoinette. The epitome of fashion excess, Marie Antoinette shifted from one novelty of dress to another, causing many a lady of Versailles to hover on the brink of financial disaster trying to keep up with her. Even the lowly cushion became an accessory of sorts, albeit a hidden one, for when Marie Antoinette was "with child," the ladies of the court took to wearing skirts stuffed with pillows to mimic the look of pregnancy. ". . .'skirts of the season' were created with titles such as 'fourth month skirt,' etc., their voluminousness adjusted to the progress of the Queen." [31] The astounding hairdos that had become a mainstay of the earlier French Court continued to be embellished by this "mistress of excess." As Vertes observed, "The frigates launched by Marie Antoinette's hairdresser were the last to be added to the Royal Navy. A giddy, selfish monarchy sank with them."[32]

On a more subdued note, buttons of the 1700s, featuring pastoral scenes, flowers, and even risque drawings, were works of art, the wearer serving as a human art gallery. This elevated the simple button to a status it had rarely achieved before, making them not only functional but an ornamentation with the power to exhibit a surprising depth of inventiveness—and daring. An accessory that hid yet another accessory was the stomacher, a decorative false front designed to cover the fashionable open bodice of the latter half of the 18th century. Ladies coquettishly placed small bottles in a special "stomacher pocket" that nestled between their breasts. These were filled with water and fresh flowers, thereby elevating even tiny vases to accessory status.

The polonaise gown made its appearance during this period, and was later shortened to a more popular version that had a decorative apron, or aprons, attached. "The polonaise was worn with a small hoop, which was gradually replaced by a false rump (the forerunner of the nineteenth-century bustle) which was a padded cork contraption that fitted at the back of the waist." [33] Moving to the head, ladies' hats in the latter years of the 1700s often had three huge feathers that curved forward and "nodded" as the wearer moved—a regal gesture akin to a Queen's arm movement as she greets her subjects. *Lunardi* hats were also popular. These were monstrosities of soft material covering a gigantic wire foundation.

After and during the French Revolution yet another "revolution" was underway. Women had fought beside their men and as Vertes commented some hundred and fifty years later, perhaps with a philosophical eye to the future ". . .these women of the people never submitted to the discomfort of Fashion. They were clothed only, not dressed. They worked hard, they were the equals of their men—which is to say, wretched and oppressed."[34] Being ruled by the dictates of fashion was *out* and peasant-type outfits and inconspicuous demeanor took over where excess had left off. During the Reign of Terror that followed, the only accessory women could add to their simple "uniform" was a humble sash.

Although not of French origin, and conceived an ocean away during the time of the Colonies' own battle for independence, equestrianism spawned an innovative accessory. Ladies and children carried masks on long sticks to protect their faces from the sun as they galloped along. These masks were equipped with a silver mouthpiece to clench between the teeth so the face would continue to be shaded while hands remained securely clasped on the reins. During this century, sticks of another kind became an important method of expressing individuality. These were the walking sticks and canes few gentlemen, and even many ladies, would not leave their homes without. Prussian Emperor Frederick II carried the walking stick to its ultimate with an ivory cane embedded with 93 rubies spiraling its length all of which served as a magnificent depository for field glasses—the "vault" thereby having greater value than its contents. Voltaire and Rousseau were purported to own dozens of walking sticks in styles to match their outfits, and each had a shoe collection that was equally extensive. Not to be outdone, ladies utilized the cane for more than mere ornamentation, and their walking sticks frequently included whimsical items like music boxes, mirrors, and vials of perfume.

In France, the death of Robespierre flung open the "wardrobe doors," and French women could again enjoy greater freedom of dress. This time "west" came to "east," and for some unfathomable reason, British hunting clothes consumed the interest of Frenchmen. As might be expected, they added a "continental" interpretation, resulting in hunting clothes with elongated tails accented by boots in all manner of strange shapes. For dress in general ". . . collars rose to great heights behind the head and neckcloths became so voluminous that they sometimes rose over the chin and even concealed the mouth. Wigs were abandoned and the unpowdered hair was worn in a wild mop sometimes brushed forward over the forehead. Few more bizarre silhouettes have ever been seen than those of the French *Incroyables* of the 1790s."[35]

There were compensations, small though they were, for this period saw the introduction of little handbags called "reticules" or "ridicules" that, when flimsy fabrics became popular, replaced the garment pockets normally used for holding one's special grooming needs. Indeed, by the close of the century, clothing for women of the period again became a fashionable means of expression and a revealing sheath dress of sheer muslin, harkening back to the Greeks and Romans and tied with ribbons under the bosom, heralded the beginning of a new classical period. These fashions continued throughout Napoleon's reign, although they were somewhat more controlled and less revealing.

Napolean did, however, encourage the flaunting of extravagant jewels, and his bride Josephine also indulged his penchant for "the lady in white." At one ball ". . . she was 'a vision in misty white . . . with a narrow lame border like a rivulet of gold round the hemline of the pleated skirt, a gold and black enamelled lion's head on each shoulder and another as a clasp on a gold belt.' (The costume is described by Laure Junot.)."[36] In 1809, following the divorce Josephine so dreaded, ". . . an inventory of her wardrobe . . . listed no less than 676 dresses, 49 court costumes, 252 hats and head-dresses, 60 cashmere shawls, 785 slippers, 413 pairs of stockings and 498 embroidered chemises."[37] Although France's dominance of fashion had dimmed during the Napoleonic wars, their end revived that country's primary position in couture, and England, now in the midst of its Regency period, was also captivated by sheer white gowns, even though they were totally unsuited to the British climate.

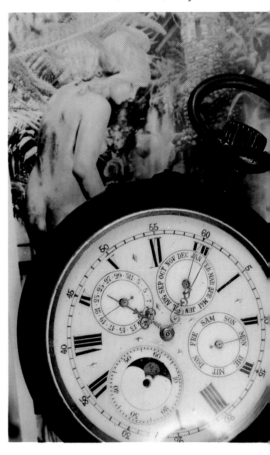

French pocketwatch, circa 1888.

From George (the King) to Beau (the Brummell)

Born in 1762, George, Prince of Wales—later to become King George IV—exerted his own "far out" sense of style and fashion power early on, much in the manner of the Macaronis before him. Details of a court ball he attended at the age of eighteen record that "Frizzled, powdered and curled, the prince appeared in radiant pink satin with a waistcoat bedizened with gems of pink paste and a mosaic of colored foils and a hat blazing with 5000 metallic beads."[38] The standard was set, and other young men of the court could now fervently devote themselves to the overblown excesses of male *dandyism*. George was also credited with being responsible for a 5-inch wide shoe buckle, starting a fad that soon became a mainstay of male dress. His influence continued throughout his reign into the 19th century, helping to cement the dandy's image: that of a man who was ". . . heroically consecrated to this one object, the wearing of clothes wisely and well: so that others dress to live, he lives to dress."[39] And so—for good or ill—men, once again, held their own in the recording of fashion history.

The illustrious George Bryan "Beau" Brummell epitomized the lengths to which the more tastefully restrained forms of "dandyism" could take one. His name has become a permanent part of the lexicon of fashion—with the *nom de plume* Beau Brummel assuming universal significance far beyond that of mere "fashion foppery." In spite of what many considered his insolent snobbery, Brummell cannot be faulted for the contributions he made to male grooming. He instigated cleanshaven chins, short hair, devotion to personal hygiene, and the necessity for clean clothes. His accessories were limited mainly to ". . . snuffboxes, monocles, gold-handled canes and matching fobs," (and he wore) '. . . either laced boots or light pumps, the last revealing a brief expanse of embroidered silk stockings. The extraordinary gleam of his boots, he let it be known, was achieved by applications of the froth of champagne.'"[40] Simplicity was the byword when it came to jewelry, however, for he decreed that the truly dedicated gentleman should wear only a signet ring and diamond stickpin.

Brummell's cravat was an artistic square that wrapped around the neck and tied in a bow or knot in the front. Now a cravat knot was a time-consuming piece of business and could necessitate patiently standing in front of a mirror for as long as two hours in an attempt to tie it "just right." The cravat knot also became one more item of apparel that, by its very design, signified class, thereby separating the elite from the masses. Despite his foibles, Brummel deserves much credit, for the power he wielded caused a sartorial metamorphosis, giving credence to the underplaying of male dress and the importance of proper tailoring.

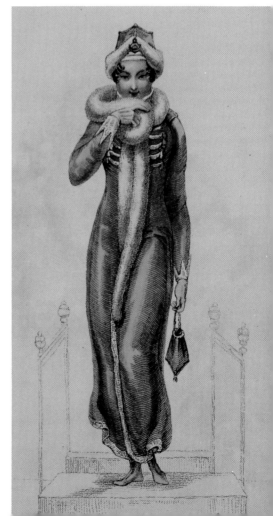

This walking dress from 1831 bears a striking resemblance to "the look" 100 years later.

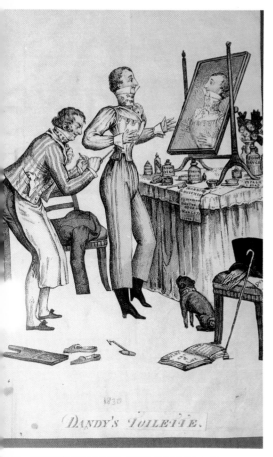

DANDY'S TOILETTE.

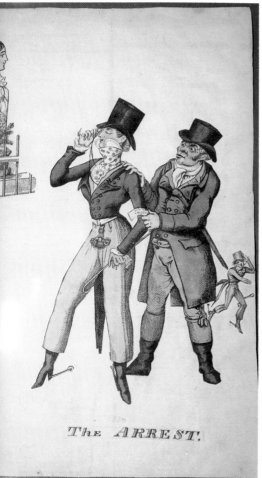

THE ARREST.

19th Century England

How much male fashion needed the calming influence of Beau Brummell became startlingly evident after Brummell fled Europe in 1819 to escape his creditors (apparently being a "fashion plate" was not an inexpensive avocation!). Immediately, the more conservative dress he had affected with such aplomb began to change, and caricaturists had a "field day" with the results. Not to be outdone by the French, "The top hat had swelled out at the top until its crown was wider than the brim, the visible ends of the shirt collar came up almost to the eyes, the stock or cravat grew tighter and higher, the shoulders of the coat were padded and the waist nipped in with the aid of a corset . . ."[41] Their pants ballooned about them in voluminous folds and were held in place by straps under the instep. By the mid-1800s, it was considered unseemly for men to wear flamboyant clothing or bright colors, and not until well into the next century would men once again preen their "fashion feathers".

No discussion of male accessorizing would be complete without mention of a mainstay of male social status that has traditionally captured attention and respect—military decorations and medals. They were, in many respects, an example of accessorizing at its finest. These masterpieces of the jeweler's art, especially those created in Europe during the nineteenth century, were a "badge" of each individual's existence—from courage and valor in battle to fellowship with one's comrades. As works of art, they stand alone in their elegance of design and workmanship, and they remain coveted family heirlooms and collectors items even today. Not to be outdone, English women wore their own patriotic accessories—but discreetly—and expressed their grief at the death of Lord Nelson by donning Trafalgar garters, inscribed with the nationalistic admonition, "England expects every man to do his duty."

On the Threshhold: The Victorian Era

For women, the focus of skirts shifted yet again and by 1820 had returned to their former fullness. Sleeves were weighted with material, and the overall result of this restrictive wear, as opposed to the freedom of movement that preceded it, molded the English lady into the staid image she presented during the mid-1800s and the Victorian era. With Queen Victoria as its figurehead, respectability in decorum and dress became the hallmark of the times. Man exhibited his hard-working status in the elaborate luxury of his home, ". . . and his wife now dressed in keeping with the furniture, like a well-upholstered armchair (as William Morris despairingly noted.)"[42]

Bringing a whole new look, and attitude, to fashion, another monumental revolution was underway—this one introduced paper patterns and sewing machines to "ordinary" women of the day. Both heralded the beginning of the ready-to-wear trade, an advancement that would eventually change the face of fashion, for before long women would be able to purchase their dresses "ready made" instead of hiring a dressmaker or tediously sewing them by hand. In the meantime, however, persons on the "lower" rungs of the social ladder could finally emulate their "betters," causing those at the top of this fashion pyramid to change direction and style with a fervor that could never have been possible before. It set the fashion and couture world spinning.

One change shortly thereafter saw skirts expanding once again, but this time to the rear. The staple crinoline was replaced by the bustle, which, as most artificial accoutrements before it, soon became disproportionate and ugly, taking a bizarre turn when the "Langtry model" both literally and figuratively *shot* onto the scene. Named for Lily Langtry, it consisted of metal bands on a pivot that could be raised when one was seated and then sprang magically into place when one stood up. Looking back from his vantage point in the 1940s, Vertes mused, "Still women remained the meek captives of their voluminous skirts—though by now the main bulk had moved to the rear. Our grandmothers resembled snails, carrying their house behind them."[43]

Low-cut dresses defied the prudity one is apt to associate with the Victorian era, and by the end of the century skirts had become even more tight and restrictive. Some of the accessories of this period were equally bewildering, especially when hats and dresses were decorated in a macabre manner with stuffed or imitation birds, butterflies, centipedes, and even mice. In pleasant contrast to what they pinned to their hats or shoulders, evening wear saw jet beads, pearls, and long fluttering trains aglitter with sequins, as well as ostrich feather fans and boas. Shoes had high heels and were fastened with lace or buttons. Gloves were a "must," and elbow-length suede ones, with rows of tiny buttons ascending the arms, were a particular favorite. The rules of etiquette were assiduously followed, including even the seemingly simple application of gloves. For, as the *Ladies Home Journal* decreed in an 1892 edition, "The putting on of one's gloves in the presence of a man is quite permissible." Whatever was the world coming to?

Ties and bows at the neck also gained favor, and many sports-minded females affected male dress, proudly wearing copies of men's caps and their stiff white collars. In athletics, the male of Victorian times made his own fashion statement—of sorts. For example, "For the new sport of cycling . . . an extraordinary costume was devised: tight-fitting knee britches, a very tight, military-looking jacket and a little pillbox cap. The really smart wearer of this outfit carried a bugle to warn pedestrians of his approach."[44]

And, thus, one might properly conclude that even a bugle, if you "played" it right, could qualify as a fashion accessory.

Under less strenuous conditions, men wore capes and smoking jackets, and collars rose even higher under the chin. "In one pocket he placed the timepiece that was the measure of his station in life. If rich, his watch was heavy gold. For the man on the lower rung of life's ladder, it was a silver Ingersoll costing $1. Through an open buttonhole of his vest he looped a heavy watch chain, anchored in an opposite pocket by a penknife or some other heavy object."[45] Although most males dressed conservatively, no less than Benjamin Disraeli boldly displayed his colorful plumage when he appeared at a party in "...green velvet trousers, a canary coloured waistcoat, low shoes, silver buckles, lace at his wrists."[46]

Earlier in the century, the military was involved in a strange anecdote involving another accessory—the umbrella. The story goes that the Duke of Wellington was more than mildly upset when he viewed his troops on the battlefield and saw, with horror, that they held umbrellas over their heads to keep their uniforms from getting wet. The Duke quickly "... sent a message firmly stating that he did 'not approve of the use of umbrellas during the enemy's firing and will not allow gentlemen's sons to make themselves ridiculous in the eyes of the army.'"[47]

The umbrella gained important accessorizing status as the century progressed, losing some of its original intent in the process. In order to make a proper impression, these "rain protectors on a stick" had to be furled in just the right way, which was a time-consuming process. Consequently, "... if it looked like rain the fashionable man of the late nineteenth century simply hailed a cab."[48] The lady's parasol also served a dual purpose, for although women carried them as fashionable protection from the sun, they were admonished not to cover their faces (the better for gentlemen to see them) and instead dangled the parasol provocatively from one hand. Parasol handles were made of precious materials like ivory, and the parasol itself was often covered with delicate laces, colorful fabrics, or flowers. Some models sported an ingenious hinge that could be adjusted according to the sun's placement, thereby enabling the dome to move in whatever direction necessary to offer the most effective shade.

Unfortunately, as in past cultures, even *people* became accessories during this period. The Southern lady had her servants following her "... dressed in descending degrees of finery according to their position, while the English lady liked to be seen with an Indian footman, gorgeously attired, walking ahead of her and a servant leading an ornamental dog following behind." [49]

Led by Emperor Franz Josef—who, with his aristocratic bearing and garb replete with gold and braid trims, created a resurgence of interest in the sartorial glories of the "man in uniform"—and his wife, the Empress Elizabeth, class distinctions in manner of dress began to slowly disintegrate. "In his ... book, 'A Nervous Splendor, Vienna 1888/1889,' Frederic Morton writes, 'In earlier centuries, high fashion had been yet another aristocratic privilege. It separated blueblood from the commoner. But then, more and more, ambitious burgers began to emulate what hitherto they had only admired. Gradually fashion became commerce, professionally created, cannily merchandised, widely broadcast, tensely practiced. It was as widely reported on, as greedily read about, as any interesting war.'"[50]

The Melting Pot

The examinations of life in the mid- and late 1800s would be incomplete, and seriously so, without a synopsis of the monumental changes taking place in the United States and their eventual effect on lives throughout the world. For this was a land where much was happening with lightning rapidity. The European influence had, of course, made itself felt across the ocean, and American women and men were also susceptible to the dictates of the French and English as they waited expectantly for word of the latest fashions. Nevertheless, by its very existence, the *New World* created an American culture with special needs, for its inhabitants were no longer completely in sync with their European brethren.

Here was a rare blend of individuals whose influence throughout the 19th century, and into the next, was a force with which to be reckoned. There were characters on this virgin "stage" as diverse in their roles as the rugged cowboy to his Indian nemesis, and hoop-skirted Southern belles to hearty pioneer women. In big cities and tiny hamlets, on farms and open prairies, there appeared a melting pot of cultures unlike anything seen before, for it represented the diversity of immigrants from lands around the world. The so-called "working" people—the laborers and ranch hands, farm wives, and shopkeepers—bore little resemblance to their European counterparts, and they unwittingly wielded more long-term power than they possibly realized. Their voice was heard. "Fashion" had changed direction. It was no longer the exclusive domain of the elite. There is no stronger evidence of this than the revolutionary addition to male and female wardrobes that had its beginnings in the late 1800s and resurfaced during the following century. It was destined to become, in one form or another, a staple of nearly every individual's wardrobe, worn more frequently, and in greater numbers, than any other article of casual clothing, bar none. In 1850, Levi Strauss, a Bulgarian immigrant,

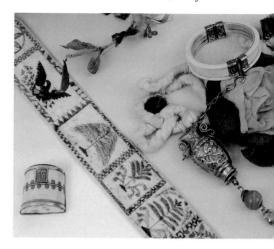

A silver and ivory pendant that was originally a game piece, a silver-hinged ivory bracelet, and a needle holder necklace, all Chinese from the late 1800s, frame a scrimshaw corset busk to keep milady's back straight.

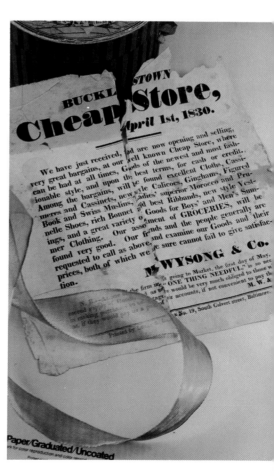

introduced to eager California "gold rush" miners a coverall made from sturdy tent material. Variations on his basically simple design were added, deleted, and embellished over the years, but that now-generic term *Levis*, or the all-encompassing "jeans," actually had its beginnings long before the "flower children" of the 1960s thought they'd uncovered something avant garde. They'd simply resurrected a garment that grizzled occupants of California mining communities had coveted a century before.

It was during this same period that our all-American cowboy hero began his trek through the pages of American cultural history, and what he wore in the late 1800s and early 20th century has enjoyed continuing popularity, raising the simple cowboy to cult status around the world. Hats were a mainstay of the cowboy's attire. Nevertheless, each geographical area had its own distinctive look. "Whether a hat was uncreased, creased, rolled rim or stiff was dependent on the time, region, and prevailing style." [51] Bandannas and vests were also a part of the cowboy's lore. From solids to polka dots and plaids, the vest became a measure of the cowboy's individual taste. Even the standard bandanna developed an individuality of its own. "Everyday bandannas were made of brightly dyed cotton, while expensive silk neckerchiefs were bought for those special occasions in a cowboy's life, like community meetings, dances, and picnics."[52] The cowboy saga is uniquely American. He too strove to fashion his own special niche when surrounded by others so very like him in dress and lifestyle, and as a group, and individually, it is safe to say that he succeeded—for the idolatry of the American cowboy is destined to just "keep on goin'"!

Another figure of this pioneering period also became larger than life—the native American Indian. The casual dress of Hopi Indian women influenced fashion in the early 20th century, and the simple Indian moccasin has inspired innumerable variations over the past hundred years. Be it a fine old saddle or a hand-wrought silver and turquoise cuff, people of other countries and other cultures continue to fall under the hypnotic spell of "cowboys and Indians." From the staid British to the exuberant Italians, an appreciation of the legends of the Old West lives on.

On both sides of the Atlantic, the late 1800s ushered in a new era of freedom, which individual needs and conditions demanded. While the birth of couture is usually associated with the French, it was an Englishman, Charles Frederick Worth, who in Paris in the mid-1800s set the evolution of couture into motion. The popularity of his fashion theories is evident, for Worth's clientele eventually grew to such enormous proportions that at one time he had 1,000 workers hand-sewing his garments. Worth was the first designer to use "live" models to showcase his clothes, " . . . but they had to wear full-length, black leotards, since it was considered improper to wear the clothes next to their skin." [53] Casual clothing was becoming more important than ever before, although among the elite, opulent dress and accessorizing were not soon to be displaced. Nevertheless, the Victorian period was drawing to a close, and the world hovered expectantly on the brink of a "new day."

Three fine glass bead purse figurals. On left, a romantic scene crowned by a French jeweled frame, with stones in green and blue surrounded by enameled flowers. 8" x 11". Center, a majestic bird with sweeping tail. The French frame has brown stones and enameled flowers. 6" wide x 10" long. A fine Victorian beaded floral purse. Measuring 5-½" x 10", it has a divided, diagonal background of cream and pale blue. The frame is marked "Made in Czecho-Slovakia." Courtesy of Veronica Trainer.

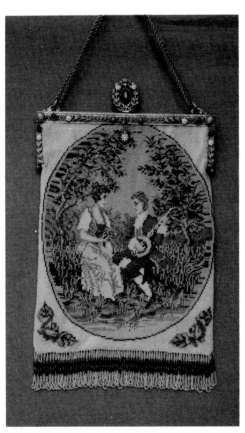
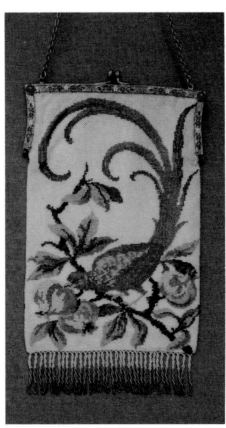
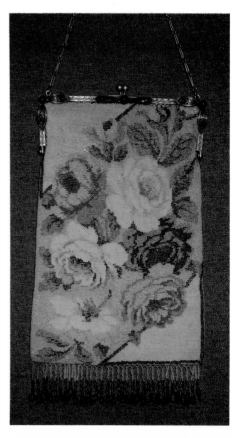

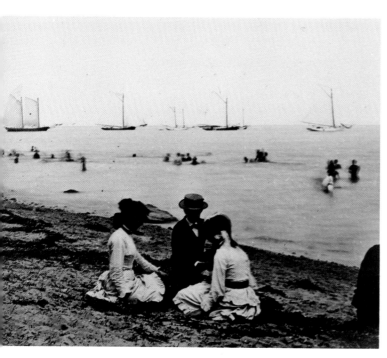

Forced to wear these cumbersome day clothes, there was little frolicking on the beach at Martha's Vineyard in the late 1800s.

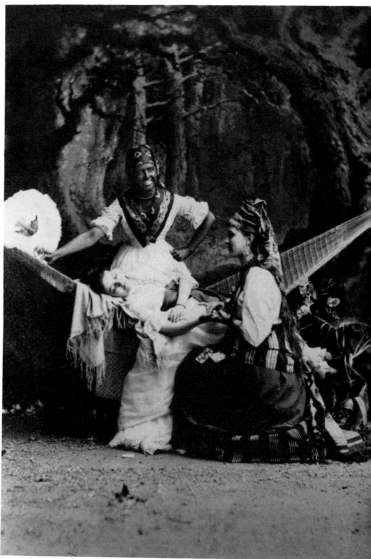

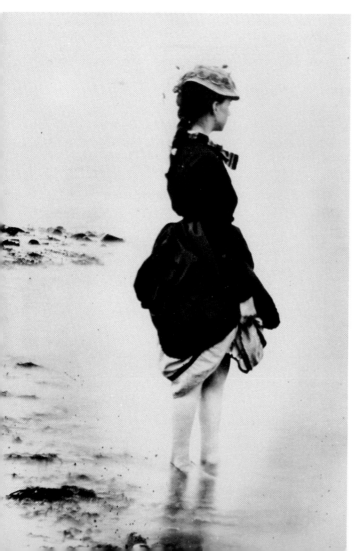

Having a ball! Mrs. Henry Leavitt (reclining), Miss Ada Thayer, and Miss Edith May. From photo album entitled "Fancy Dress Ball, New York, 1875." Courtesy of The Newport Historical Society, Rhode Island.

It's summertime at Oak Bluffs, Martha's Vineyard in the late 1880s, but there's no "coolin' down" in these duds . . . even the dog looks "all pooched out"!

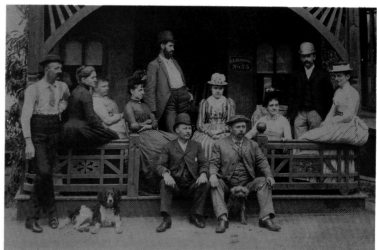

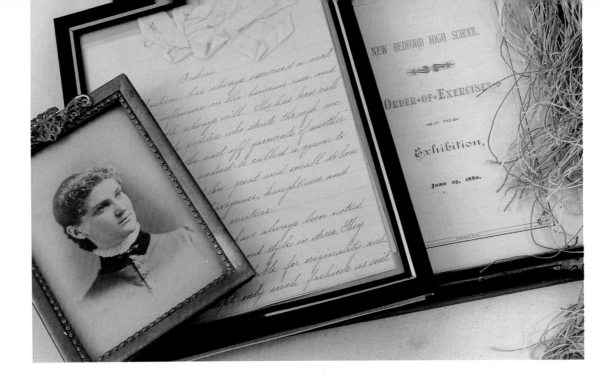

Testimony to the changes in attitudes was recorded in the words of a relatively naive source. Entitled simply "Fashion," the following was written by Caroline Otis Pierce and given as a commencement address to the New Bedford, Massachusetts high school class of 1880. It provides an innocent, but surprisingly mature view of fashion as seen through the eyes of a young lady about to embark on her life's journey.

Fashion has always exercised a most powerful influence on the human race, and undoubtedly always will. She has been called "a fickle goddess who struts through one country in the cast off garments of another."

She may indeed be called a queen to whom high and low, great and small do homage. Gossip, extravagance, haughtiness and ostentation are her courtiers.

French ladies have always been noted for their good taste and style in dress. They are especially remarkable for originality and, as a rule, adopt only such fashions as suit their face and figure. I have somewhere read long wristed gloves were devised by a French woman to conceal a scar upon her arm. Doubtless many of our fashions had their origin in some such purpose.

Fashion's devoted subjects willingly submit to her laws, while a few denying her right to rule are constantly fighting against them. It is perfectly right for me to follow the fashions moderately and to spend proper thought and care on his appearance. Many people yield too readily to her dictates. If they would stop a moment and analyze some of them I am confident we should not see so many of our friends dressed in such extreme fashions that we scarcely know where in nature to class them.

As one travels through various countries it is both instructive and interesting to note the different ideas of the inhabitants concerning their apparel. The German ladies put on good clothes for fine occasions. It is said they do not know what dress means. A number of ladies in Deipuc have formed a society under the name of "Simplicity" to oppose the extravagance of fashion in dress and ornaments. The members have pledged themselves not to wear false hair, trains, tunics, or any double skirts. All their dresses are to be plainly trimmed.

Philadelphia ladies are said to have a particularly delicate and refined style of dress. Probably this is due to the Quaker element of society whose quiet simplicity of attire has an effect on the dress of all classes.

How many of our ladies from whom we naturally expect nobler aims go to church merely to show their fine clothes and obtain the latest styles. We hear people talking of "Feminine Scrutiny in Church." Persons of this character fix their eyes upon the approaching one, stare solemnly into her face and then dropping them to her feet commence to travel up again. The flounces are examined, the eyes linger at the most striking article, the bonnet, and if the examination proves unsatisfactory the chin is tossed in the air and they anxiously await the next newcomer.

As we take up the latest fashion book and hastily look through its fascinating pages we see no particular style is exclusively "the fashion." At the present time one has more liberty in his ideas of dress. Simplicity is a quality much sought for and not only promises satisfaction but indicates refinement of taste.

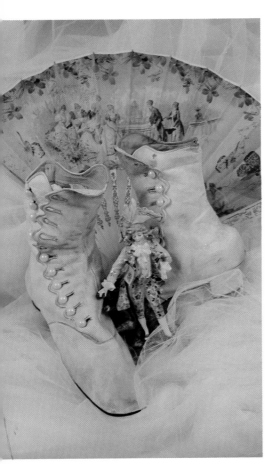

A German "dandy" figurine admires an ivory-handled fan and soft kid boots, both from the 1850s. Collection of Gloria C. Malloy.

All that has paraded down fashion's runway in the past will give the reader new insight into garments and accessories of the 20th century, itself now poised to welcome yet another. Somehow, a modestly pointed shoe and backbreaking stiletto heels, bobbed hair and flapper skirts, rhinestone-studded hose and cats-eye sunglasses appear innocently harmless by comparison. Indeed, the 20th century has been remarkably good to us. As you will see, the decade-after-decade journey to the threshhold of the year 2000 has been a kaleidoscopic ride on the whirling wheel of fashion.

1 Vertes, Art & Fashion, p. 54
2 Vertes, Art & Fashion, p. 55
3 Laver, Costumes & Fashion, p. 23
4 Laver, Costumes & Fashion, p. 15
5 Batterberry, Fashion, p. 41
6 Batterberry, Fashion, p. 35
7 Batterberry, Fashion, p. 59
8 Batterberry, Fashion, p. 54
9 Batterberry
10 Batterberry, Fashion, p. 58
11 Batterberry, Fashion, p. 57
12 Laver, Costumes & Fashion, p. 47
13 Yarwood, Encyclopedia of World Costume, p. 70
14 Yarwood, Encyclopedia of World Costume, p. 61
15 Webb, The Heritage of Dress, p. 19
16 Laver, Costumes & Fashion, p. 72
17 Dorner, Fashion, p. 13
18 Dorner, Fashion, p. 99
19 Laver, Costume & Fashion, p. 74

20 Dorner, Fashion, p. 17
21 Laver, Costumes & Fashion, p. 87
22 Laver, Costumes & Fashion, p. 119
23 Laver, Costumes & Fashion, p. 102
24 Laver, Costume & Fashion, p. 106
25 Laver, Costume & Fashion, p. 112
26 Laver, Costume & Fashion, p. 112
27 Dorner, Fashion, p. 25
28 Cassin-Smith, Costume & Fashion, p. 124
29 Vertes, Art & Fashion, p. 58
30 Dorner, Fashion, p. 49
31 Thesaurus of Anecdotes, p. 129
32 Vertes, Art & Fashion, p. 80
33 Cassin-Smith, Costume, etc., p. 118
34 Vertes, Art & Fashion, p. 59
35 Laver, Costume & Fashion, p. 152
36 Dorner, Fashion, p. 31
37 Dorner, Fashion, p. 31
38 Batterberry, Fashion, p. 211

39 Batterberry, Fashion, p. 212
40 Batterberry, Fashion, p. 216
41 Laver, Costume & Fashion, p. 162
42 Dorner, Fashion, p. 32
43 Vertes, Art & Fashion, p. 60
44 Laver, Costumes & Fashion, p. 204
45 Churchill, Remember When, p. 20
46 Dorner, Fashion, p. 89
47 Dorner, Fashion, p. 56
48 Dorner, Fashion, p. 57
49 Dorner, Fashion, p. 57
50 The New York Times Magazine, Nov. 25, 1979
51 Ball, Cowboy Collectibles and Western Memorabilia, p. 17
52 Ball, Cowboy Collectibles and Western Memorabilia, p. 7
53 The House of Elliot, Jean Marsh, BBC-TV, Arts and Entertainment Network, August 9, 1992.

Part Two: The Twentieth Century

IN GREETING THE NEW CENTURY, "THE NEW YORK WORLD CHOSE TO BE
MORDANT, 'THE 1800s ARE GONE FOREVER', IT SAID, 'AND BRISK, BRIGHT, FRESH,
ALTOGETHER NEW 1900 GREETS EVERYBODY TODAY—GOOD FOR A CLEAN
HUNDRED YEARS BEFORE 2000 COMES AROUND AND EVERYBODY NOW ALIVE IS
GONE . . .'"

"Remember When" Alan Churchill

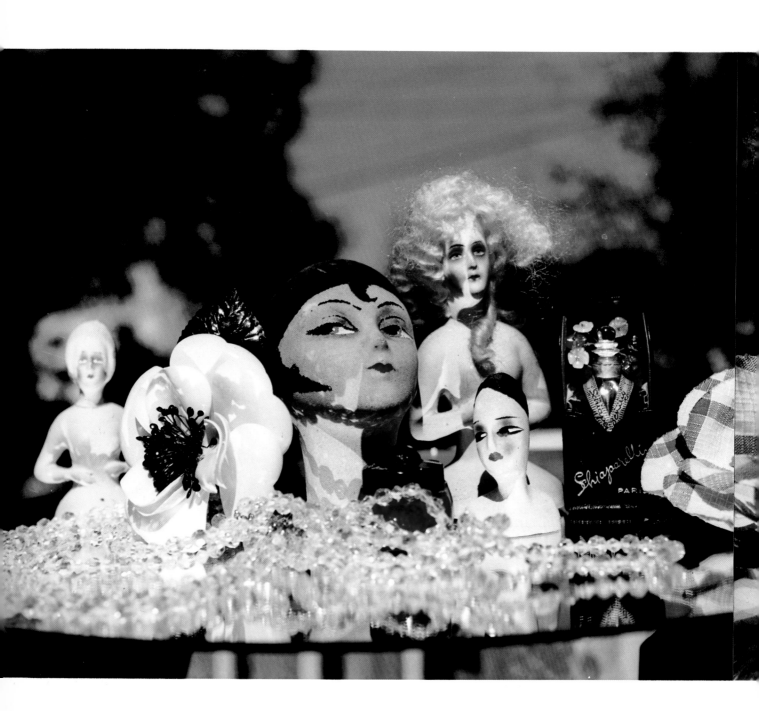

"What to wear...what to wear."

These were the ten decades that probably more than any other were destined to revolutionize the shape of fashion. For in no other century was there a greater opportunity to influence and change the predilections of the world's inhabitants.

The 20th century widened communications and, in turn, narrowed boundaries. It brought us radio, movies, phonograph records, and television, and expanded the audience of live theatre. The art of photography was refined. Magazines and newspapers flourished and, along with books, reached a larger mass audience than was ever possible before. Trains streaked across continents, and airplanes, constantly increasing in sleekness and speed, turned vast expanses of ocean into mere puddles. Telephone wires transported the human voice in the twinkling of an eye. Computers created a communications revolution, and facsimile machines conveyed written messages from state to state and country to country in only seconds. Space travel began, and "the man in the moon" actually became "the man on the moon."

For what more, pray tell, could New Year's Eve revelers in that split second between December 31, 1899 and January 1, 1900 have asked?

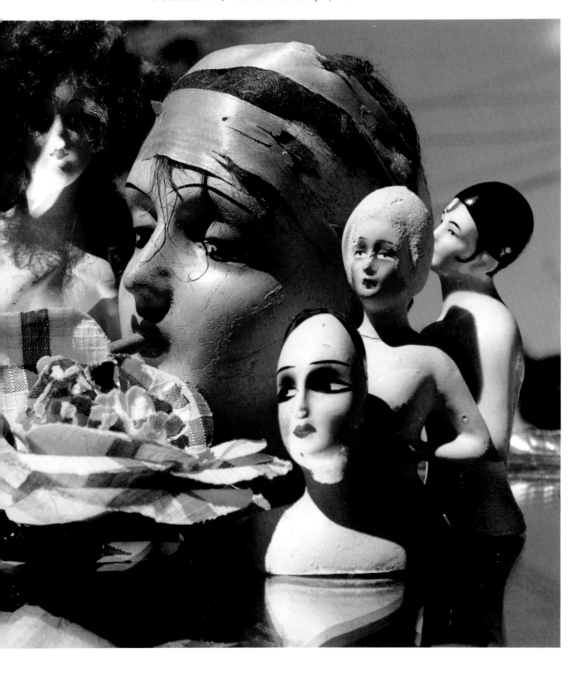

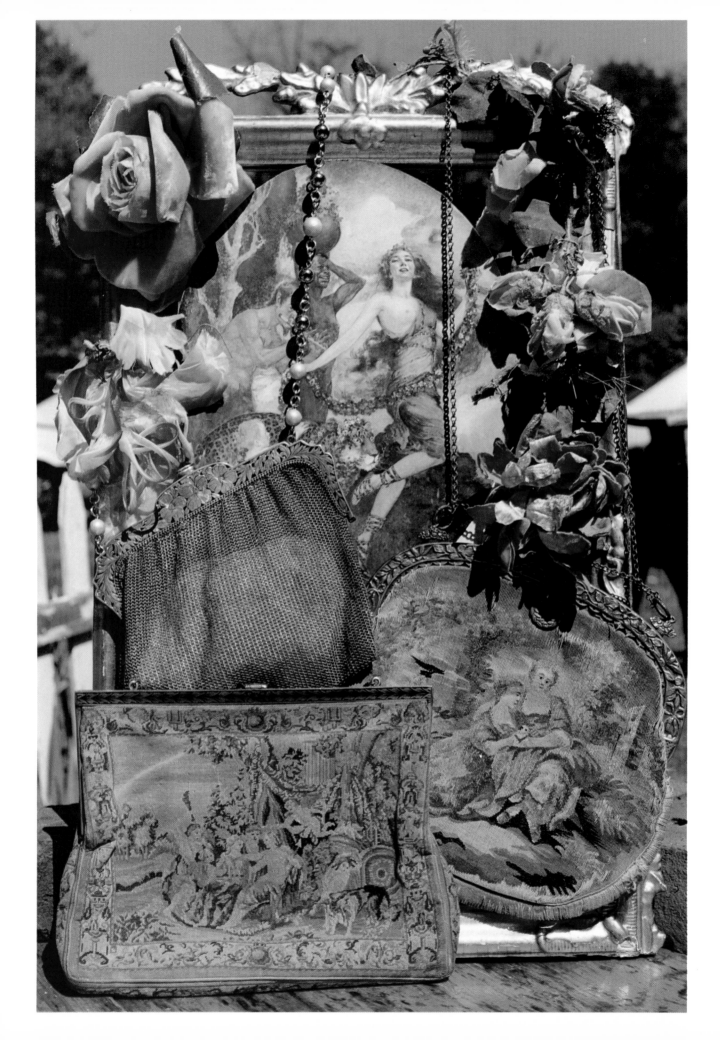

The Turn of the Century

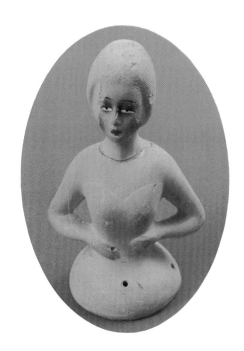

MAINLY IT IS THE EXTREMITIES OF FASHION THAT DISTORT GOOD TASTE.
Marcel Vertes

The clock ticks, the hands move, hearts beat faster . . . the 20th century is here. " . . . already, high spirited Americans were calling the new year Nineteen Oughty-Ought, or even Naughty Naught."[1]

Hats! Hats! Hats! They were, in all their overblown glory, the fashion accessory of the 20th century's first decade. Enormous, festooned with flowers and feathers, bows and ruffles, a woman could hardly appear inconspicuous in one. To view them now can only make one ponder how heads could possibly be held erect under the weight of such questionable creations. Undoubtedly, as in times past, everyone tried to "outdo" everyone else, until hats grew to cumbersome and seemingly unmanageable proportions. That the female population paid little heed to an article in the July 1900 issue of *The Woman's Home Companion* is evident when viewing the overpowering hats of this period, most of which negated common sense. The article pleaded, "Don't get an eccentric shape; beware of monstrosities of outline in felt, straw or braids. Avoid the use of large masses of feathers—of course you will not wear dead birds or their wings, or their fragile aigrettes . . . and be a little chary of too many bright flowers massed near your face." Sound advice, but destined to fly in the face of fashion as the decade continued.

Yet another torture chamber was endured in the name of fashion: the corset. "We forget the corset that the Paris dressmakers hid craftily under materials that were light and filmy. But the woman who wore it could not forget, because it gave her the vapors; often she came near fainting, so relentless was its grip. She was never more completely the slave than in the years that preceded the First World War."[2] It was the "health" corsets (a misnomer, if ever there was one) that resulted in the strange S-shape women's bodies took on, and understandably so, for ". . . in a laudable effort to prevent a downward pressure on the abdomen (they) made the body rigidly straight in front by throwing forward the bust and throwing back the hips."[3] By the end of the decade, the bust-line receded, and the hips no longer needed to be thrust out like self-styled bustles. In fact, as hats got wider, hips appeared to narrow, changing the silhouette even more.

On the plus side, lace collars decoratively adorned evening dresses, and gloves, usually to the elbows, were worn by the mannered ladies of the day. For evening, decorative fans fluttered demurely and jewelry appeared in abundance. As the July 1900 issue of *The Woman's Home Companion* entreated, ". . . you must be careful about your shoes and gloves, daintily immaculate as to the band of snowy linen or the film of lace, chiffon or muslin at your throat and wrists, your veil if you wear one, your handkerchief and purse. All these must be fresh and carefully chosen. Shoes and gloves, you need not be told, are of first importance. They should fit hands and feet, being neither too large nor too small, but leaning toward ease, as a tight shoe is unendurable, while a tight glove makes the hand ugly and shapeless, as well as uncomfortable."

Although the Edwardian mode of dress exerted some influence during the first years of the new century, as the decade progressed its style was soon rejected by the younger generation as too restrictive, and a more straight and flowing line eventually took its place. With it came bursts of bright colors (although young, unattached females were generally seen only in white and could not affect the more vibrant look until they were safely married). Even stockings, which peeked seductively beneath the shorter hemlines, were in shades designed to attract the eye and complement the outfit. Skirts with split hems both front and rear came into vogue, revealing another layer beneath, and around 1910 it became a form of pantaloon. Influenced by French fashions, purples, blues, taupes and smoky hues were considered especially attractive for ladies suits—an addition to female wardrobes that swept the fashion scene and has remained, in one form or another, ever since.

Embroidery, beading, and fringe added accessorizing interest to the dressier fashions, like tunics, which also enjoyed popularity for a time. In some instances, these decorative items became a convertible accessory that could easily be removed and placed on another garment. Accessorizing with fur on muffs, cravats, and detachable collars, was also popular. Linen collars were worn with the standard, uniform-like shirtwaist dress that was eagerly adopted—with variations in fabric and detail—by most women of the period, and much admired for its comfort and versatility. It has remained a faithful standby ever since.

When questioned as to preferences in clothing, young women in the early years of the decade were reported to rank shoes first, gloves close behind, then neckwear, hats, underwear, jewelry and ribbons. With the exception of underwear—which under certain

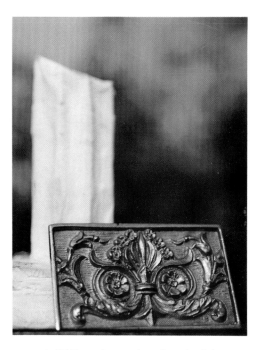

A 1990's papier mache column by Jake Torem provides a stark backdrop for a Victorian French pin from Didier Ludot, Paris.

circumstances would possibly qualify—it's interesting to note that all were *accessories*, giving credence to the long-held observation that women place great emphasis on wearing items of clothing that affirm their individuality while adding interest to their outfit.

The psychological effects of certain modes of dress were already being scrutinized by those prone to delve into the deeper implications of milady's wardrobe. As early as 1907 it was written that, "Feelings of lightheadedness are the results of filmy clothes, and one girl of eighteen said that whenever she had a garment of this consistency she always wanted to dance." Conversely, the writer went on to observe that "... heavy clothes bring about mental depression."[4]

Although most matrons employed the services of dressmakers for their clothing, many women, especially young shop girls and servants, sewed and cared for their own garments. As outlined in a *Ladies Home Journal* article in June of 1903, instructions for maintaining them were rigid. "The girl making her own clothes must keep her tailored and street suits in good repair, well brushed and pressed, hang her jackets on a stretcher covered with old muslin, fold her gloves and veils, dispense with all cheap geegaws, and avoid all unusual colors, if she desires to appear well dressed."   What was worn on the beach during this decade became another story—this one of liberation. Annette Kellerman, the champion long-distance swimmer, changed swim attire for all time by sporting a practical one-piece bathing suit sans the skirts, stockings, and monumental "cover-ups" that women previously endured while seeking a semblance of relief from the blazing sun. Although certainly not revealing by later standards, this new beachwear was daring for its day, and created no small measure of comment, both pro and con.

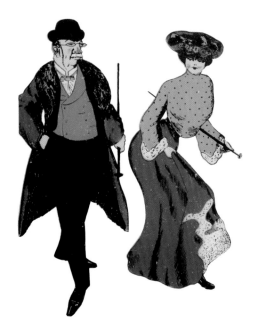

Motoring prompted other fashion necessities if one was going to be in tune with the "latest." Simplicity was the by-word and, as the name implies, the purpose of long dusters was self-explanatory. Big hats, held tightly in place by wide ribbons or veiling wrapped around the head and chin, protected hair from the elements. The automobile was here to stay—and the modern woman was ready to meet the challenge of the road.

The French designer Mariano Fortuny began his long and illustrious trek through fashion history during the close of this decade. Known for his understated garments and delicately pleated materials, his concept of fabric and style has stood the test of time. Among his accessory creations were scarves of the most artful design. No longer an uninteresting piece of colored fabric, Fortuny's became works of art when strategically draped over garments of all types, creating a relatively new field of "modern" accessorizing that has become a staple of the fashion industry.

Another mainstay of scarf-making, along with handkerchiefs, had its beginning when Arthur Liberty opened his shop in London in 1875. It wasn't until 1904, however, that the venerable *Liberty of London* began producing scarves bearing their name. Fashioned from highly distinctive prints that have become their trademark, each continues to be prized for its beauty and understated elegance. The popularity of even simple scarf designs was drastically enhanced by an "invention" that eventually freed women from elaborate and time-consuming hairdos and motivated more and more of them to include scarves as a vital accessorizing tool. Although it took another decade to assure its acceptance, the Parisienne permanent wave, heralding short, wavy tresses, made scarves the perfect new head covering.

Men's fashions, however, had not "loosened up." Stiff collars and cuffs still impeded comfort. "Waistcoats were now made to match the coat, except for the white pique waistcoat worn later with the black suit. Knotted ties worn with turn-over collars started to gain popularity."[5] But one male accessory overshadowed all others. One of its major manufacturers was the Hamilton Watch Company. Founded in 1892 in Lancaster, Pennsylvania, its name was in honor of Andrew Hamilton, who, with his son James, laid out the plans for Lancaster on land granted to him by William Penn. The pocket watch, that mainstay of a gentleman's wardrobe in the late 1800s and early 1900s, was the Company's "flagship" product. An epidemic of fatal railroad crashes, many caused by faulty timepieces, resulted in the manufacture of 1.6 million railroad watches by Hamilton between 1893 and 1957. Since they were recognized as the most accurate, the public's fears were allayed, and before the new century had begun, a name synonymous with dependability was born—a dependability so unquestioned, that during World War I General Pershing used a Hamilton to time the movements of his troops.

At the same time, Hamilton also supplied a limited number of strap watches to officers in the trenches, marking the beginning of a trend away from pocket watches to wristwatches—a somewhat easier way to tell time than the ritualistic removal of a bulky pocket watch from one's vest pocket, and a sure winner in a time-and-motion study! Sensing an untapped marketing opportunity, Hamilton introduced their first lady's timepiece around 1908, and with the market booming for both ladies' and gentlemen's wristwatches, styling and case designs became extremely important in the years after World War I.

The emphasis of fashion was shifting, but in his own inimitable way it was the irascible Mark Twain who gave us a glimpse of the *casual male* to come. Twain found life sans collar and tie to be more to his liking, and frequently visited friends and neighbors without them. Mrs. Twain, on the other hand, considered the practice distasteful and, after one such occasion, she forcefully expressed her displeasure at her husband's defiance of the social graces. He of the rapier wit sought to assuage her—or, more likely, point out the foolishness of her argument—by packing both articles of clothing carefully into a box and having them delivered to a neighbor with the following note: "A little while ago I visited you without my collar and tie for about half an hour. The missing articles are enclosed. Will you kindly gaze at them for 30 minutes and then return them to me?"[6]

Twain was no stranger to flying in the face of convention. It is doubtful, however, that even his prescience could have hinted at the magnitude of imminent world events, and the revolution in fashion that was to accompany them.

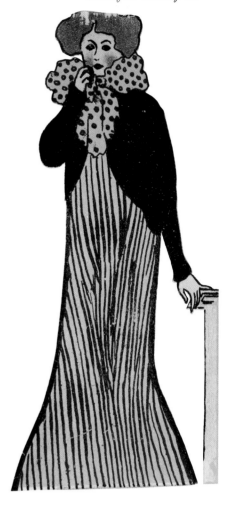

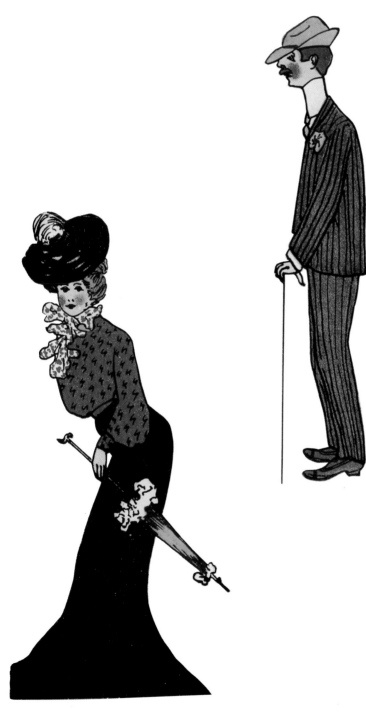

These early 20th century European figures (probably French or German) display the witty, artistic style of the comic strips that captured the public's imagination several decades later.

1900—1910
[1] Churchill, "Remember When" p. 8
[2] Verte, Art & Fashion, p. 62
[3] Laver, Costume & Fashion, p. 213
[4] Cassin-Smith, Costume, etc., p. 195
[5] Thesaurus of Anecdotes, p. 129

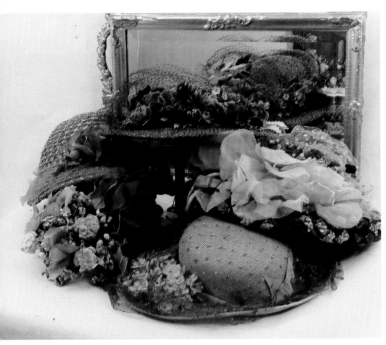

A collection of vintage straw and floral hats are both fragile and powerful. The sky blue straw laden with flowers is from the turn of the century. Courtesy of Alyson Torem French.

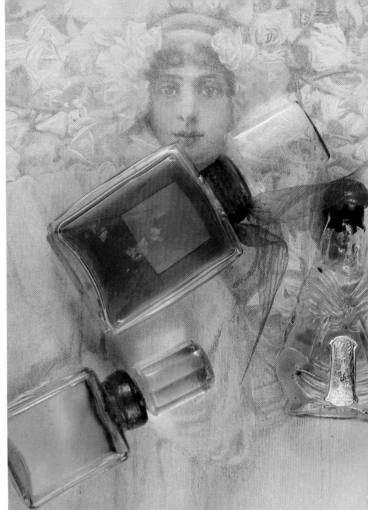

This lovely lady graced a vintage 1897 magazine. The perfume bottles reflect the age of Victoriana.

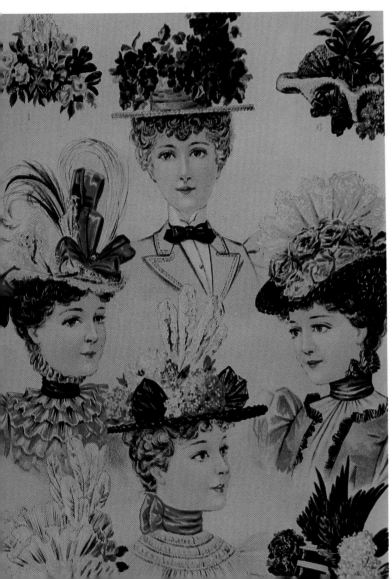

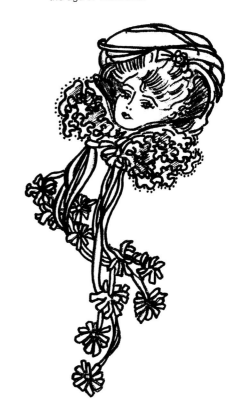

Fashion hats as featured in a 1904 issue of *Delineator*.

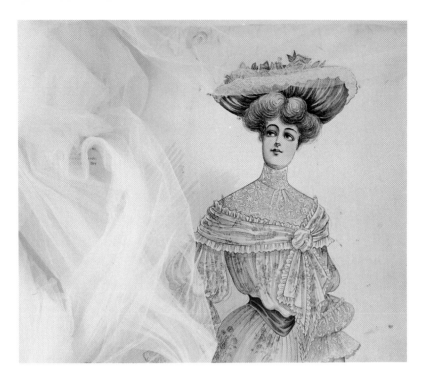

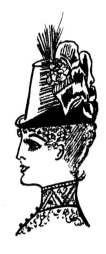

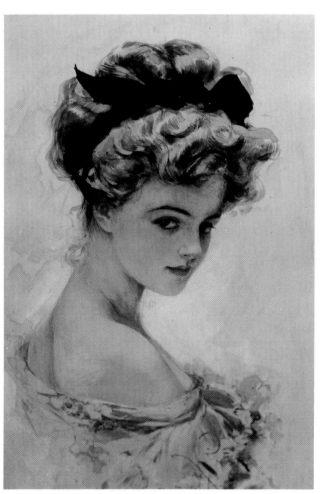

"Her Eyes Were Made to Worship."
Harrison Fisher (1875-1934). Gouache,
watercolor on board, 17″ x 12″.
American Beauties cover. Courtesy of
Alan M. Goffman, The Fine Art of
Illustration, New York.

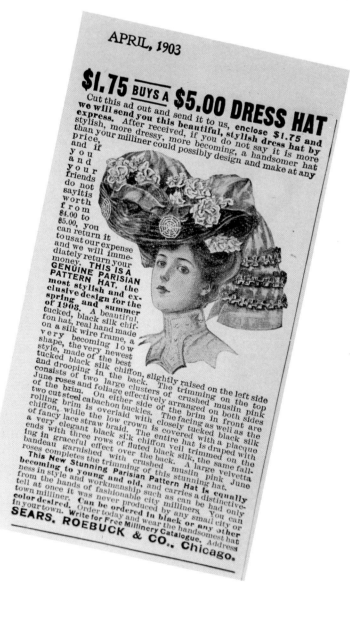

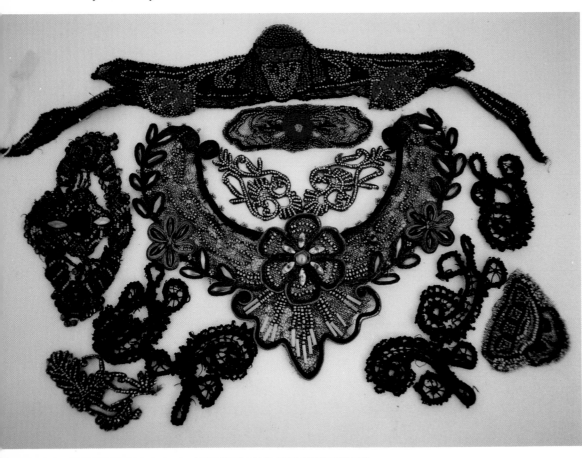

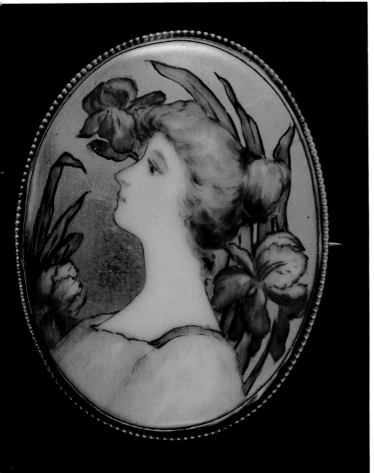

"Frosting on the cake" . . . turn of the century beading and delicate macrame.

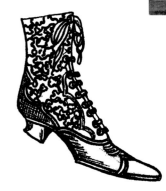

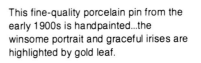

This fine-quality porcelain pin from the early 1900s is handpainted...the winsome portrait and graceful irises are highlighted by gold leaf.

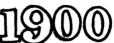

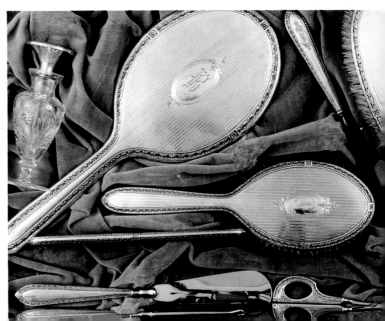

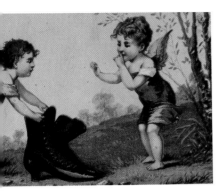

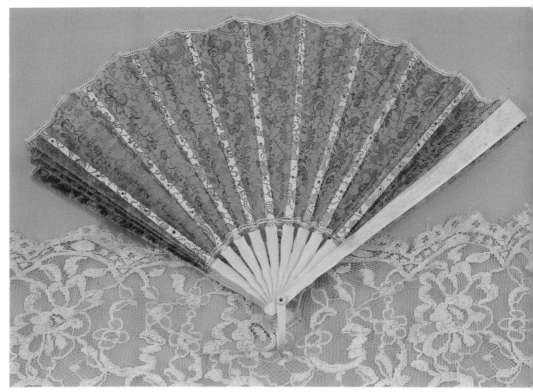

A fan with 18K gold leaf. Courtesy of
Golden Heart Antiques.

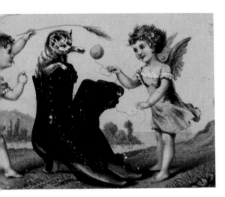

Victorian to the core—the cat in the
shoe . . . with angelic cherubs.

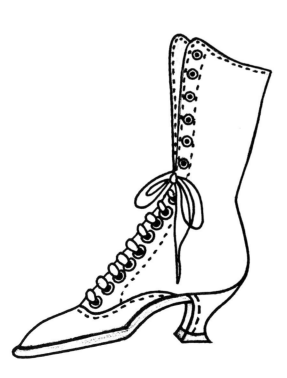

This 10-piece sterling dresser set from
International Silver Company in original
velvet-lined presentation case features
an etched crystal parfum with sterling
stopper.

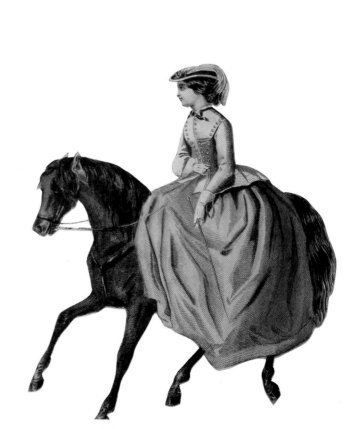

Side saddle!

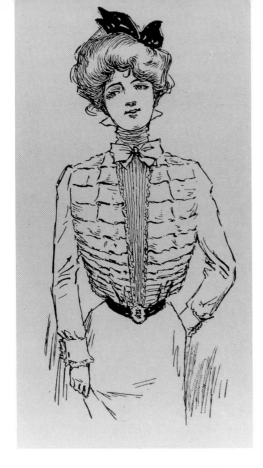

From the *Ladies Home Journal*, 1900.

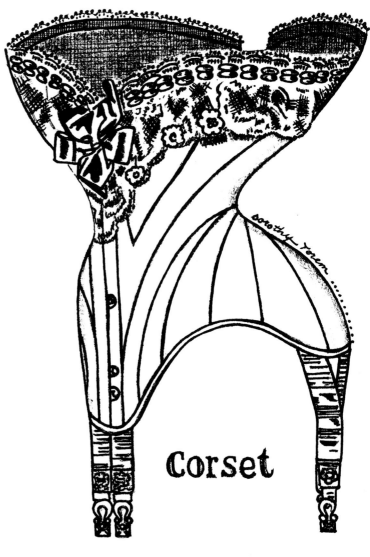

Corset

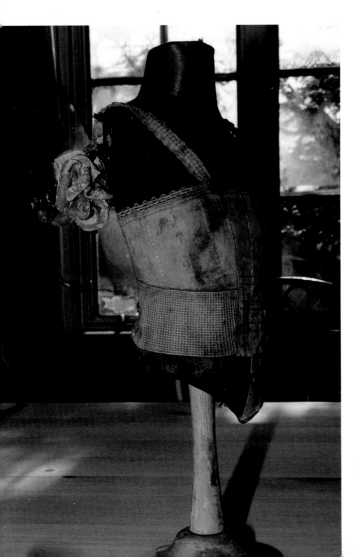

A miniature dressmaker model, dated
1910.

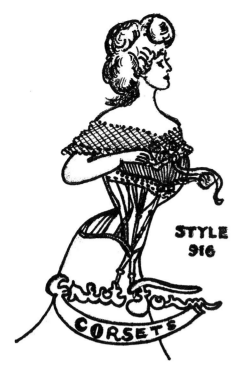

STYLE 916

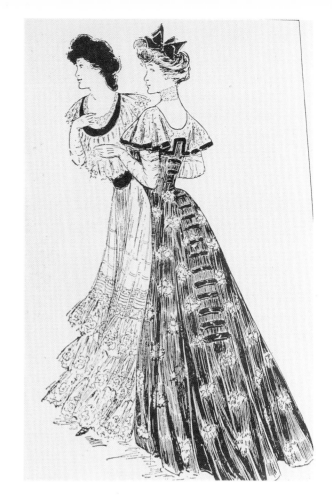

Vogue, 1907.

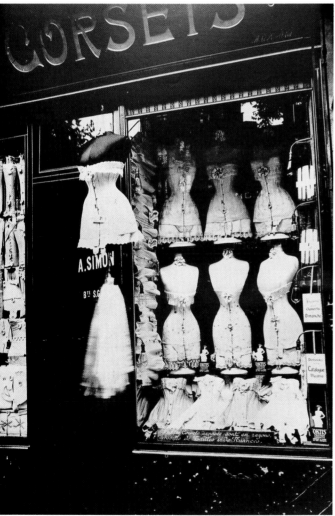

This window of an early 1900's French corset shop features "breathtaking unmentionables" with dimensions decidedly not for the "faint at heart."

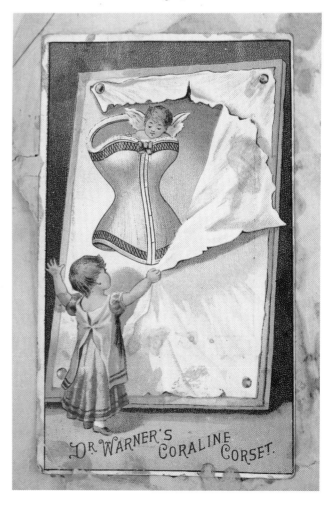

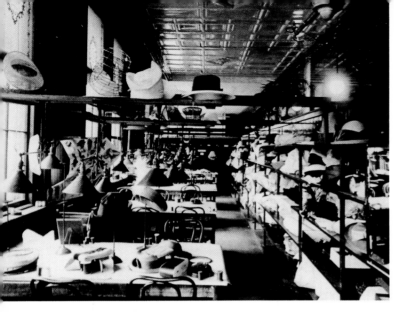

Millinery salon.

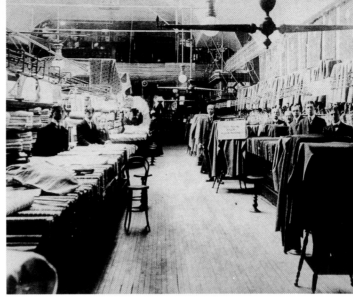
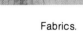

Fabrics.

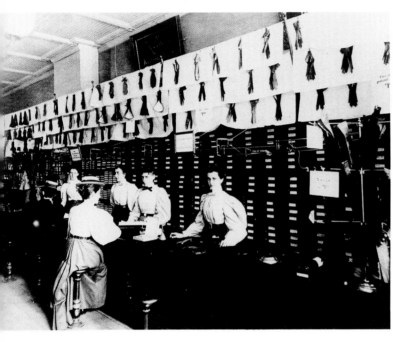

Gloves.

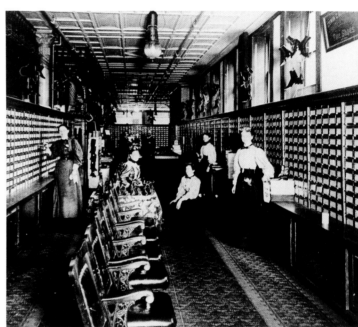

Shoes.

Inside the Forbes & Wallace department store, Springfield, Massachusetts, 1900. Courtesy of the Connecticut Valley Historical Museum.

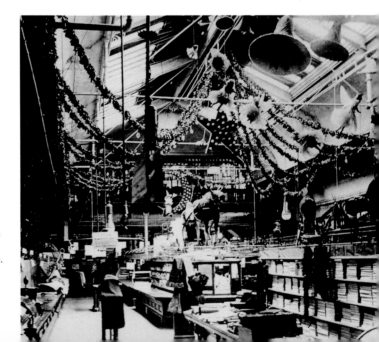

Deck the halls...Christmas at Forbes & Wallace, 1902. Courtesy of the Connecticut Valley Historical Museum.

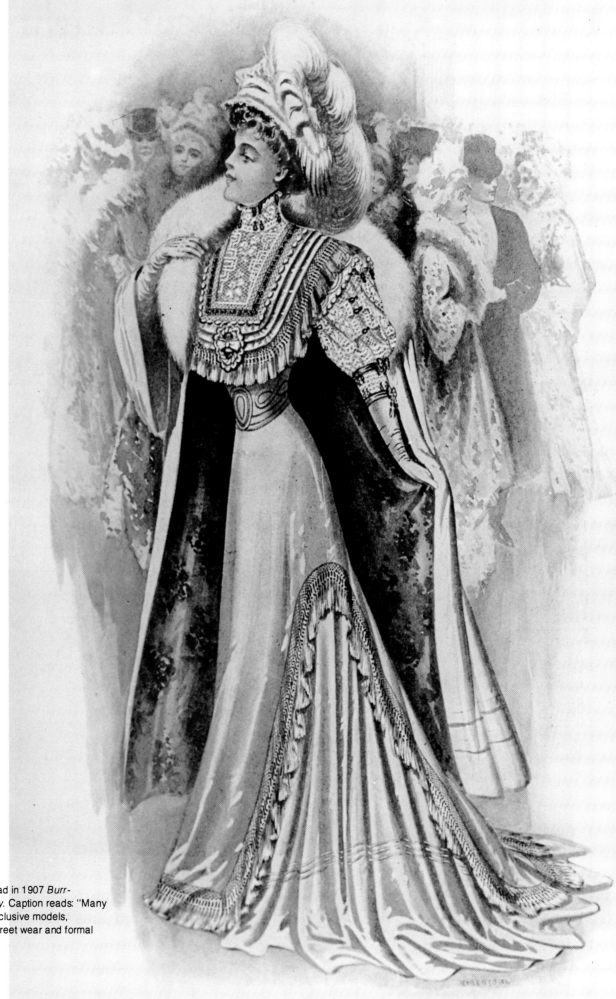

Lord and Taylor ad in 1907 *Burr-McIntosh Monthly*. Caption reads: "Many attractive and exclusive models, appropriate for street wear and formal dress."

Postcards from 1902 and 1907 bring us
the wit of the times—and an
exaggerated view of the fashions!

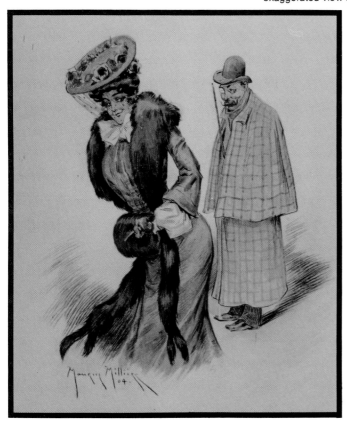

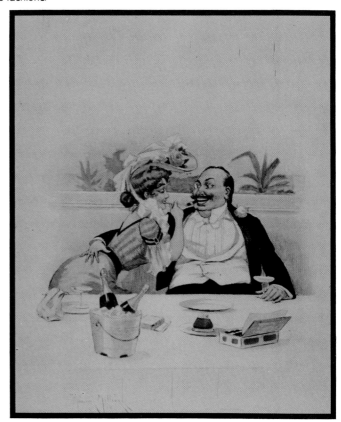

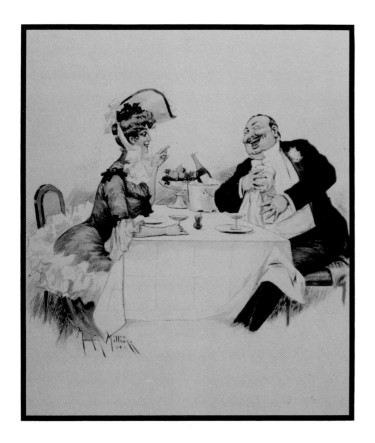

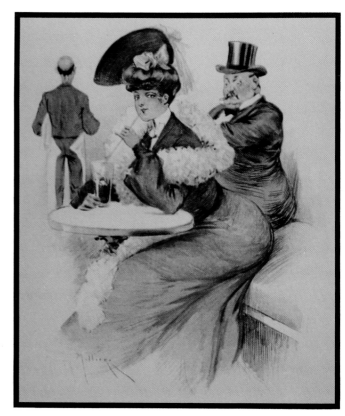

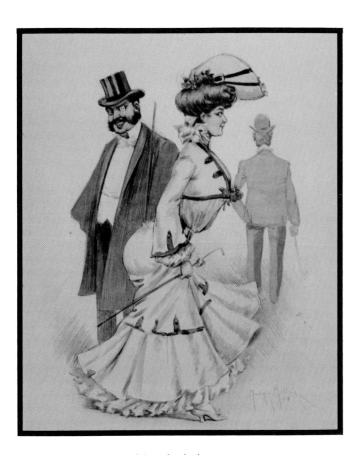

A knowing look

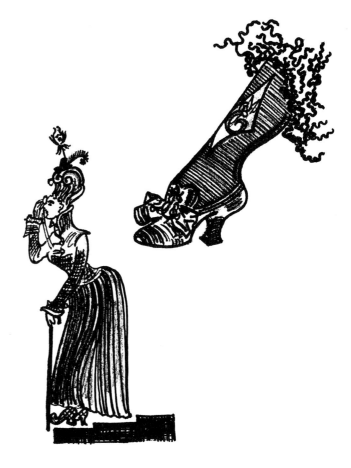

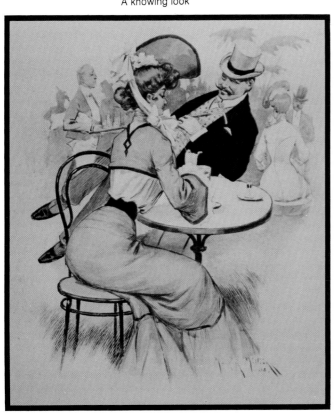

Demure and delighted.

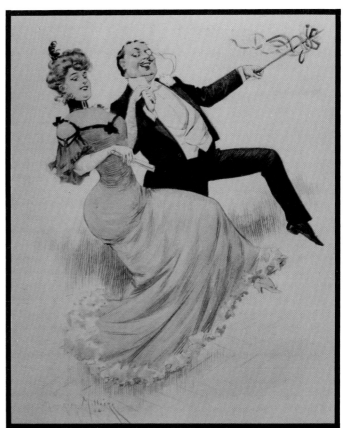

A romp

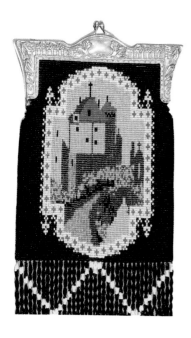

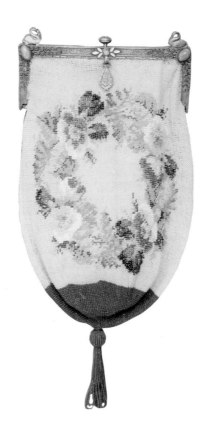

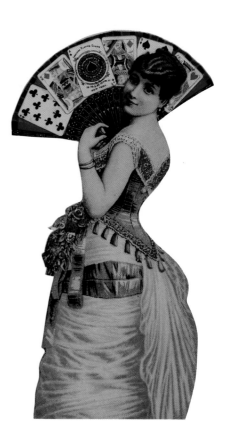

This Victorian glass bead purse is
decorated in an interesting castle scene
in vibrant hues. The silverplated frame
has bold, Art Nouveau designs. 6″ x 11″.
Courtesy of Veronica Trainer.

Pansies float softly on this Victorian
beaded purse. The French frame is
jeweled and enameled. Courtesy of
Victoria Trainer.

"If you play your cards right . . ."

Beaded pouch bag . . . flowers, houses,
trees and even a wispy tassel.

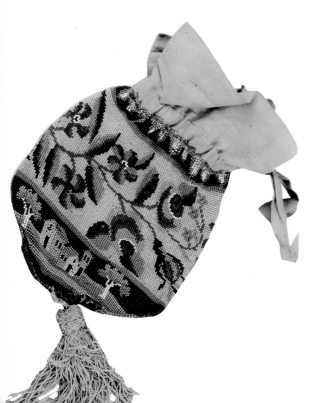

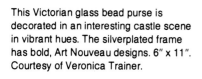

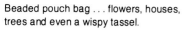

Smell the roses! Beaded floral bag with
800 silver frame. Courtesy of Victoria
Trainer.

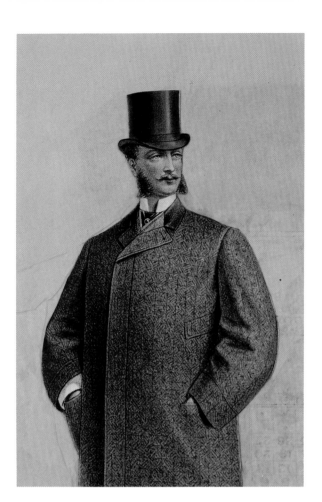

"I'm suave and debonair . . . and warm in wool!"

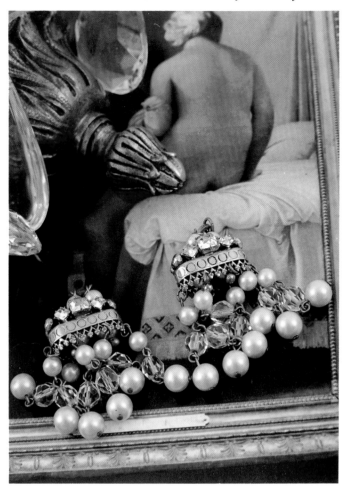

Out of that shower cap, into some clothes... and on with the earrings. These Victorian beauties are of 14K gold, with pearls and rose-cut diamonds.

Buttons and bows . . . Set of Pims military regalia buttons.

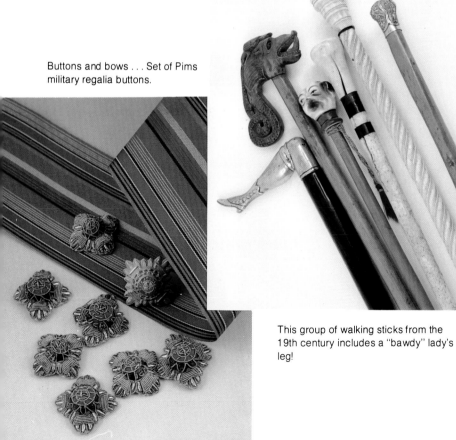

This group of walking sticks from the 19th century includes a "bawdy" lady's leg!

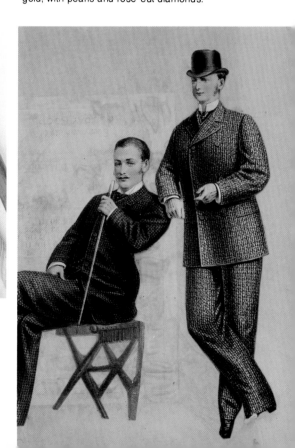

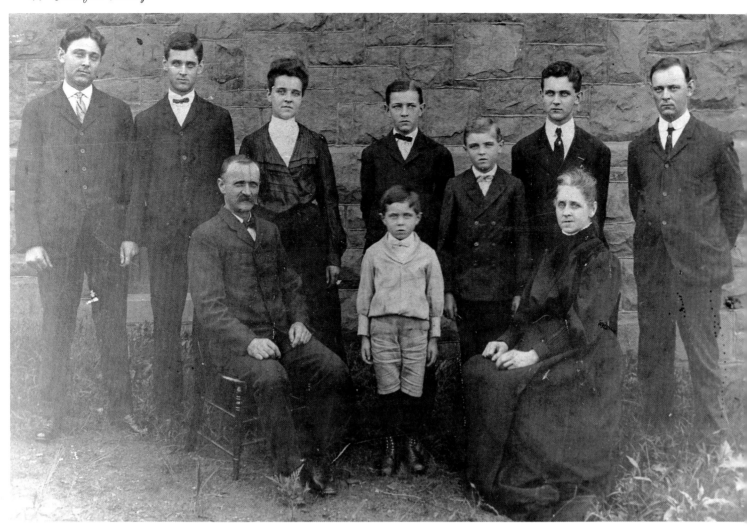

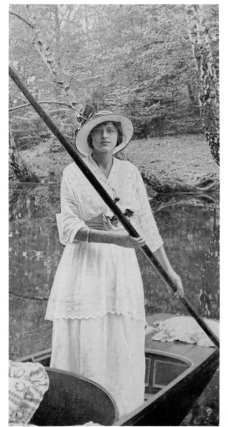

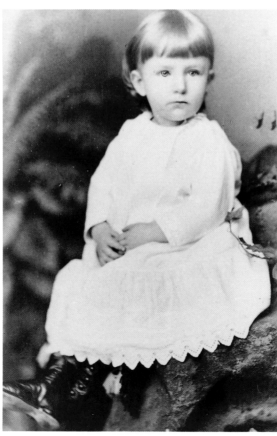

Faces and Places

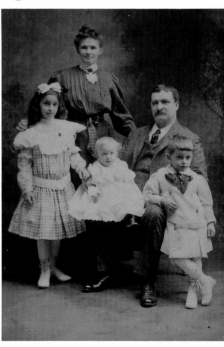

The Ladies' Home Journal June 1903:

"Linen underwear that wears well. Made from ideal material—a vegetable fiber—pure linen; woven in the ideal form, an open mesh . . . has real absorbent properties; takes up perspiration rapidly, evaporates it just as quickly, leaving the skin cool, dry and comfortable."

"Girls between six and fifteen still continue to wear the regulation sailor suits . . . with them are worn sailor-hats in coarse straw with a simple ribbon band for trimming."

Sears Roebuck & Co. Consumer Guide, Fall, 1900:

English Lavender Smelling Salts. Refreshing. Invigorating. For faintness, headaches, etc. In pretty glass stoppered bottles, a useful and handsome ornament for the dressing table. Price each $0.50. Per dozen $2.00.

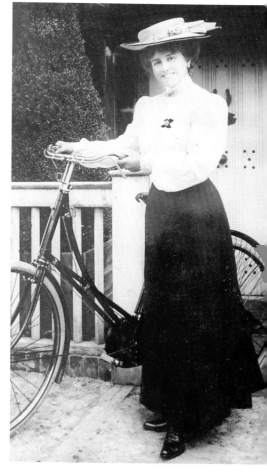

A gentleman's stem-wind watch for 98 cents . . . guaranteed American made and a very good time piece.

Sterling silver curling iron, length 7 inches. Price 85 cents. If by mail, postage extra, 6 cents.

Sterling silver mounted garters, set with handsome ruby, fine silk web. Very handsome. $2.00.

Ladies' changeable silk vesting top shoes. A $3.50 shoe for $1.95.

Ladies' fine imported all-wool jersey leggings. Knee length and with ribbon top. Color black. Per pair $0.65.

Ladies' mufflers: While ladies frequently wear the same size and style mufflers as the gentlemen do, we present . . . an especially pleasing article of fine quality in raised striped effect . . . Light colors such as delicate pink or blue. Price $1.50 each.

Cashmere mufflers. Large size, dark and medium colors. Plaid, stripes and fancy figures. Price per dozen $2.80. 25 cents each.

Cowboys' extra fine heavy weight Saxony wool sombrero with 4-½ inch crown and 4 inch brim with wide single buckle embossed leather band and leather binding. Band is embossed in beautiful floral and novelty patterns in variegated colors. Price $1.50.

The Eugenia wave. This is a new and very becoming wave for middle aged and elderly ladies, made of the best quality natural curly French hair; easily dressed and cared for. Price each $4.00. Grey and blonde $6.00 each.

A very full 10 inch demi-plume made from extra quality real ostrich feathers. Fine fiber and handsome curl. Very rich and glossy in appearance. Price each $0.55.

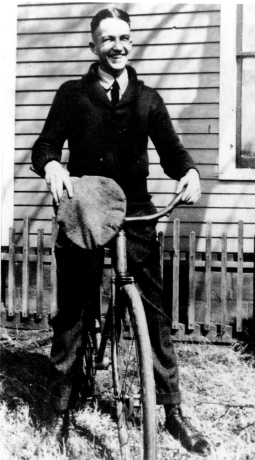

Ladies' chambray sunbonnet made of good, fast color chambray. Laundered bow strings in back and full cape. Colors black, navy, light blue, pink and cardinal. Price 25 cents.

A very stylish Velvetta hat with tucked brim slightly drooping in the front and back, a beautiful crown of velvetta, and trimmed in light blue tafetta rosettes. Two quills on either side complete this very nobby hat. Can be ordered in black and colors. Price each $1.55.

Stylish cape made of fine seal plush neatly embroidered with black soutache and beads. It measure 30 inches in length and 125 inches in sweep. Lined throughout with silk radome and interlined with wadding. Bear fur edging around the large storm collar and in front. The embroidery is one of the newest designs. Price each $9.35.

Mens' medium shape stiff hat. An excellent hat that will give good satisfaction. Price each $1.49.

Fancy silk embroidered elastic web suspenders. Braided mohair ends, gold sliding buckles and drawer supporters. Assorted patterns, very handsome. Per pair 35 cents.

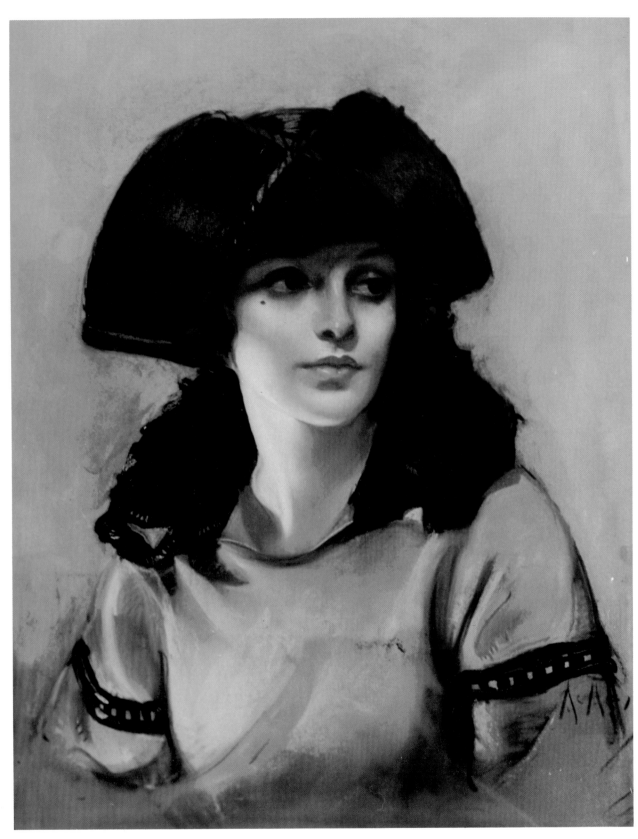

"The Fur Collar," Neysa McMein (1890-
1949). Pastel on paper, 19-½" x 26".
Courtesy of Alan M. Goffman, The Fine
Art of Illustration, New York.

The Teens

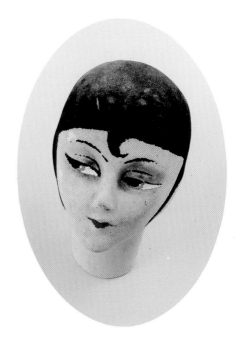

STUDENTS OF SUCH MATTERS ASSURE US THAT FASHION ALWAYS GOES COMPLETELY MAD ON THE EVE OF GRAVE CRISIS... WE HAVE ONLY TO RECALL THE YEARS THAT PRECEDED THE FIRST WORLD WAR, WHEN FASHION ABANDONED HER RELATIVE CALM FOR A SERIES OF SOMERSAULTS THAT SHOCKED CONSERVATIVE SOCIETY.

Marcel Vertes

The decade that began in 1910 laid the groundwork for much of what would follow in the ensuing eighty years. In fashion, it was a quite surprising time—somewhat like a reluctant bather tentatively dipping his toe into the cold and roiling surf, pulling it back in alarm, and then moments later, like a playful child, plunging in with hapless abandon. As we shall see, this "testing of the waters" spawned some interesting results, along with all the vagaries of fashion one might expect.

Although the tendency to less restrictive clothing had mercifully begun, one of fashion's most torturous devices appeared in 1910. Called a *hobble strap*, it was in effect an accessory of the period, albeit a hidden one. Necessitated by hobble skirts (their name creates a word picture that tells it all), these garter-like straps enabled the wearer to keep her ankles tightly together, a necessity for the protection of life and limb. The simple act of walking was threatening enough, but getting in and out of vehicles, or merely sitting down and standing up again, became an art. This aberration was probably intended to convince women—and men—that ladies were meant to walk in the manner of foot-bound Oriental women. It's unlikely the wearer was convinced, or that the gentlemen—who watched in horror as their wives and lovers were deprived of a normal gait—were enchanted by women hobbling through the streets like wind-up dolls. Condemned by the church and medical profession, the hobble skirt's "reign of terror" was short lived.

Contributing to the demise of the hobble skirts was the genius of Paul Poiret. A Frenchman born in 1879, Poiret was more than a couturier—he was also an artist, a designer of theatrical costuming, and a man of superior vision. Poiret was responsible for airy, Persian-inspired garments, including the audacious harem-style pantaloons, fetchingly topped with short, ballerina-style skirts, that were introduced by his wife at an enchanting gala they hosted in 1911, aptly titled "The Thousand and Second Night." His friend, artist Raoul Dufy, assisted with the fairy-tale decor, recreating what must have been a breathtaking scene to satisfy the most fanciful imaginings of any aficionado of the "Arabian Nights" legend.

Poiret's artistry, coupled with a newfound fascination for the Russian Ballet and its Oriental flavor, combined to make these exotic fashions an instant success. Accessorized by wide cummerbunds and turbans of exquisite fabrics like gold lame, frequently with aigrette plumes seductively fastened with jeweled clips, each melded into a gossamer look of comfort and beauty . . . a far cry from the restraint of hobble skirts. Although Poiret is reported to have foreseen women becoming more masculinized by wearing trousers, Vertes did not view Poiret's pantaloons as an attempt to give women the freedom of pants; instead he saw them as a step *away* from equality and a push backward ". . . to the insidious silk cushions of the harem."[1] Poiret, understandably, would not have agreed for, as he saw it, "'I do not impose my will upon fashion . . . I am merely the first to perceive women's secret desires and fulfill them.'"[2] Harem trousers weren't only confined to the atmosphere of home, and certain daring individuals even ventured onto the public streets with these gossamer "nothings" peeking seductively beneath the hem of their regular skirt. This behavior was deemed "unseemly," but that didn't stop the adventuresome from opening *new frontiers*, no matter how short-lived.

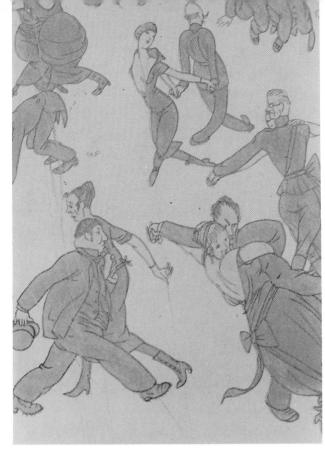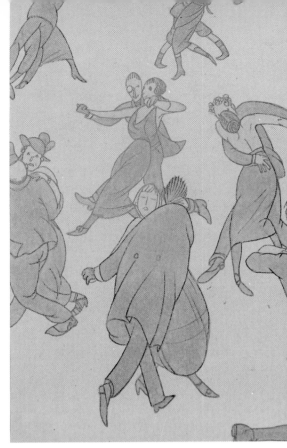

La Vie Parisienne, 1919. A. Vallee. "I dance; therefore I am."

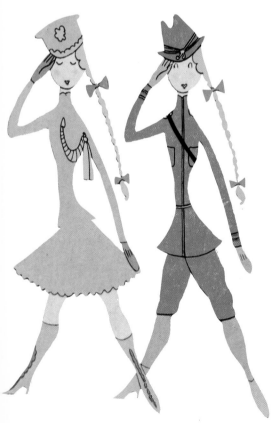

Fast on the heels of one fashion "no-no" came another. This was the V-necked dress. Tame by today's, and certainly previous day's, standards it was not viewed as such then. In fact, it created quite a stir. As usual, theologians and doctors were the chief critics. The clergy denounced it as unseemly and the medical profession branded it a health hazard, which seems ludicrous considering the revealing cleavage and topless couture of centuries past. Women, of course, paid no attention, and the V-necked dress was here to stay.

Although large hats remained in fashion early in the decade, many were less rigid than their predecessors, with crowns encircled by delicate flowers, and soft ribbons tied femininely around the wearer's chin and face to hold the hat in place. After 1915, hats became smaller, however, and tricorne, sailor, and pillbox models gained favor. Even children's hats of the day mimicked the larger adult styles, and being "dressed in mummy's clothes" was no longer for play time, as attested to when one views these oversized—and comically overpowering—hats on little girls of the mid-decade. For their mothers, "Day shoes were black or brown, buttoned or laced, low or high-heeled. Dressy slippers were made of bronze kid and evening slippers of satin or brocade. Evening pumps were in patent leather or calf and were ornamented with flat bows."[3]

Evening headdresses, in the French fashion, featured helmet-like ropes of beads and pearls, some with a semi-circular, feathered halo surrounding the head. Overall, it was a "look" that with one glance embodies the fashion image and proclivities of the social scene of the day. This image extended beyond the mere trappings of fashion, for it served to permanently enshrine its subjects in the stylized works of the illustrators and designers who, with supreme elan, converted it into an art form that has rarely been duplicated for sheer audience appeal. More traditional fashion illustrations of the day featured evening wear accented by ornate sashes, plumes, and hip-length ropes of pearls and beads, and for daytime strolls, long-handled parasols, an important accessory that served a dual purpose—it complemented the outfit while protecting its wearer's face from the harmful, and cosmetically undesirable, rays of the sun.

The seductive yet ladylike look to be gained from a simple scarf was revealed when "On a 1913 menu cover for the Savoy Hotel, fashion artist George Lepape suggested how important scarves were to become. Around the head of a dancing woman in a white pleated crepe dress, he wrapped a black silk scarf that covered her ears and billowed out exuberantly for yards behind her."[4] One of the masters at interpreting the "look" of the contemporary woman was Erte—the brilliant Russian artist and designer, whose idolatry of the beauty, power, and mystery of this elusive woman is so dramatically shown in his ethereal designs. In an editorial contribution by Erte for the March 1919 issue of *Harpers Bazar* (for it *was* Bazar then and not Bazaar), he expressed his feelings about women and fashion. "You ask my opinion on fashions. I do not recognize the mode. I love the luxury and beauty of fashions, and I believe that feminine clothes should serve to adorn woman's charm—not to conceal that which is beautiful. In short, woman's costume should be individual."[5]

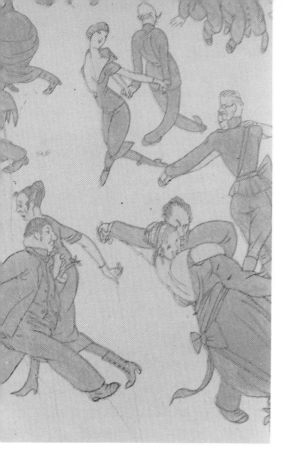
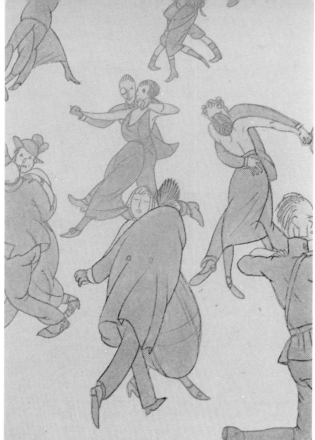

Erté was an artist and fashion genius, able to bring innovation to new heights. In 1915 he designed a coat featuring a belt that extended into a long piece that overlapped in front, was fastened with buttons, and became a hand-warming and decorative muff, thereby creating an accessory that was an actual part of the garment. The concept was practical, but nonetheless enchanting, as were the gloves that appeared in the December 1918 issue of *Harper's Bazar*. How, one wonders, could the mere illustration of a pair of gloves take on the appearance of something out of a gossamer fairy tale? One glance tells it all. Embroidered in shades of green and violet, they were tied with flowing ribbons of narrow kid—an exquisitely feminine rendering that transformed a simple accessory item into a work of art!

Heir to the horse-drawn carriage, the motor car continued to evoke a separate set of requirements for "proper attire when on the road." Cars, in fact, went hand in hand with fashion commentary: "In 1913 New Yorkers liked their extravagant but undependable foreign automobiles. They admired the season's new hats with eighteen-inch feathers; and its new dresses, draped in the manner of wet canvas . . ."[6] Interestingly, both *Vogue* and *Harpers* utilized evocative captions to focus on a variety of different items featured in the same edition, such as "'The time has come, designers say, to talk of many things, of shoes and furs and lingerie and if one flares or clings, and where the waistline ought to be and whether hats have wings'"[7] or in a less poetic vein "'When is a lampshade not a lampshade? When it is a hat . . . in blue cloth with wooly flowers growing on it and worsted tassels hanging down.'"[7]

The addition of elaborate beading to all manner of dress became an important element of the garment. There was a resurgence of interest in jet beads and mother of pearl, and even simple items like glass and wood were utilized. The head once again commanded attention, but as we have seen, woman's "crowning glory" was more apt to be covered (to the displeasure of some) with turbans, sprays of feathers and gems, and decorative headbands. Even suspenders were worn by ladies, although they gained a far different look than their male counterparts by the use of elegant fabric and ornamentation of all kinds.

The pannier was revived in 1913-14 and, as reported in the *Ladies Home Journal* of January 1914, "Ivory-toned print d'esprit was draped to form the pannier and overblouse, with angel sleeves and three frills of white tulle with one big rose at the side front . . . almost always a rose, but dyed, sometimes as nature never did. Even black ones are worn." Wraps were all-important, some cut in one piece, made of deep shades of plush or fur fabrics and gracefully draped to one side with a fashionable diagonal closing. It should be noted that prior to World War I, American couture was a relatively unknown player in the scheme of fashion, and American women were forced to rely on French fashion influences that, unfortunately for those hungry to keep up with the latest trends, had already been through one European season before finally making their eagerly awaited appearance in the United States.

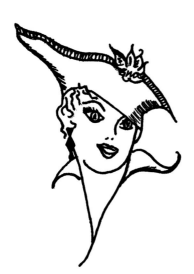

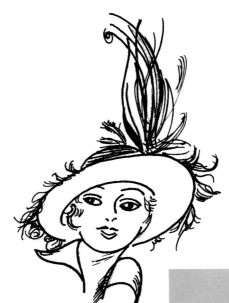

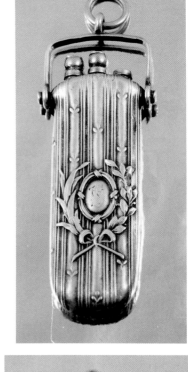

With the advent of the "great war," skirts regained the fullness of past years, at the same time getting shorter, which probably explains the abundance of fashion photographs and illustrations of the time that featured long-legged dogs. The inclusion of these animals in the famous illustrations of George Barbier, for example, "...echoes not only the more 'leggy' fashions, but also the many references to dogs which were made by wartime fashion journalists who considered the animals to be accessories just as subject to the whims of fashions as the clothes themselves."[8] An interesting observation, and certainly one with merit—thus adding a new category, at least for this century, to lists of "strange" accessories—man's best friend, the dog. Fashion and society reporters were not oblivious to this trend, and felt that proper coverage should include all aspects of the "overall" look of its subjects, from dogs (which they roundly criticized if they clashed with the "look") to the state of the subject's complexion.

This was not the first venture of dogs into the world of fashion accessories, however, for ornamental dogs had been an acceptable part of the "look" during the 18th and 19th centuries. In certain societies, including the British, tiny lap dogs were considered the ultimate pet for the mistress, who was then viewed as totally indolent, thereby creating what she considered a pleasing picture as she lolled around her boudoir or sitting room. In fact, this fascination became so great that ..."Toward the end of Edward VII's reign *Punch* declared, '"The cult of the toy dog has reached a stage when ladies have to look at the little darlings through a microscope."'[9]

As for men of the period, "...kings may have fallen and republics gone by the board... but neither age nor time could quell the renewed mode for the 'shiny top hat and the neatly tailored cutaway suit." It was probably safe to assume that dogs, at least the "fashionable" canines, were for ladies only, since this gentlemanly garb would have appeared somewhat foolish with the master tethering an afghan hound. Just like women's, men's fashions came ... and went. A case in point was the double-breasted men's waistcoat that gained some acceptance in 1915 but, with their rolled collars and rather strange shape, were soon viewed as unattractive and summarily dismissed.

Shortly after America's entrance into the First World War, a British couple named Vernon and Irene Castle brought about their own revolution in ballroom fare—and fashion. Dances like the "turkey trot," the "bunny hug" and "Castle walk" took the country by storm. They required ease of movement and flexibility, and to match the rhythmic abandon of these new steps, Irene Castle daringly shed her corset and bobbed her hair. American and European women—for more reasons than merely dancing, truth be known—eagerly followed suit. Next to go, as skirts got shorter, were petticoats, thanks again to Irene. The relaxing of fashion standards had a patriotic end as well: American women eagerly contributed a mountain of discarded steel corsets weighing about 28,000 tons, enough to build two battleships. "Good riddance" most of them must have sighed, taking—for the first time in many moons—a good, deep breath!

This new freedom was all in keeping with the avant-garde movement, tinged with European flavor, that around 1913, found expression in Greenwich Village. This tiny section of New York City took on a new identity, and the United States had its own "Left Bank" to match its Parisienne "cousin." Writers, artists, musicians and other non-conformists started a wave of Bohemianism that attracted much attention. By the end of the decade "The Village" had become a mecca for young people, and the "look" was casual ... with an artistic bent. Consequently, smocks with big floppy bows became popular among the daring, with berets and sandals completing the picture. One brave fellow became a "fashion" martyr, and scandalized the media. "Poet Harry Kemp...won newspaper notoriety by daring to stroll the streets without a hat. Next he appeared without a necktie and with his collar informally open."[10]

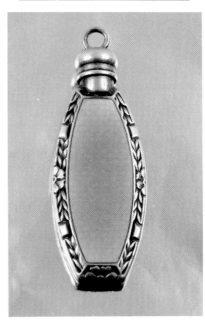

These elegant sterling perfumes are British hallmarked.

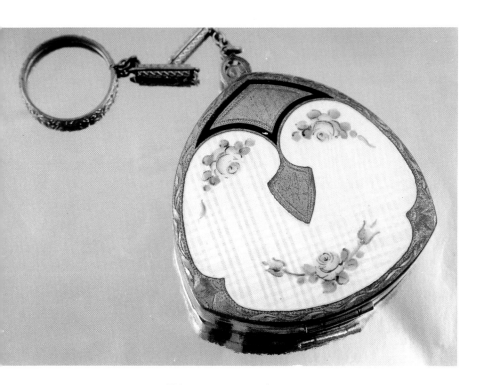

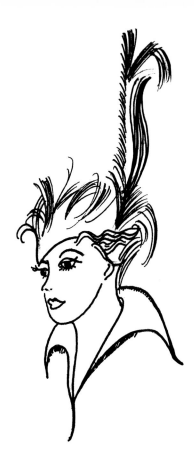

This enameled purse/compact could be
attached to a belt or bag.

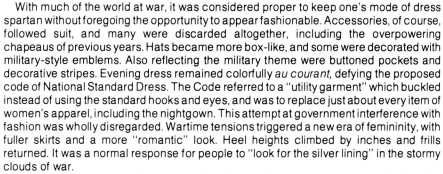

With much of the world at war, it was considered proper to keep one's mode of dress spartan without foregoing the opportunity to appear fashionable. Accessories, of course, followed suit, and many were discarded altogether, including the overpowering chapeaus of previous years. Hats became more box-like, and some were decorated with military-style emblems. Also reflecting the military theme were buttoned pockets and decorative stripes. Evening dress remained colorfully *au courant,* defying the proposed code of National Standard Dress. The Code referred to a "utility garment" which buckled instead of using the standard hooks and eyes, and was to replace just about every item of women's apparel, including the nightgown. This attempt at government interference with fashion was wholly disregarded. Wartime tensions triggered a new era of femininity, with fuller skirts and a more "romantic" look. Heel heights climbed by inches and frills returned. It was a normal response for people to "look for the silver lining" in the stormy clouds of war.

The importance of color in all areas of fashion and design was recognized by the first appearance, during World War I, of the Textile Color Card of America. The names were appealing, and indicative of the mood of the times . . . blue violet became "heron," leaf-green "thyme," pale grey "mist," and "blossom" was a pinky violet. "These quiet colorings were called 'sympathetic hues,' suggesting the mental tone of the world under the stress of war."[12]

As the decade edged toward the 1920s, skirt lengths became the daring news of the day. "The handwriting was already on the wall," for although skirts would rise and fall at the whim of designers and the public, never again—at least in this century—would it be considered acceptable for daytime attire to brush the floor or billow in great trains beyond (although some of the styles of the late 1940s and 1960s came close). This revolution in fashion took its first tentative steps during the *Great War,* and when soldiers returned from the front they were no doubt delighted to see that female skirts were shorter than when they left.

As skirts climbed higher, the focus turned to footwear. The stiff, matronly black shoe, a wardrobe staple, understandably fell from favor, and those in colors like gray, blue, pearl, and bronze took its place. In order to meet the hem of the shorter skirts, most were more boot than shoe. Apparently the drastic change to shorter hemlines was enough for any proper lady to deal with and, at least at the beginning of this conversion, displaying one's ankles was still considered somewhat risque.

Another revolution was underway as well—this one on the retail front. A mainstay of 20th century existence, the department store, with it's ready-to-wear, off-the-rack fashions, had its beginnings around 1918. The repercussions of the enormous, ever-expanding business of fashion and accessorizing would prove to be a mind-boggling leap forward for the retailing industry. However, due to the obvious need for this burgeoning business to cater to the rapidly changing fashion scene and the vagaries of female tastes, these fledgling specialty stores were forced to offer only fabric lengths or partially finished garments, rather than the racks of items that would be available in later years. In fact, until around 1920, customers were unable to buy anything but the most simple finished pieces in stores.

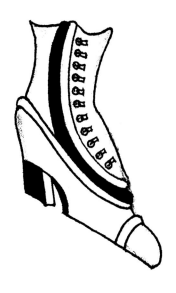

1910—1920
[1] Vertes, Art & Fashion, p. 81
[2] Batterberry, Fashion, p. 268
[3] Cassin-Smith, Costume, etc., p. 194
[4] Baseman, The Scarf, p. 12
[5] Blum, Designs by Erte, p. viii f
[6] Vogue, Sept. 15, 1940, p. 70
[7] "The Golden Age of Style", p. 37,
[8] "The Golden Age of Style," p. 60
[9] Dorner, Fashion, p. 58
[10] "The Golden Age of Style," p. 66
[11] Churchill, "Remember When," p. 157
[12] "Historic Costume," p. 234
[13] "Vogue History of Fashion," p.10

During this decade of change, women continued their determination to participate in sports rather than to merely watch from the sidelines. Before shorter lengths appeared, the female penchant for bicycling made it necessary for manufacturers to deal with the long skirts that were then *de rigueur* for women by putting nets over the back wheels so this billowing mass of fabric couldn't become entrapped in the spokes. These nets remained, even as skirts edged higher, for shorter or not, they still fell below or near the wheels. It would, unfortunately, be some time before women could enjoy the freedom of wearing shorts, slacks, or skimpy skirts when bicycling.

Like the dances of the Castles, tennis required that women remove their corsets or at least wear looser, more comfortable undergarments. This enthusiasm for bicycling, tennis, badminton, croquet and the like spawned a myriad of casual accessories that went far beyond what was needed on the "fields of play," ". . .such as the close fitting hood attached to the coat collar, which could be unbuttoned and pocketed . . Pockets were now adopted on a wide scale for women's attire. One American hosiery manufacturer even offered garters with flap pockets—a safe place for money and jewellery."[13]

When it came to stockings, Alan Churchill observes in *Remember When* that the decade's females had few choices. "Her stockings were probably black or beige cotton, unless she was that one woman in two thousand who owned silk stockings." All that would change in the 1920s, however, when this luxury item finally found its way into the hosiery drawers of the woman of average means and changed her look forever.

That same woman would also "kick up her heels" inside those silk stockings as the second decade became the third. A new day was dawning, and women everywhere seemed eager to welcome it. But without those fashion and social innovators whose ingenious ideas bloomed at the most unexpected times in the most unexpected ways, that new day might very well have ended as simply another black and starless night.

Early perfume and sachet bottles. (Richard Hudnut, the cosmetic giant, was the father of Rudolph Valentino's wife, Natasha Rambova.)

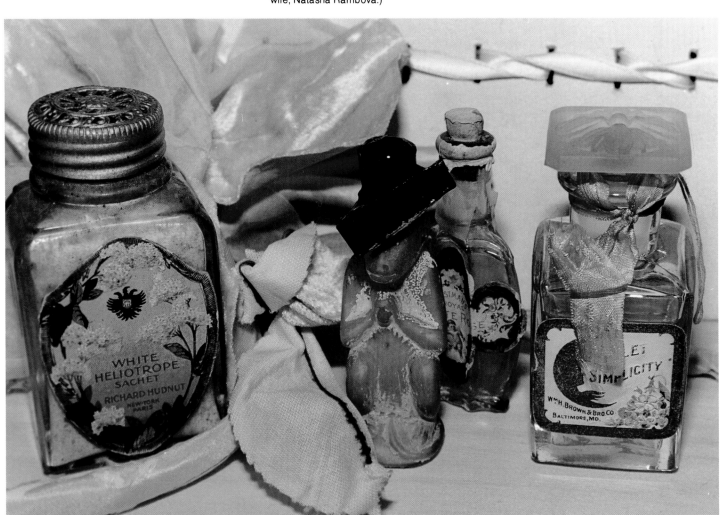

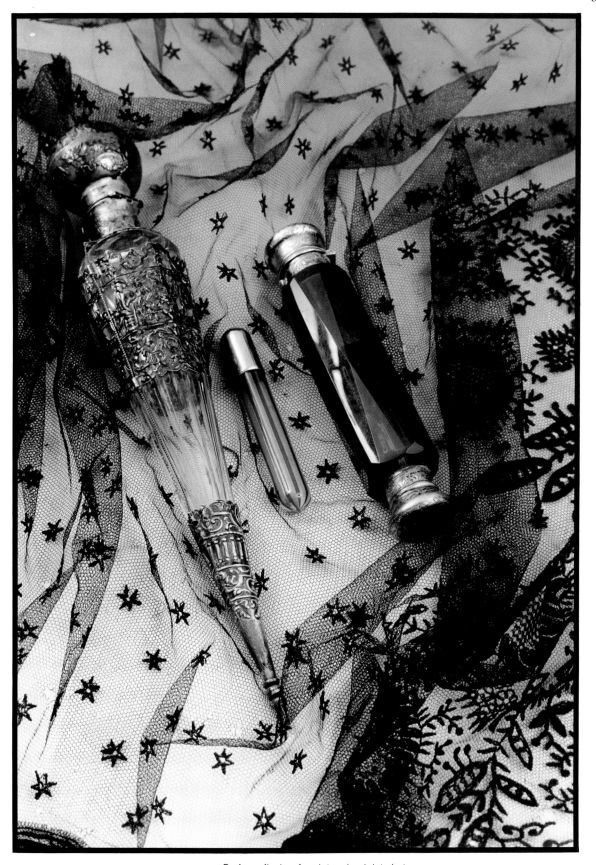

Perfume flasks of undetermined date but
most likely from the late 19th or early
20th century. The stately beauty on the
left is of German origin. Collection of
Gloria C. Malloy.

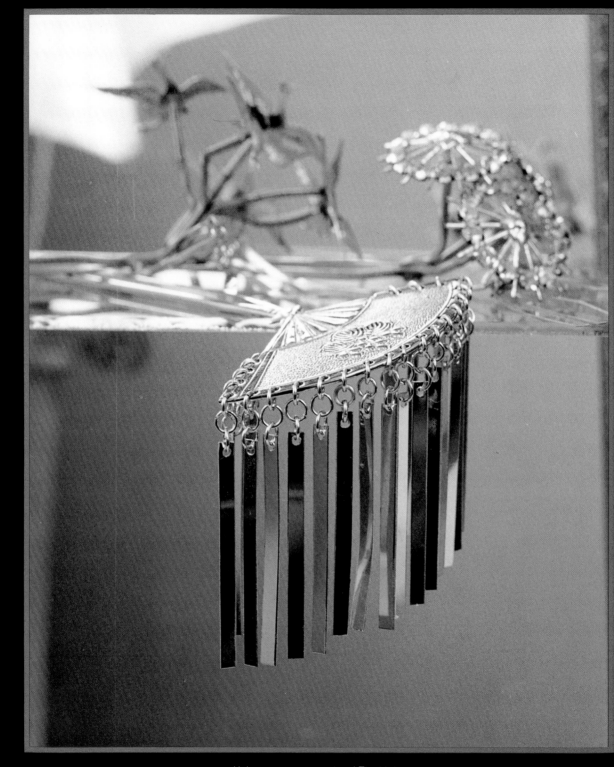

Hair ornaments to enchant! The birds
trembled and the pinwheels bobbed as

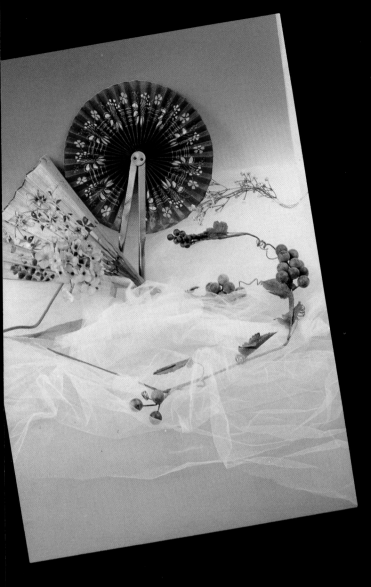

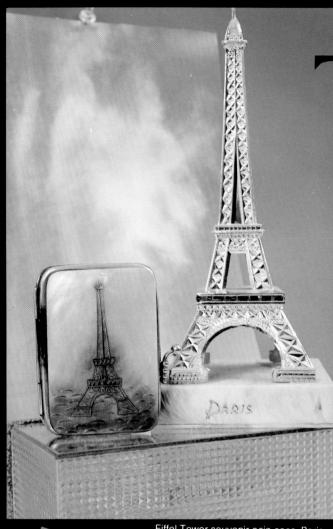

Eiffel Tower souvenir coin case, Paris.
Courtesy of Joan Orlen.

Early 1900's paper fans. Note metal
frame that folds.

The Language of the Fan

Carrying in right hand, in front of face: Follow me.
Carrying in left hand: I desire your acquaintance.
Twirling in left hand: I wish to get rid of you.
Drawing across forehead: We are watched
Drawing across cheek: I love you.
Twirling in right hand: I love another.
Closing: I wish to speak to you.
Drawing across eyes: I am sorry.
Resting on right cheek: Yes
Resting on left cheek: No
Open and shut: You are cruel.
Dropping: We are friends.
Fanning slowly: I am married.
Fanning fast: I am engaged.
Open wide: Wait for me.

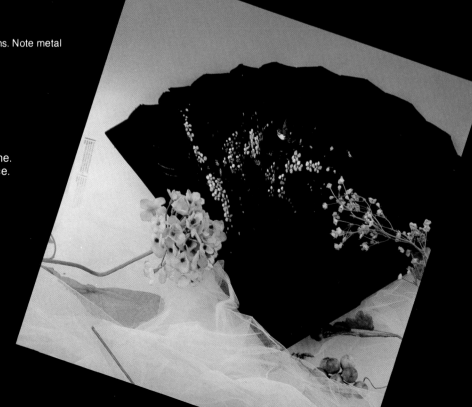

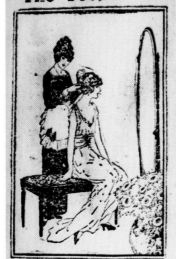

FORBES & WALLACE

The Proper Care of the Hair

Especially during the summer the hair is apt to become dull and dry. Make it a habit to visit our hairdressing specialists frequently to keep your scalp in a normal healthy condition.

Yvette Henna will color gray, faded or bleached hair to its original or any desired shade and leave the hair soft and glossy, box $2.00

Switches Transformations, Bangs, Curls, Pompadours, Wigs and Gray Hair Goods attractively priced.

The Diana Facial Massage is the most remarkable cleansing process we know of. This massage is new and leaves the complexion in a wonderfully healthy and attractive condition.   Personal Service Shop, Second Floor

FORBES & WALLACE

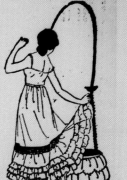

Summer Tub Silk Petticoats
In Complete New Varieties

Introducing models specially designed to our order—the most practical and desirable styles that you could wish for.

With special-made double panels and linings to make them shadowproof, and flounces of just the right fullness.

Washable White Tub Silks and Washable Satins in flesh and white, including double panel styles, tailored or lace trimmed flounces, at...................$3.98

One style in Tub Silk with scallop finish, lined throughout, at..........................$4.48

White Tub Silk Petticoats in double panel styles, with tucked and hemstitched flounces, including extra size models, at.......................$4.50 and $4.98

Special at $2.98

Several dozen Petticoats of Washable White Silk, with shadowproof cotton front and back lined panel, made with shirring and wave ruffle finish.

Petticoats, Second Floor

Courtesy of the Connecticut Valley Historical Museum.

Hair today, gone tomorrow! Advertisement for the Personal Service Shop, Forbes and Wallace department store, Springfield, Massachusetts. Courtesy of the Connecticut Valley Historical Museum.

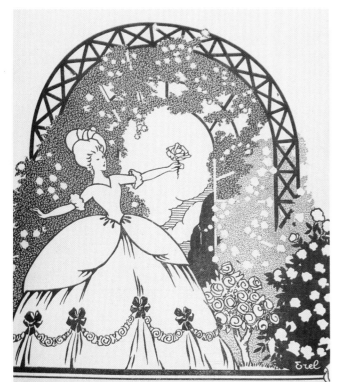

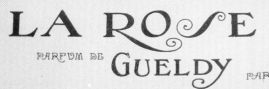

Perfume ad from *La Vie Parisienne,* 1919.

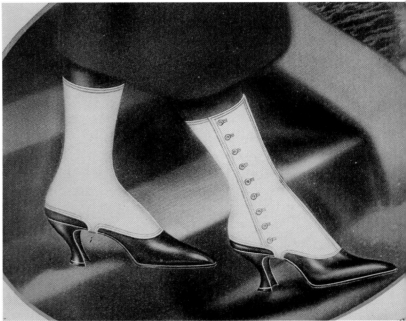

"Ankles Away" with these spats for the ladies. Advertisement for Standard Spats by Rauh. *Harper's Bazaar,* October, 1920.

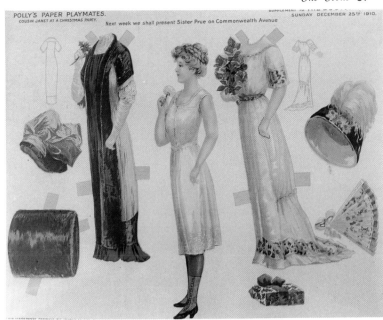

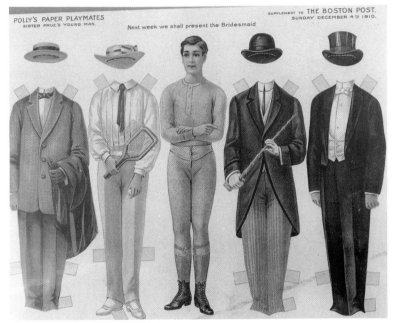

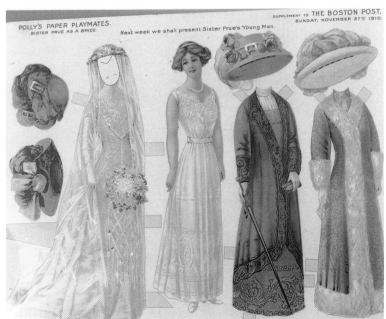

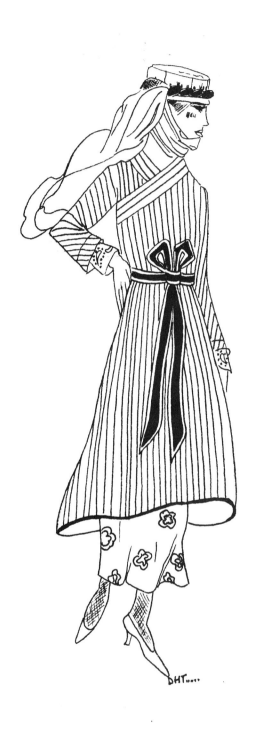

Polly's Paper Playmates from 1910.

Spanning the decades. Porcelain, hand-painted cupid buttons find the "real" Cupid. The shy young lady seems unsure!

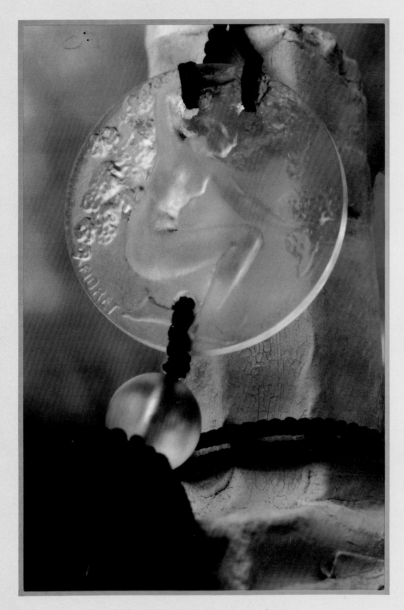

Moonlight may become you . . . but so
would this translucent Lalique pendant.

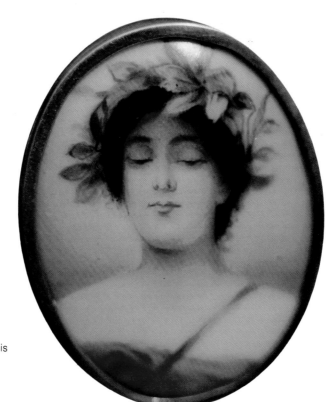

Magnified to show detail, this hand-painted porcelain Art Nouveau brooch is framed in sterling.

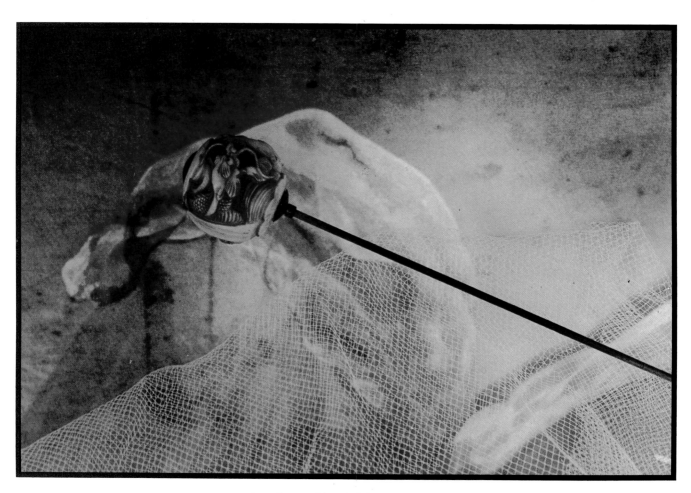

An early carved ivory hatpin.

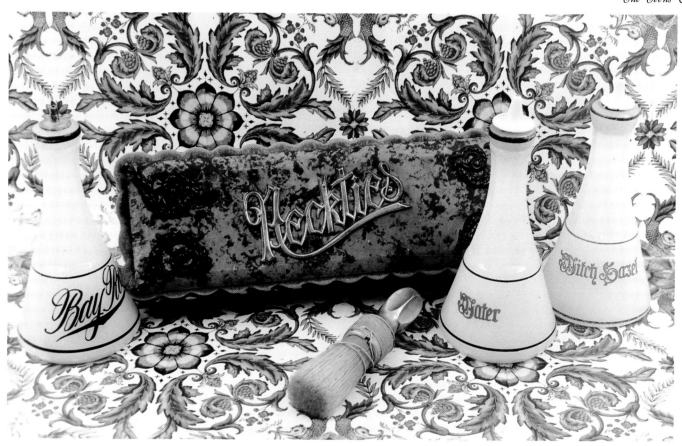

A gentleman and his neckties are never parted. This faux tortoise celluloid container is surrounded by a toilette set and pewter shaving brush.

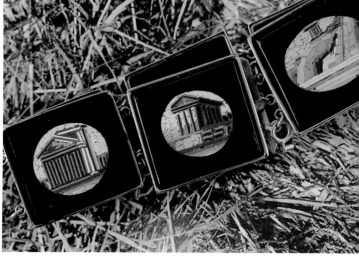

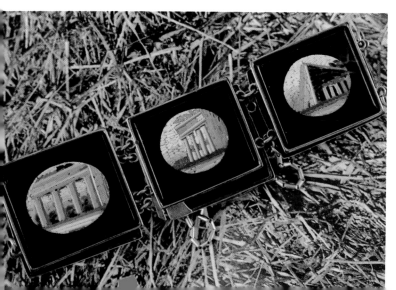

Classical influence. An 18K gold and micro-mosaic bracelet.

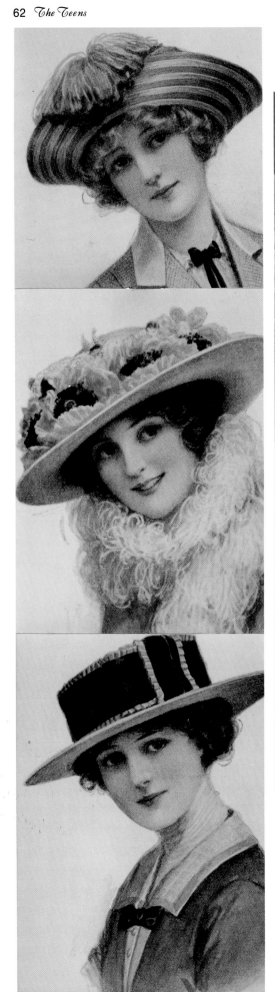

Fit for a bride...shell flower wedding headpiece from 1918.

"The Girl's First Hat" . . . and each and every one a beauty. Designed by Laura Samuels. Edwin B. Halsey (in the center), and Ora Cne. *Ladies Home Journal*, 1913.

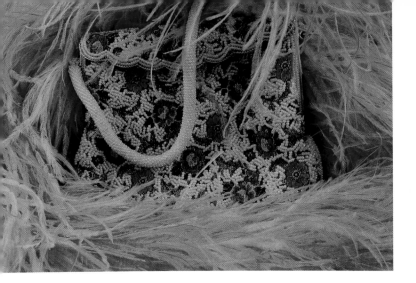

French beaded bag early 1900s
belonging to Leslie Gray's grandmother.

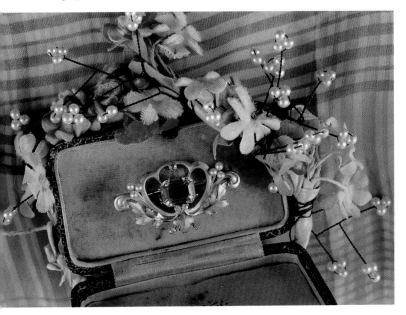

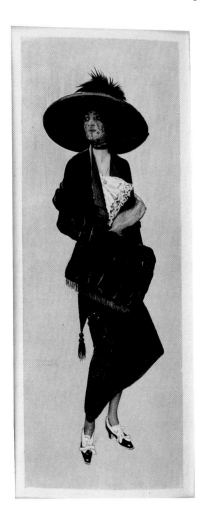

The height of fashion...a hand-colored
drawing by Rafael Kirchner.

A brooch with a large emerald cut
peridot in a 14K gold Art Nouveau frame
with Champlevé enamel, cultured pearls
and diamonds.

Two lovely cameo ladies, framed in
sterling silver.

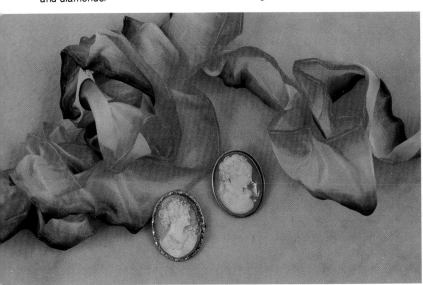

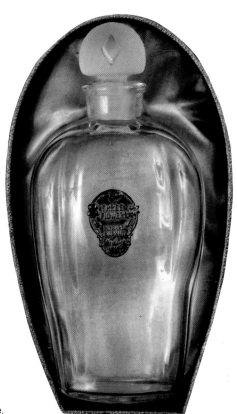

Richard Hudnut perfume "Three
Flowers" in beautiful "coffin" case.

Faces and Places

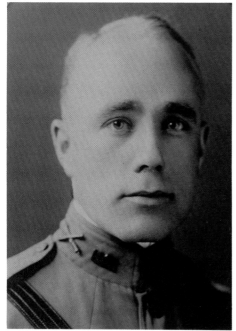

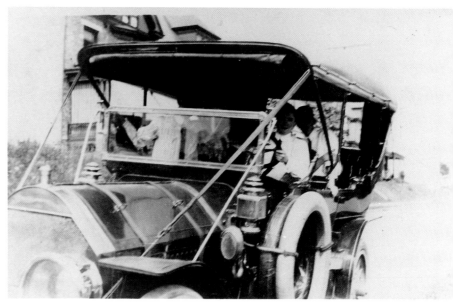

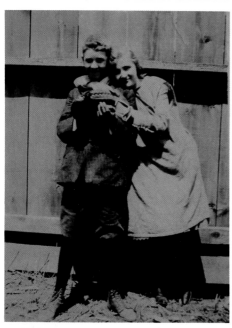

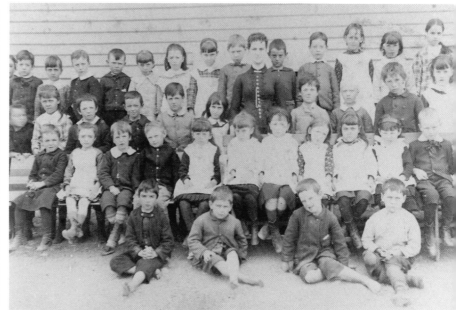

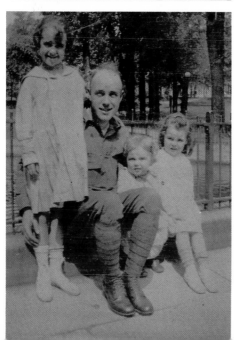

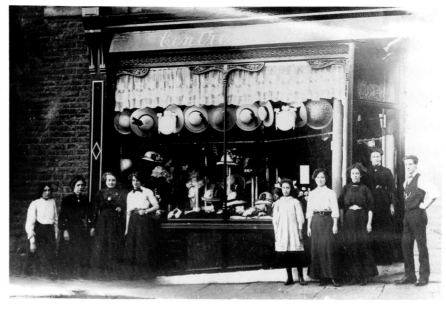

From Periodicals of the Times

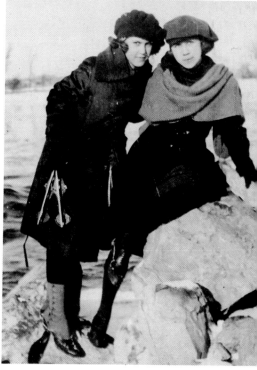

The Designer (The Man and His Clothes), October 1913:

"Don't be led into temptation and be persuaded to select any style of suit that is be-buttoned to the point of excess. Certain designers with overgenerous souls are apt to look upon a sleeve as the ideal place to plant buttons. I would advise you to steer clear of this sort of thing. It verges on the freakish."

"We all know the comfort of the soft double collar. But alas! We all know how very difficult it is to make it look presentable either by means of a safety-pin or by the addition of little tabs with studholes. We have all groaned inwardly at our soft collars when they have looked like limp rags around our necks."

"To tell the truth when your jolly clown stuffs his hands deep into his capacious pockets and extends them wide, he does acquire something like the new silhouette—narrow at the foot, full and drapy over the hips, loose and baggy in general.

"There are the 'tier' skirts . . . In lace and soft, sheer materials, the flounces or tiers are often plaited or gathered . . . It is the same idea of having the silhouette wider at the hips, and quite narrow at the foot."

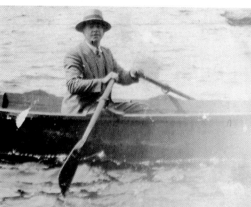

"You see sash-ends tied loosely at the back of cutaway coats; you see them coming from underneath the flounces of tier skirts . . . you see them . . . tied around the waist, with a huge bow at back."

"An Uncle Sam disguise always provokes much merriment for fancy dress and masquerade parties . . . The trousers are made of red and white striped materials, the coat of blue with white stars cut out and sewed on, and collar and reverse of red and white stripe. The dickey is also striped red and white . . . the collar is white, and the tie dark blue with white polka dots. A skull cap is given to which the hair may be sewn, or a wig may be worn."

"Pique, galatea, linen, gingham, rep, poplin and percale are appropriate materials for making the very sturdy boyish dress for little boys from one to four years old. The broad tucks give them long straight lines, and the bloomers included in the design make it a dress for real boys."

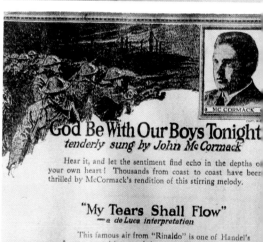

"Solid gold ring, twin Topaz setting. $2.75
Solid gold signet ring. $3.50
Solid gold cameo brooch. $3.50"

"Why not choose corsets which will make the most of your figure? Why not wear modish models which produce the 'long, lithe lines' demanded by the present vogue? . . . The season's models of American Lady Corsets, producing the smart low bust, the unrestricted waist, the long straight hip, the altogether graceful, willowy, svelte figure, are the correct foundation for the season's gowns."

"Let the beauty candidate remember: Always put the toes down first—to show the soles of the shoes is to be ungraceful."

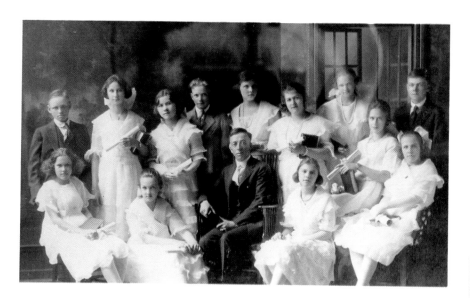

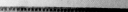

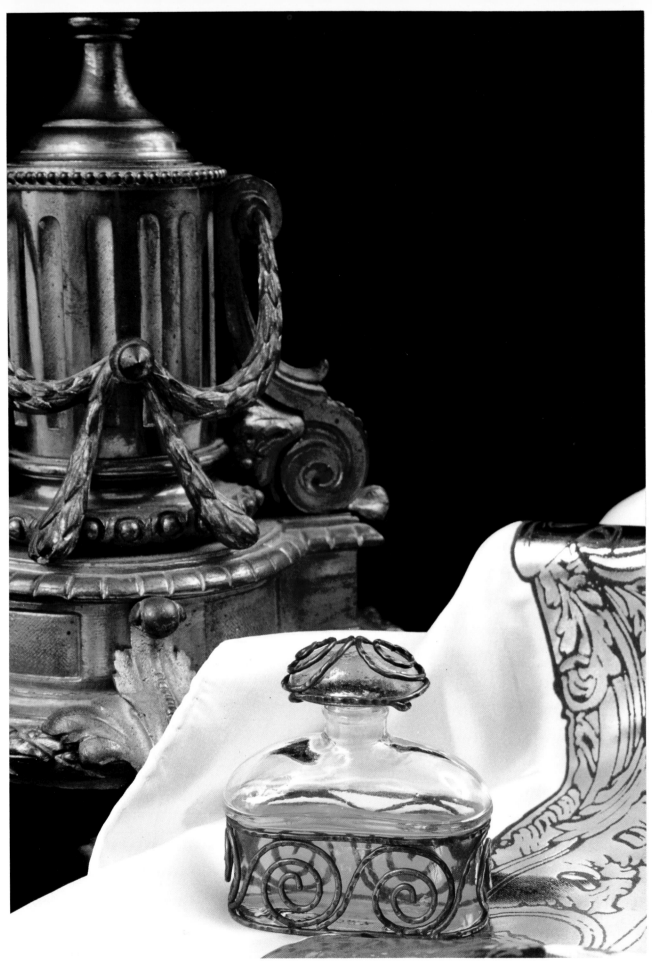

A rare treasure...on another treasure!
Perfume Le Balcon by Paul Poiret, on a
1990's Vivienne Westwood scarf.

The Twenties

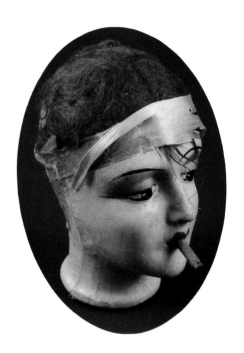

FASHIONS CURIOUS LITTLE TRICKS ARE USEFUL IN DISSEMBLING THE IMPERFECTIONS OF NATURE. THEY ALSO SERVE ADMIRABLY THOSE WHO WISH TO STAND OUT FROM THE CROWD.

Marcel Vertes

Contrary to the rambunctious mental picture usually associated with the "roaring twenties," the early years of the decade saw very elegant, feminine fashions, and it was only in the final five or six years that the flapper—and what most consider the look of the 1920s—burst onto the scene.

The early 1920s were, to put it mildly, unsettled times. It is often observed that such conditions raise skirt lengths, although there is a dichotomy here, since it has also been noted by fashion historians and others that in particularly hard times skirts descend closer to the ground, as was the case a decade later. Perhaps there is a subtle difference in fashion's treatment of the skirt, depending on whether the unsettled times are political or economic, although there were many, other than politicians and economists, who influenced fashion.

Chief among them was one of this century's most auspicious contributors to the art of couture. Her name was Gabrielle "Coco" Chanel, and she was directly or indirectly responsible for many of the remarkable revolutionary changes ushered in during the Twenties. Her march through the annals of fashion had begun in the previous decade, and the mark she left was like an indelible stamp that could never be washed away. Chanel's influence was destined to be far-reaching and would continue unabated throughout the 20th century.

Chanel's expertise at accessorizing complemented the wide range of styles she made fashionable by being in complete harmony with the casual look many women readily adopted. Her couture designs were a delightful combination of boyish *and* feminine, and Chanel's imaginative accessorizing skills were masterpieces that could stand alone. Her hats were simple yet saucy, and floppy bow ties at the neck, much like those of Greenwich Village a decade earlier, gave their wearer a gamin-like appeal, although Chanel's inspiration was culled from childhood memories of French schoolchildren. Suntans and short bobs were a natural adjunct to the look, contributing mightily to the fashion revolution that was already underway following the end of World War I.

The fairyland of Paul Poiret was no longer in sync with these sweeping changes, but he refused to be intimidated. Commercially out of step, he continued to create his works of art, including designs that now seem uncanny forerunners of the "easy" fashions so popular decades later, and which could certainly not be ignored. He was a visionary, changing fashion with his daring designs—like the suit with corduroy trousers that he introduced in 1925. Other designs included long, loose-fitting jackets, short cross-over ones with one-button closures, and dramatic, sweeping cocoon wraps. His garments demanded accessories—fans and feathers, cummerbunds, braided and embroidered buttons, fur pieces and, of course, hats—from cloches and turbans to broad-brimmed beauties.

In the past, Poiret's forward-thinking genius had "scooped" many of his contemporaries. In 1911, long before Chanel or Lanvin, he had introduced his own fragrances, under the tradenames *Rosine* and *Martine*, and with individual scents labeled—in typical Poiret fashion—with names like Maharahjah, Alladin, Borgia, and Fanfan la Tulipe. "At a single stroke he would extend the field of fashion to include perfume, cosmetics and interior design and . . . he was the only Paris couturier to market perfume for another ten years."[1] The popularity of this venture continued into the 1920s, with the results developing into masterpieces of design.

The bottles themselves, along with their marketing presentations, were supreme works of art. In one instance, each flacon was wrapped in a beautifully colored handkerchief designed to match the mood of the buyer, blending the color with the fragrance. And, as the *piece de resistance*, a wide ring designed to slip over one's glove secured the handkerchief to the container it covered. Other bottles were of metal with bold designs in *bas relief* and topped with huge ivory stoppers. The exquisite patterns of Poiret's powder boxes were visually astounding, their heavy tassels covering large dome-shaped lids, like treasure chests begging to be opened. Even in marketing skills, he was a step ahead. To promote his perfumes, at one couturier showing—in what was probably a warm and airless pre-air-conditioning salon—each female attendee was presented with a fan that wafted one of Poiret's scents from a disc identifying it by name as she fluttered it in front of her flushed face.

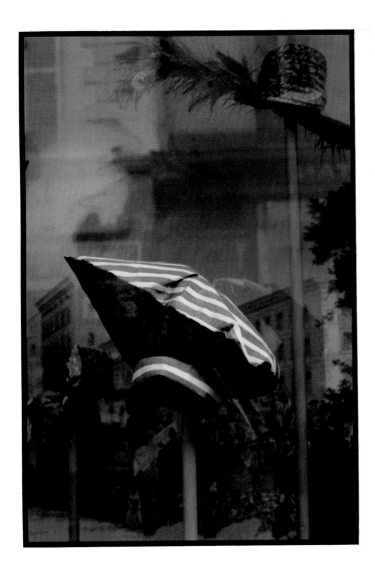

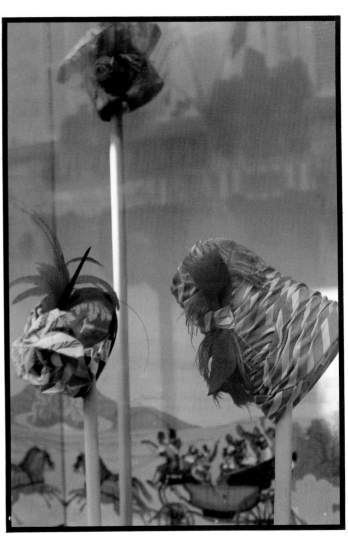

Parisienne street scene -windows of a
Left Bank antique shop featuring vintage
designer hats.

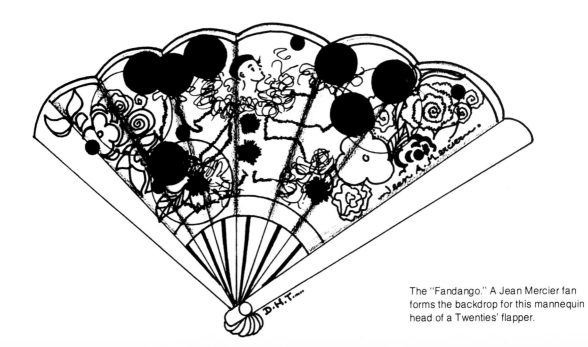

The "Fandango." A Jean Mercier fan
forms the backdrop for this mannequin
head of a Twenties' flapper.

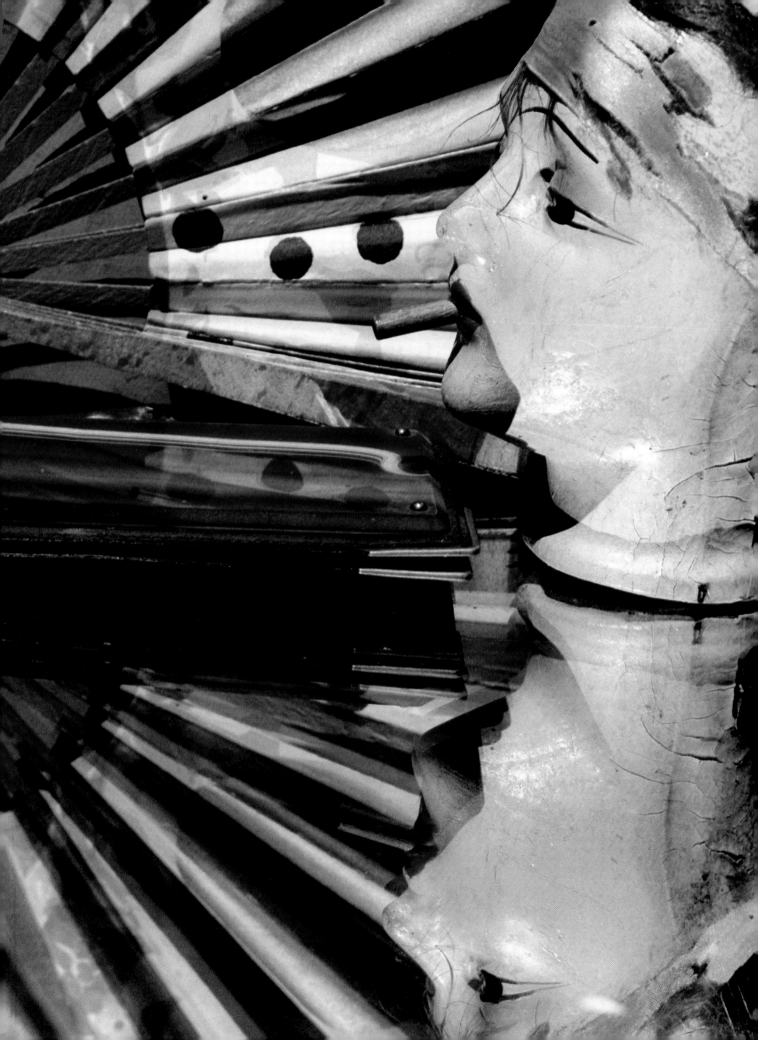

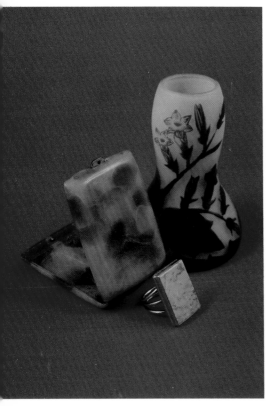

Celluloid cigarette case from the twenties, and a large turquoise finger ring in 18K gold.

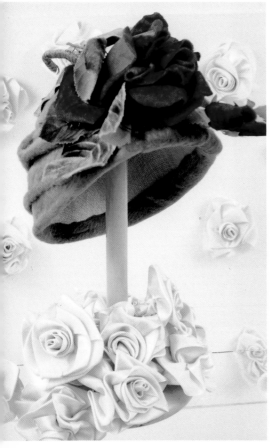

When one reflects on the 1920s, a single glorious image most often comes to mind . . . the artful grace and style of Deco jewelry. Whether of precious metals and gems or purely costume, these designs have left a magnificent legacy in the history of jewelry and design. It was a look unexcelled for its purity of line and startling beauty, and much that followed in later decades was a reflection of the grace of these unique and highly-stylized works of art. Flappers had their long ropes of pearls and beads, but the genre most attributed to the 1920s will always be dominated by the stunning look of Art Deco—in fashion and interior design.

In a much simpler vein—although perhaps more complex in its social implications—was the keen interest that developed among the "horsey" set for riding clothes and the accessories necessary to give the fashionable woman that "hunt-country" look—like crops, boots, and flat-topped hats. But another mode of transportation somewhat advanced of the horse and even the motor car also became a symbol of "keeping abreast of the latest" for the high-society set. The airplane, that exciting mode of transportation for the adventuresome, brought with it a separate concept of fashion for the "new women" of this "new age." *Styl*, the German Art Deco magazine, commented, ". . . 'just as surely as the woman of yesterdays were born to drive in a limousine, the woman of today was born to fly in an aeroplane.'"[2] Fashions had to follow suit and ". . . they wrote about the latest fashions of the air, such as 'fur-lined mink-trimmed suit of thick suedes,' and a 'tight fitting casque' worn with 'soft boots strapped in puttee fashion' and a 'specially designed coat, side-fastened with front slit which buttons into trousers when prepared for flight but fastens flat when alighting.'"[3]

One of the more curious accessories to be found in Europe during this time was the domino mask, which had been worn for centuries in Venice and became an interesting and unusual part of the social scene of the 1920s—epitomizing its very twists and turns. It was a mysterious, almost cultish article of fascination and, at times, repugnance. As Erte observed in an article for *Harpers*, "In Venice until the fall of the Republic it was commonly worn in the streets. There reigned in the enchanted city at this decadent epoch a strange corruption of manners, and the mask was a necessity. At every entrance hung the black domino. Rich and poor alike donned it, in order that they might sally forth enveloped in anonymity." Erte, the divine sensualist, envisioned his own masks, not black—and, to his eye, ugly—but masks of beauty and individuality, for he continued, "Imagine then a mask of pearls which cover the upper part of the face . . . Or a mask of black aigrettes . . . and the embroidered veil which shows only languishing eyes . . ."[4]

The June 1921 issue of *Harper's Bazar* featured an equally scrumptious confection from Erte of drawstring purses that carried "fanciful" to new heights. Titled "The Fragile Bisque Doll Finds a New Role," the descriptions read:

"To carry with her evening costume and so provide a carryall for her little nothings, Erte makes Madame a bag of silver tissue and semi-precious stones . . . The matron who would be correct may carry a doll dressed exactly like herself. The skirt of mauve and white taffeta, embroidered in orange is an efficient handbag. Even the hat is not forgotten." And finally, "Frills of black and white taffeta form the doll's petticoat and in turn a bag for the debutante. The doll's face is hidden by her bonnet. The balloon is really a jade ball attached to a thick chain."

Erte's eye for the dramatic was also delightfully illustrated in his drawings of December 1923 for *Harpers* showing a long ermine scarf and a giant muff of otter fashioned into an enormous bow; another muff is described thus: "Little ermine tails fall like showers of icicles from the ends of this fat round snowball of a muff. Bands of moleskin around the ermine strips hold them together. One wears this muff with an ermine jacket, for black and white is very smart."[5]

Far removed from Erte's French confections, the discovery of the tomb of Tutankhamen in 1922 opened more than a sarcophagus—it released a Pandora's box of fashions with an intriguing Egyptian air. Scarab jewelry lent itself admirably to the Deco influence already underway. Perfumes and exotic scents imparted their own special mystique to the aura of the "modern" woman of this "modern" age. It marked the beginning of a realization of what Paul Poiret had daringly pioneered a decade before. Scents and cosmetics could become an enormously successful adjunct to fashion— separate and lucrative industries onto themselves.

The 1920's cloche in all its glory! This beauty is of panne velvet and decorated with breathtaking French roses.
Courtesy of Alyson Torem French.

As the decade progressed, skirts edged ever upward, waistlines dropped, and daring accessories like snake bracelets climbed the length of milady's arm. Garlands of artificial flowers decorated dresses, hats, belts and coats. It wasn't until around the autumn of 1927, however, that "... for the first time in the recorded history of the Western world, women's knees became an accepted and respectable sight in fashionable society."[6] The flapper of the 1920s, with her above-the-knee skirts and stockings rolled below, caused some in the clergy to exclaim, "Low cut gowns, the rolled hose, and short skirts, born of the Devil and his angels, are carrying present and future generations to chaos and destruction.' A few states tried to legislate short skirts out of existence by passing laws against the sale of any garment which unduly displays or accentuates the lines of the female figure.'"[7]

Cloche hats became what now can surely be viewed as one of, if not *the*, fashion statement of the decade. This helmet-like chapeau was a necessity for the *new* woman to place on her freshly bobbed hair. As reported by *Styl* it..."was the hat that 'sat right in the eyes of the new fashion and attracted all the attention.'"[8]

Men had their own role to play in the "playful" Twenties. "With the exception of evening dress, formal afternoon clothes were considered the most important in a man's wardrobe: a top hat, cutaway coat, striped trousers and of course spats."[9] This bon vivant also brought scarves to their apex during this decade and the next by draping them around his neck, or tucking them loosely inside sport jackets or coat collars. Just as females earlier in the century, women of the Twenties recognized the delights of just the right scarf and used them to great advantage with evening wear and delicate daytime frocks. In a macabre twist of fate, the life of a celebrity of the day was snuffed out in a bizarre manner by her scarf. For in 1927 Isadora Duncan, the dancer and international social butterfly, met a particularly gruesome death when the long filmy scarf that had become her fashion trademark fluttered breezily behind her fragile neck and entwined itself tightly in the whirling wheels of her touring car.

Although the average "Joe" had little need for formal afternoon clothes, he refused to be overshadowed by the youthful flamboyance of his female companions. One mainstay of the wardrobe of this 1920's "rake" was plus fours—an overstated knicker. He also wore soft trousers, perched jaunty driving caps on his sleek patent leather hair, *a la* Rudolph Valentino, and frequently clasped a wide "slave" bracelet (a fad also instituted by Valentino) around one wrist. His trousers were almost comically wide and called "Oxford bags"—so huge, in fact, that the billowing pants legs sometimes totally obscured the shoes. The extremes of this fashion came to an end by the 1930s, although modified versions remained popular throughout the decade.

"In *College Humor* Katherine Brush described male attire: 'Legs in golf stockings of blue and gray diamond pattern. Knickers, voluminous and drooping low. Coat that matched the knickers, a soft collar with a neat bow tie.' A man so attired was called a *sheik*. To match this, a flapper was called a *sheba*."[10] The collegiate look was also the rage, with oversized raccoon coats (popularized by crooner Rudy Vallee and his ever-present prop—the cheerleader's megaphone) completing this "campy" outfit. Both males and females, whether collegians or not, adopted the scholarly but casual ambiance of sweaters and white bucks and, especially for the men who walked these "halls of ivy," the pipe became a symbol of the intelligentsia.

On an earthier note, cowboys continued to play a role in fashion. The cowboy craze was so great, in fact, that it spawned a premium for listeners of Tom Mix's radio program—a bandanna, complete with the Tom Mix logo and a real-life illustration of our hero...all for ten cents and a Ralston cereal boxtop. By way of comparing the proclivities of horse lovers on both sides of the Atlantic, it should be noted that across the ocean Liberty of London began their tradition of designing a special scarf for each running of the English Derby at Epsom Downs.

In the same social vein, Cholly Knickerbocker, a journalistic purveyor of society gossip items not always to the liking of his subjects, assured his critics that whatever their opinion of him, he was ever grateful, for thanks even to his detractors, his wealth enabled him to wear a rather foolish luxury they couldn't see. "Even when people snub me, I feel like saying to them, 'Thank you for just existing. I wouldn't be wearing solid gold garter clasps if it weren't for you.'"[11]

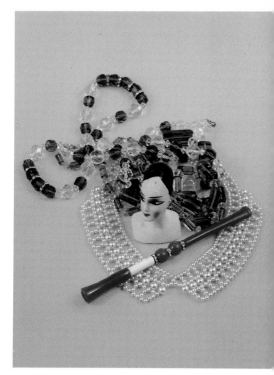

Bakelite and jeweled cigarette holder, beaded collar, and Deco rope of glass beads.

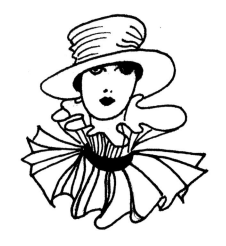

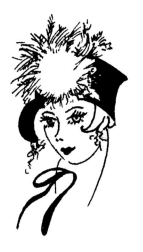

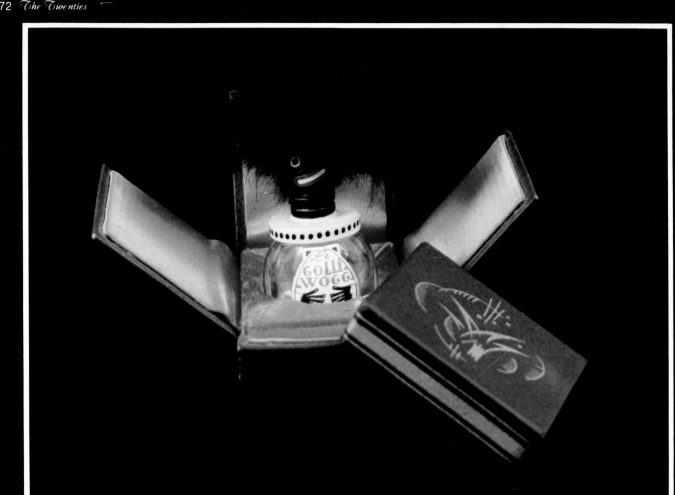

Le mint! Le Golliwog in original box.
Vigny.

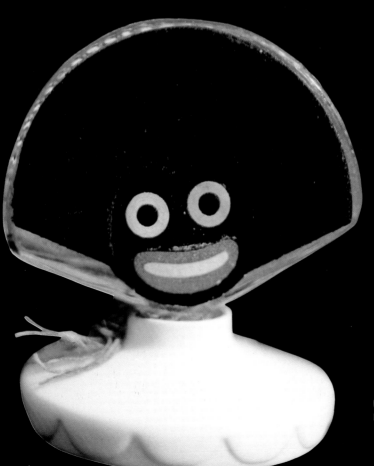

Rare micro-mini golliwog in milk glass
base with "fan" stopper.

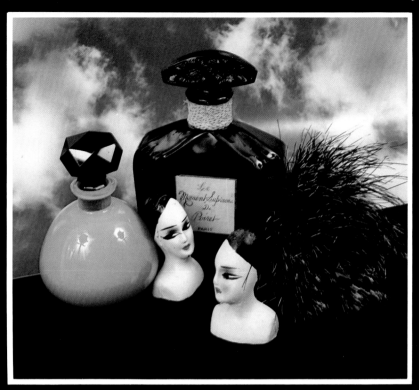

Czech bottle with cut glass stopper and
Le Moment Supreme.

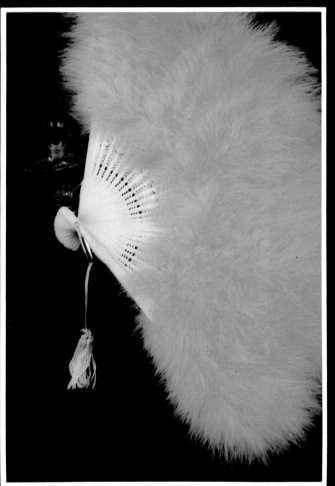

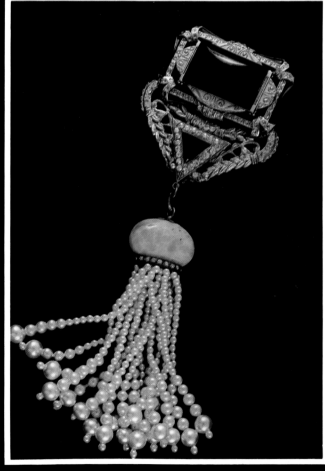

An ostrich feather fan with an early
Shalimar bottle. Fan courtesy of Jewel
Cook.

"Do the Shimmy" and "Shake your
Booty"! Tasseled brooch of sterling
silver, Peking glass, and rose-cut
diamonds.

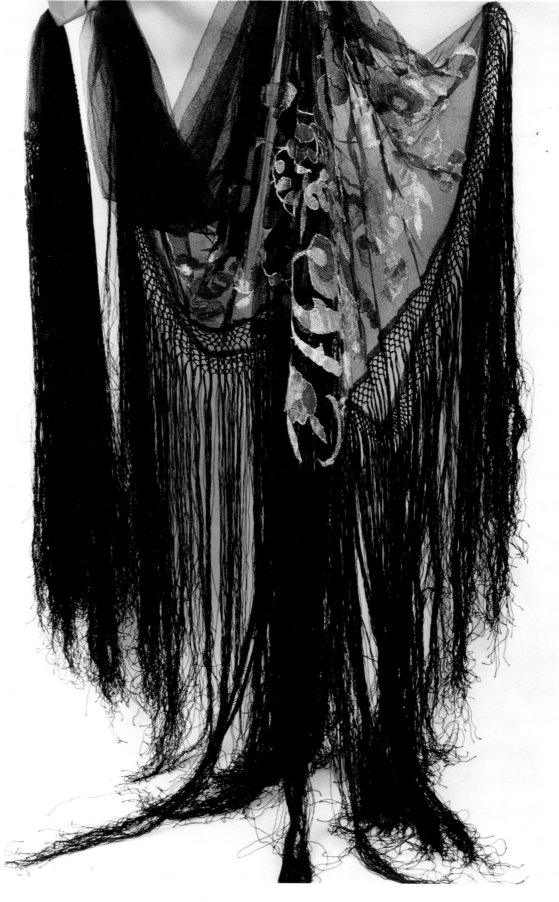

Two Parisienne fringed "piano" shawls
from the 1920s have the seductive
quality of a Poiret fancy-dress ball.
Courtesy of Shirley Clement.

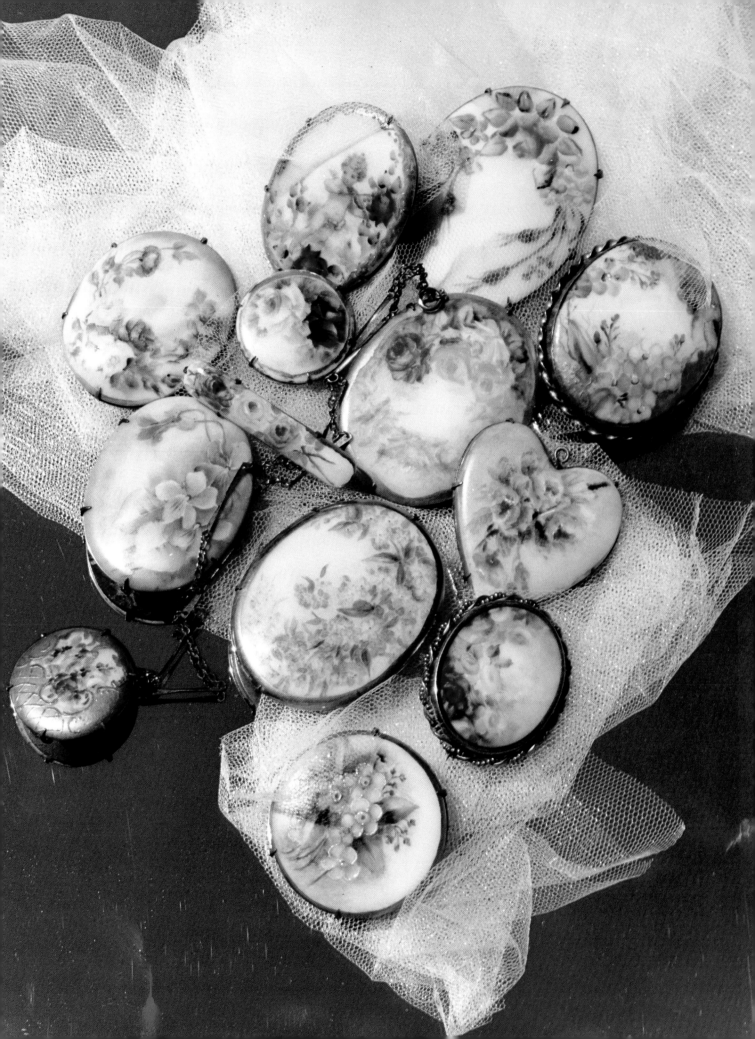

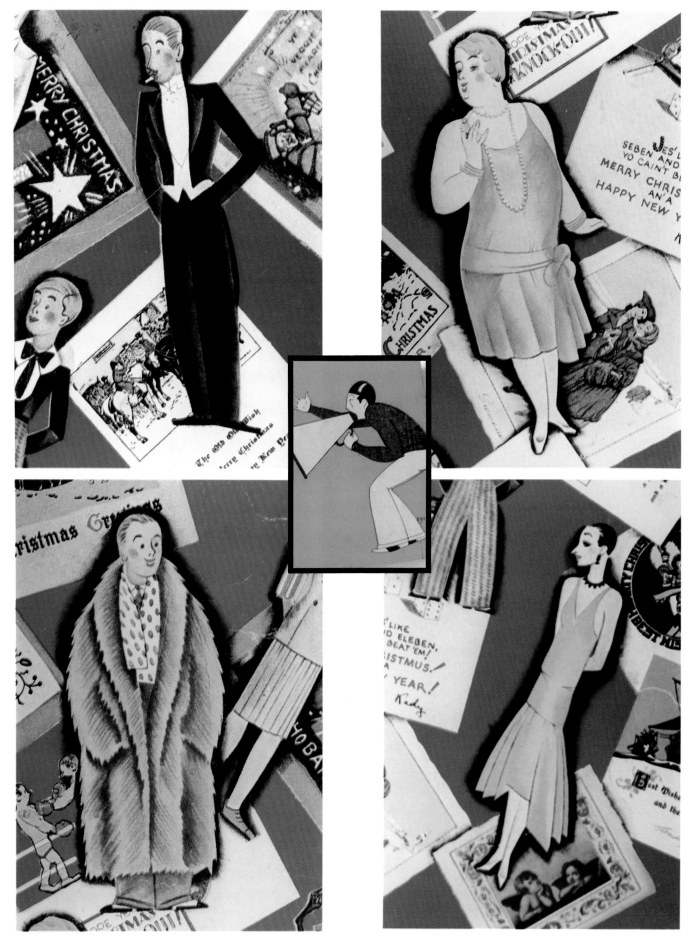

Cartoon cards . . . 1920s.

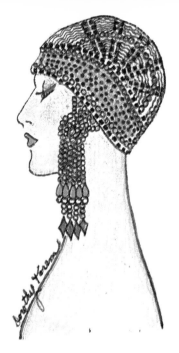

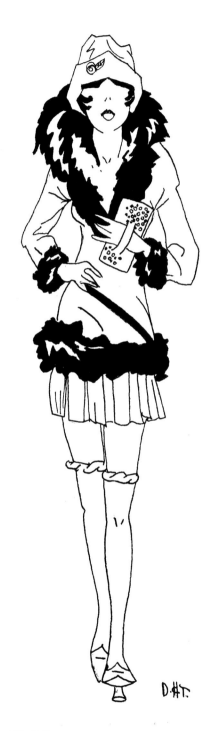

That mainstay of culture, the beauty salon, made permanent inroads as a necessary adjunct to the world of fashion during the 1920s. And these parlors of tonsorial splendor were, surprisingly, unisex. "Advertisements carried the message: 'Ladies be beautiful. Intelligence is deceitful. Amiability is useless and Virtue is vain. If you want to please the strong, sensuous, silent male, looks are your only bait—Be lovely or lose him!'"[12] And men were not excluded from being similarly insulted (at least by later standards) in these ads for mixed salons. "...'You have lost the privilege of being ugly. All you have left is your charm. So make the most of it—Get pretty or beat it.' All that was needed it would seem, was the price of ten sittings at a Mixed Beauty Salon to guarantee the desirable look of a *Lounge Lizard* or *Gimmy Girl*."[13]

Lingerie of the day became as brief as the skimpy material that slithered over it, causing flapper Dorothy Parker to quip, "Brevity is the soul of lingerie." However, the brevity of what didn't show underneath was balanced by what was considered by many to be an excess of cosmetics—at least by previous standards—on the painted face above. Thanks in no small measure to the influence of advertising, shrewd marketing techniques, and the beautiful belles of the silent movies, cosmetics established a permanent niche in women's toilettes. Lipsticks, rouges, and accessory items like vanity cases and compacts all helped create the final brush stroke that completed this picture of the 1920's "girl-woman." Her sultry, sometimes hedonistic behavior was always tempered by that doll-like, little girl look of pouting mouth, short skirts, and "Mary Janes" with heels.

Even the comic strips, followed religiously in the daily newspapers by a legion of fans, did more than just entertain. *Winnie Winkle* was emulated as the model for the fashionable well-dressed working girl, and *Harold Teen* portrayed the "laid-back" guy of the Twenties.

Although New York society matron Mrs. Patrick Campbell had indelicately puffed on a cigarette in the Plaza Hotel in 1901 and then defiantly refused when the shocked proprietor asked her to leave, it took another few decades for smoking by women to be considered socially proper, especially in public. By the time the 1920s were well underway, it had become a relatively acceptable form of recreation, and cigarette holders and cases became an important accessorizing accompaniment to the air of gaiety and self-styled sophistication that permeated the society and fashion scene. Many decades later, the cigarette advertising slogan "You've come a long way, baby," came to represent much more than mere cigarettes in the female mind. It was a slogan of liberation her "sisters" from the 1920s would have heartily supported, for the Roaring Twenties marked the tentative beginnings of greater equality for women in what had been an almost exclusively male dominated society. This was reflected in the assertion of her independence, not only in behavior and conversation, but also by her choice of garments and accessories.

Illustrations of the day caught the new and sometimes naughty look of the 1920's woman to perfection, especially in the works of artist John Held, Jr. Prior to that time, beauties like those created by Charles Dana Gibson were untouchable—stunningly haughty woman in idealized form. "Held's sheba was a caricature, although many young women of the time managed to look exactly like her. She resembled a precocious child dressed up in her mother's high heels and skimpy attire."[14]

That portrait of the "thoroughly modern" woman, along with her equally modern "sheik," sums up the look and feel of this awesome decade—the repercussions of which would reverberate, not unpleasantly, throughout the remainder of the century.

1920—1930
[1] "Poiret," p. 231
[2] "Golden Age of Style," p. 80
[3] "Golden Age of Style," p. 80
[4] "Art and Fashion," p. x
[5] "Art and Fashion, p. iii
[6] "Golden Age of Style," p. 99
[7] Churchill, "Remember When," p. 172
[8] "Golden Age of Style," p. 79
[9] "Golden Age of Style," p. 100
[10] Thesaurus of Anecdotes, p. 145
[11] "Golden Age of Style," p. 102
[12] "Golden Age of Style," p. 102
[13] Churchill, "Remember When," p. 173
[14] Churchill, "Remember When," p. 173

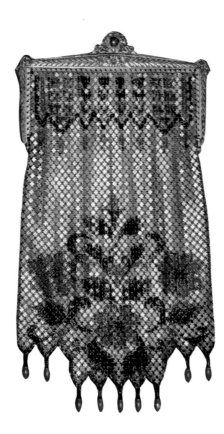

An enameled mesh purse by Whiting and Davis in a stiking Deco design of lavender, purple, orange, and green. The bottom is fringe-cut. It measures 4″ x 7″. Courtesy of Veronica Trainer.

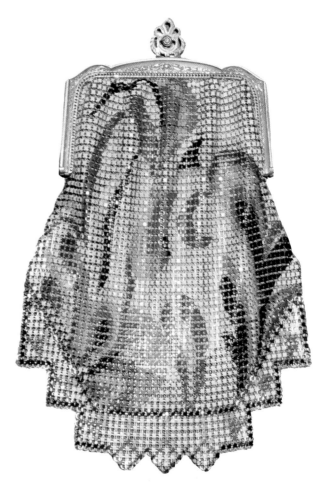

This enameled mesh bag by Mandalian is a delicate floral design in pink, green and black, with pink tear-drop bottom. The frame is silverplate. It measures 4″ x 8″. Courtesy of Veronica Trainer.

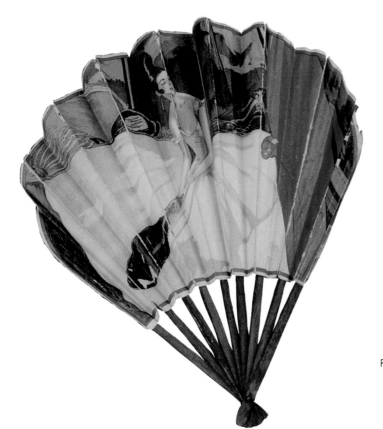

Fan Club . . . by Jean Mercier.

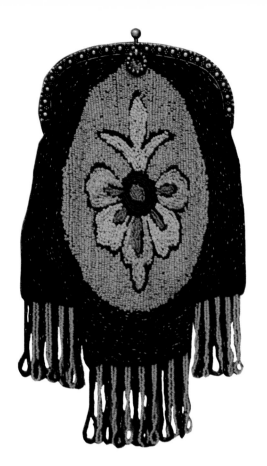

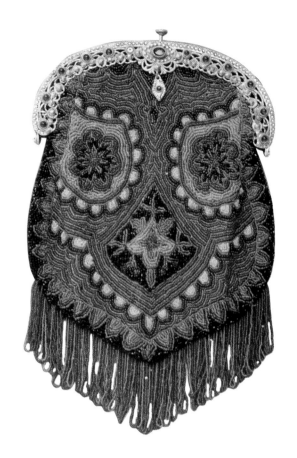

Two brightly colored glass bead bags of the Deco era reflect the gaiety of the times. The fringe design on the bag at left is unusual, with three levels of alternating yellow and black beads, and the frame is silverplated. It measures 6″ x 10″. The purse at right has a gold filigree frame accented with red stones, and is 8″ wide x 11″ long. Courtesy of Veronica Trainer.

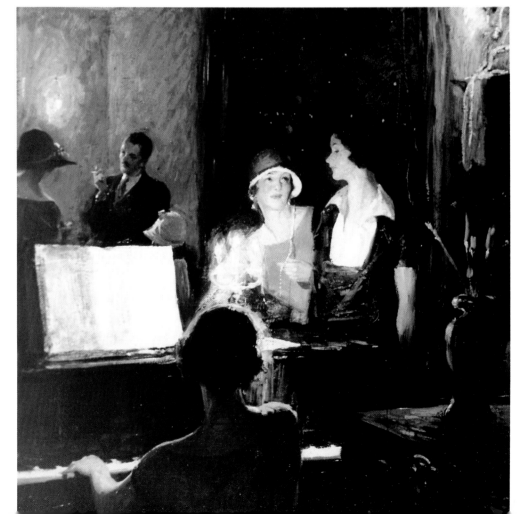

"At the Piano," Arthur D. Fuller (1889-1967), oil on board, 23″ x 22-¾″. Reproduced: *Pictorial Review Magazine*, 1925. Courtesy of Alan M. Goffman, The Fine Art of Illustration, New York.

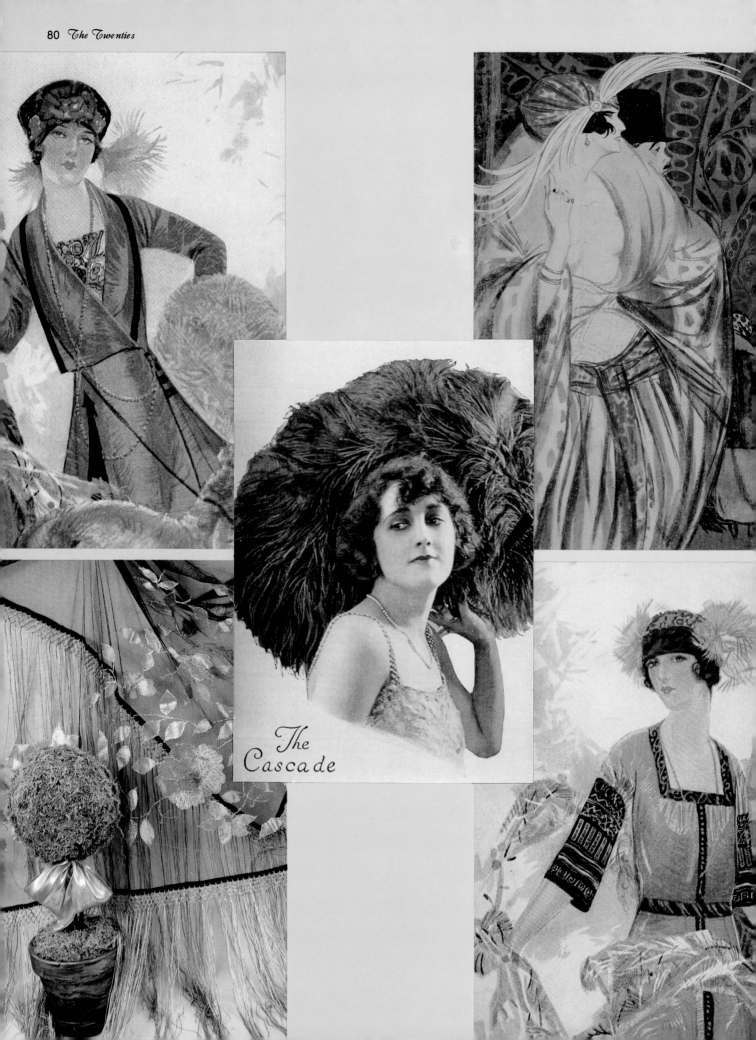

The
Cascade

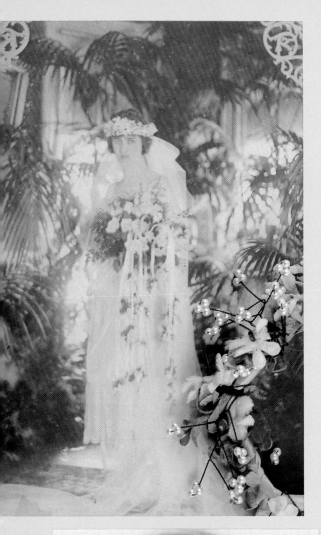

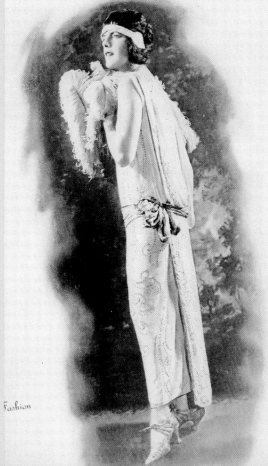

Fashion

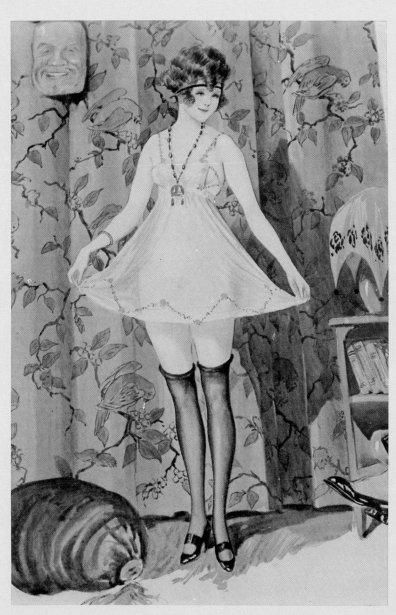

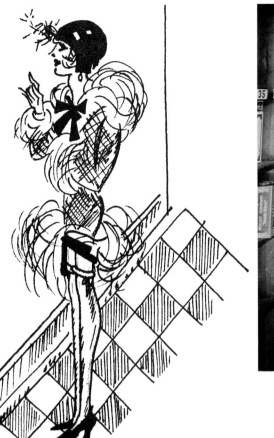

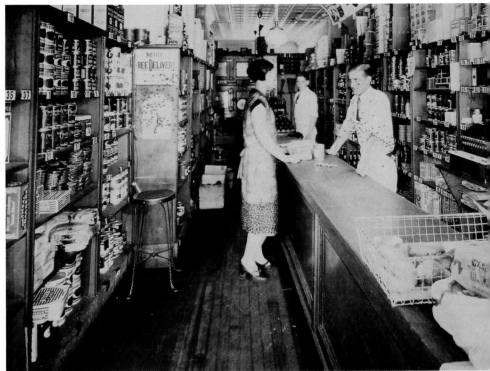

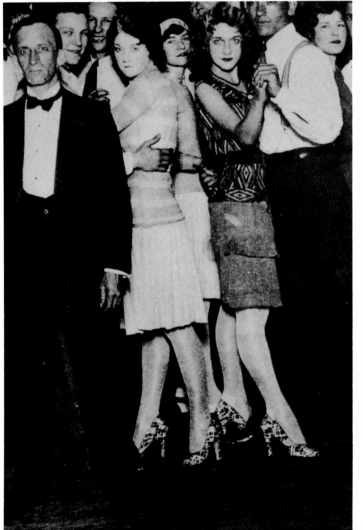

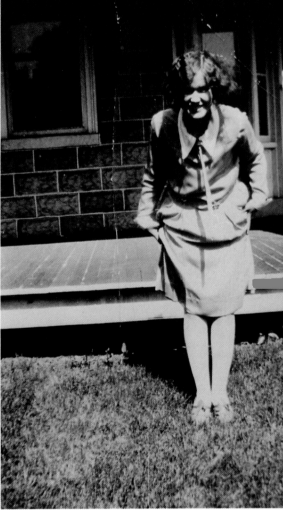

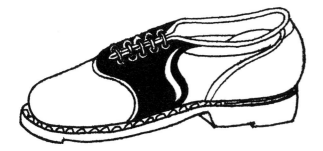

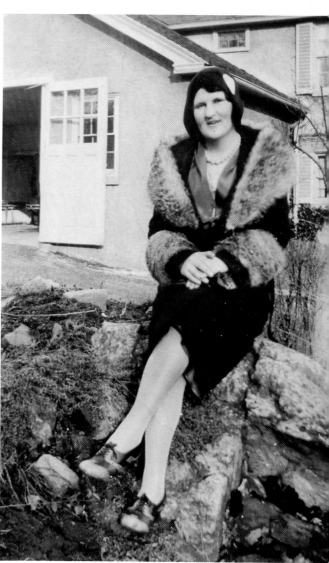

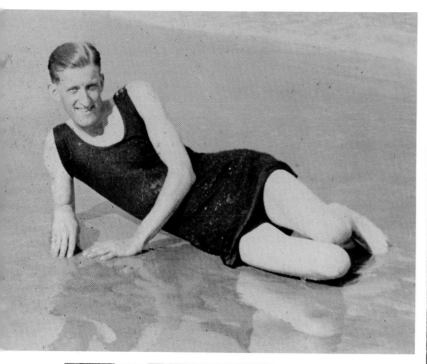

Faces and Places

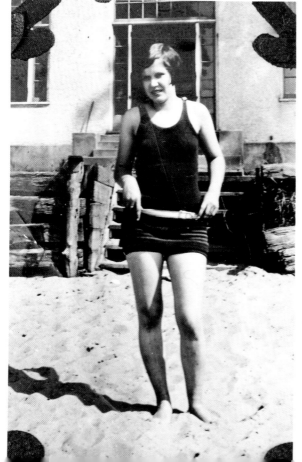

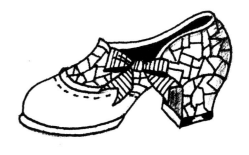

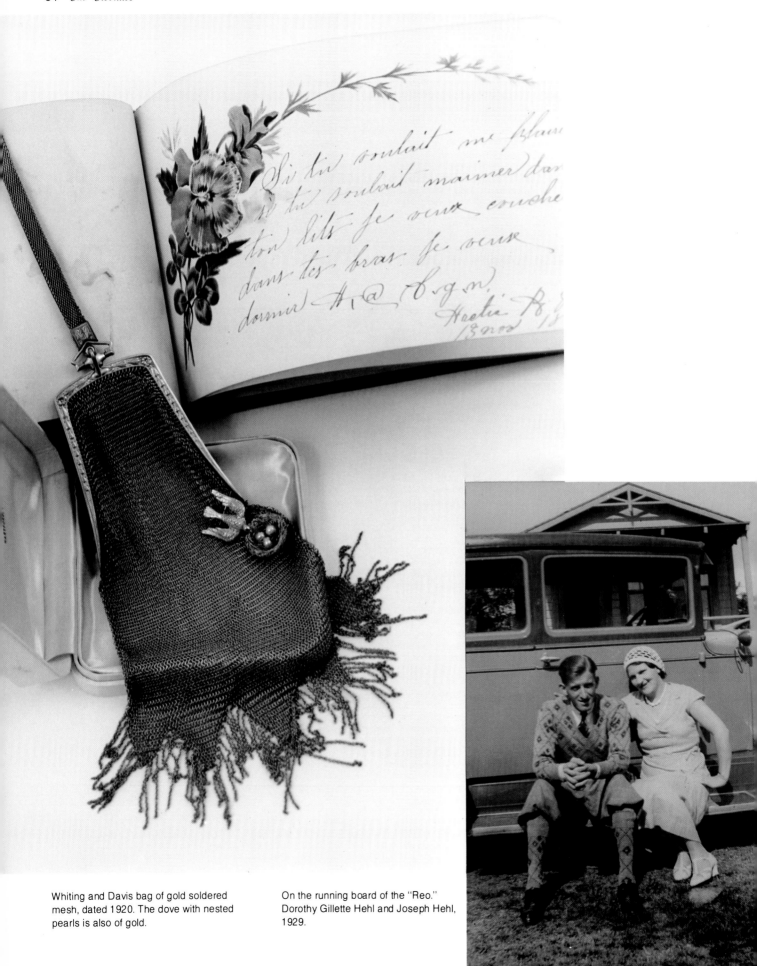

Whiting and Davis bag of gold soldered mesh, dated 1920. The dove with nested pearls is also of gold.

On the running board of the "Reo." Dorothy Gillette Hehl and Joseph Hehl, 1929.

From Periodicals of the Time

The Ladies' Home Journal, January, 1923:

"We had a letter the other day from a uniquely sour critic, who remarked that our fashion pages were an abomination; 'they filled the minds of his womenfolk with a pernicious desire for pretty clothes.'... Instead of apologizing for our fashion pages, we intend to boast of them. Their sole purpose is to promote good taste and beauty..."

"Fashion is not the will-o-the-wisp—here today gone tomorrow—that people are fond of calling it. It is a slow process of evolution, and the experienced person can predict the general lines and salient features of the next season with uncanny prescience. Witness the chemise dress and the bateau neck line, which have been the mode for at least four years. Then there are the detached or semidetached side panels on skirts, which came in during the winter of 1919 and are by no means out today. The popular side-draped skirt of this winter appeared a year ago last fall in Paris..."

Harpers Bazaar, October 1920:

"Brocaded velvet is rich and delightfully warm for chilly winter days. This robe may be had in Copenhagen, rose, light blue, wisteria or pink. $9.44 tax 20 cents"

"A pair of mules to flirt with each charming leisure hour costume. Of satin and ribbon roses in all the shades of the negligees themselves."
R.H. Macy & Co. Inc. advertisement

"'Standard' Spats... the actual standards for style and quality since 1870. With its graceful lines and smart snug fit, the Standard 'Trimline' is the accepted style for everyday and city wear with high heel pump or oxford, while the new Standard 'Sport' Spat is preferred wherever low heel shoes are worn."

Delineator, September, 1928:

"When one hears that in 1876—only about fifty years ago—the most valuable piece of jewelry displayed by the greatest jeweler in America at the Centennial Exposition was a seed pearl necklace valued at one thousand dollars, one gets a vivid impression of the swiftness with which prosperity has come to us."

"You American women are remarkable," said Patou. "Two weeks in Paris and the American woman looks as chic as a Parisian. She soaks it up through her finger tips. In a few days she is tilting her hat at a new angle. In a week, she is wearing just the right shade of hosiery and gloves. In ten days she has a new coiffure, the latest bag, a different way of holding herself, of walking—and in two weeks—*voila,* she has the true chic."

Delineator, September, 1928:

"With his flare for the individual, Paul Poiret stitched silver threads in wavy lines on the bodice and sleeves of the otherwise chastely simply black transparent velvet frock. The very full skirt is deeply scalloped."

"Off went the corsets, snap went the garters. Roll went the stockings. Women were free at last. And what funny looking things most of them were! Of course, mummies are funny looking too. Why not? Anybody would be who had been wrapped up and bound down the way women had been for thousands of years. They suddenly found themselves with a lot of things they hadn't given much attention to so long as they were under cover—hips, knees, and thighs, waists and breasts."

"In the beautiful Lalique glass of one of the windows of her dressmaking establishment in Paris, Vionnet has impressed the proverb, 'To steal an idea is to rob a benefactor'... in fact, one can be jailed for copying a dress in France—and frequently is. Imagine the condition of our cloak and suit industry if this principle were applied in America... But whereas the models of the *grandes maisons* are carefully guarded from French manufacturers, they are sold freely to American copyists with the result that unless a Frenchwoman is quite fabulously rich so that she can buy grand couturier models, she can't hope to keep up with the fashion; but the American woman can, according to her purse, buy the original French model, or a copy at any price from three hundred to thirty dollars, and the excellence of the thirty dollar model is amazing... Take the winter collections, for example: Chanel, one of the most difficult to bend to the buyer's wishes, shows on, let us say, August fifth. By the twenty-second she delivers her orders. A week later the models are in America and two weeks thereafter... the copies are on sale in the shops."

"Is Chic a French Monopoly" Marie Beynon Ray

"And how did the American woman become so sophisticated? For one thing, increased spending power had meant a tremendous increase in good taste... Ten years ago one saw in America comparatively few women who had mastered even the rudiments of good taste in interior decorations and dress. Today every stenographer has some inkling of them, and charming houses and well-dressed women are as the sands of the sea. This swift spread of good taste, covering the country like a blanket, has been brought about very largely by the press—by fashion magazines which conveyed information with unprecedented speed and accuracy. Sketches of the actual French models, sent by radio, are available but a day or so after their creation. The press in Paris is shown the models of the *grand couturiers* even before the buyers are admitted."

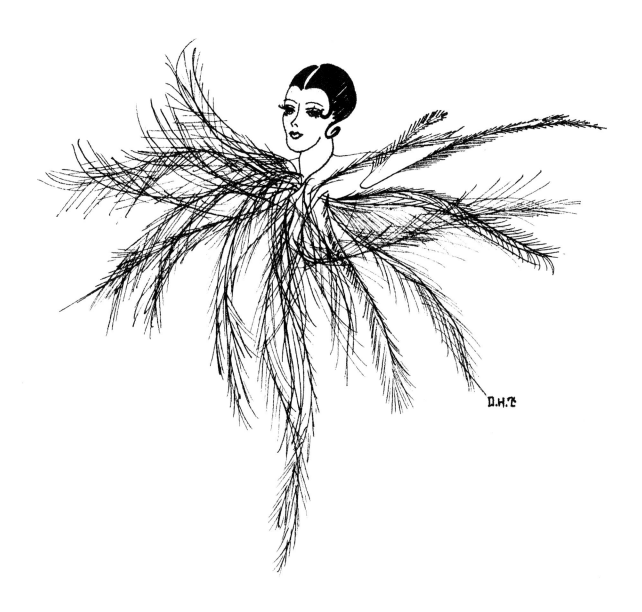

The Thirties

"WHERE'S THE MAN COULD EASE A HEART LIKE A SATIN GOWN?"
Dorothy Parker *The Satin Dress*

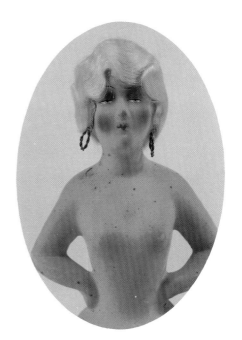

The 1930s were a time of tribulation for the United States, while the world at large ushered in an even graver upheaval—the Second World War. These differing plights on both sides of the ocean, either through the economic chaos in the United States or the threat of impending war in Europe, were reflected in all areas of life, including what people wore—and why.

In the United States, the crash of October 1929 marked the end of the "good times." The happy-go-lucky post-World War I years were replaced by the Great Depression, and the carefree lifestyles of the "flappers" and their "lounge lizards" suddenly turned into a somber dirge for survival. Short skirts had enjoyed an all too brief moment of glory, and longer dresses with austere lines took their place. The silhouette, at least at first glance, had all the trappings of a dull piece of business, especially in light of the gaiety that had gone before. But, oddly enough, couturiers elevated these elongated lines into a stylistic presentation that has rarely been equalled. As always, accessories were the "extra something" that added individuality—not only for the elite, who were privileged to haunt the salons and better shops, but even more so for the average woman who couldn't indulge in the flawless workmanship, design, and attendant cost of couture.

One of these new fashions was a sensual "at home" look, for that's where the "tea gown," considered England's contribution to couture of the 1930s, held court. Difficult to categorize, these garments resembled, on the one hand, filmy lingerie and, on the other, seductive evening attire. Those wearing them looked "picture perfect" draped languidly over boudoir chaise lounges or standing elegantly by the drawing room mantlepiece. The tea gown clung to the body when necessary, billowed elegantly as the wearer moved, and had eye-catching accoutrements like trimmings of soft furs and fastenings covered with silken flowers.

Other pre-war accessorizing fashions originated in the society playgrounds of the world, like St. Tropez, where, as Cecil Beaton—renowned designer, photographer, and fashion maven—wrote in a 1932 *Vogue* article titled "Putting on Local Color," "... one could find little shepherdess hats trimmed with impertinent bows and bouquets of oddly assorted flowers.... Even the best of friends fight in their endeavors to be the first to make their choice of the infinite variety of grotesque hats, some enormous and like a Chinese mandarin's, others nothing but berets or knitted caps as small as the Pope's birettas ..."[1] Beaton went on to caution, "The rules of suitability and practicality apply and there are many pitfalls . . . nothing can be overdone . . . you must not wear an African necklace unless you wear it with an air. You must be cocksure in your St. Tropez shepherdess hat. You must not blush when your lederhosen are remarked upon."[2]

In the world of off-the-rack fashions, daytime skirts fell to approximately 10" from the floor, and women had to contend with fabric mid-calf or lower. At least with regard to the "average fashions for the average woman," this skirt, with good reason, held little or no appeal. Small wonder that accessories were so important. With the disappearance of women's legs, designers saw fit to "home in" on another so-called "erogenous zone"—the back. The oval scooped lines of formal evening wear spawned many decorative accents, like outlines of glittering rhinestones or long ropes of pearls draped seductively behind, all of which served to make a woman's exit more provocative than her entrance.

In the meantime, waists returned to their natural place, and lines were softer and less angular. Madeleine Vionnet, the master Parisienne designer, whose cutting skills and wizardry with bias panels and flowing skirts firmly entrenched her as a major player in the history of fashion, converted the overall look to more Grecian lines, but in modern form. Along with Vionnet, couturiers of the calibre of Chanel and Schiaparelli refused to be stilled by threats of war, and their creative influence on the world fashion scene continued in the early years of the decade.

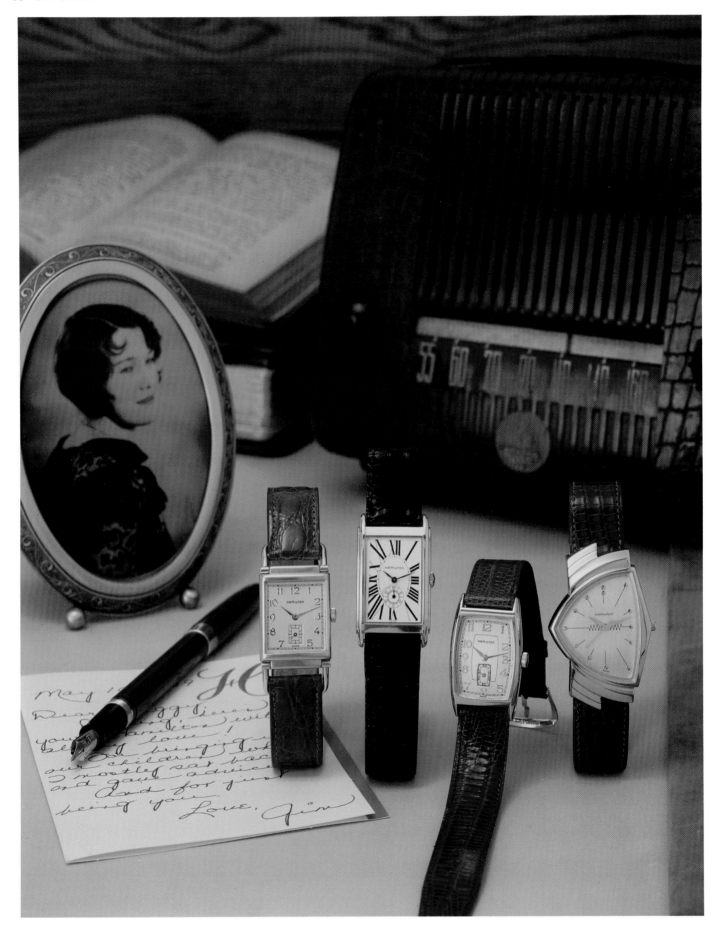

When viewing the 1930s, however, it was the bold innovation of one of these bright stars that shines like a beacon. For just as the 1920s were in great measure Chanel's, the 1930s rightfully belonged to Elsa Schiaparelli, who found her real niche during that decade. "Schiaparelli's innovations were more in the tradition of Poiret's showmanship than Chanel's grasp of modern realities but then the 1930s had had quite enough of realities."[3] However, showmanship aside, Schiaparelli also performed some very practical services. For, as Verte lovingly wrote in 1940, ". . . It was she who arrived on a shocking-pink cloud to put many things back where they belonged—including the feminine waistline, which around 1922 had slipped dangerously near the knees . . . It was she who first fastened into women's dresses that diabolic little 'Sesame' that shuts you in or out: the zipper."[4]

Schiaparelli's playful side was just what the 1930s needed. She brought new meaning and verve to the most simple of accessories—like buttons. No longer were they used merely to fasten a dress together. As in the French court of earlier days, they were wearable art—an adjunct that brought the garment to life. Schiaparelli also saw the beauty, fun, and infinite possibilities in costume jewelry and was instrumental in elevating it to acceptable status. Her jewelry was something to behold—beautiful and bold, provocative and sensual, witty and charming. At last the art of costume jewelry had begun its dizzying ascent into fashion lore. Along with a handful of other pioneers in this relatively new field, Schiaparelli helped to make it possible for women of modest means to spend little on jewelry and have much to show for it.

In a return to the Venetian masks that had captivated the international society set decades before—but with a nonsensical twist—Schiaparelli painted silly, clown-like masks on long-handled fans designed to be carried "just for fun." Although Schiaparelli's accessories were sometimes outrageous—albeit deliberately so—women were drawn to them like a magnet, for each provided a delightful infusion of devil-may-care magic. Considering economic conditions, her timing couldn't have been better.

There is little doubt that Schiaparelli displayed a special genius that made her a forerunner of many fashion concepts of the future. And isn't that one of the primary missions of couture—to have the foresight to present, at just the right time, in just the right social climate, something new, daring, and different before anyone else has thought of it? In this respect, Schiaparelli more than succeeded, but like any true *artiste*, she would have continued her work accepted or not. Other couturiers also left their mark. "But it was 'Scap,' a Roman woman with huge dark eyes and a taste for the 'tasteless' shocking pink, whose surrealistic fantasies most successfully succeeded in teasing and amusing the public."[5]

With the focus of couture encompassing the *whole* woman, proper accessorizing became an absolute necessity for the fashion-conscious female of the 1930s, a trend that was reworked, refined, and splendidly carried over into the 1940s. Fashion demanded that hats, gloves, and handbags complement the outfit—but with a much-needed "new look." "The trend is away from literal matching of accessories with the costume. Contrast and harmony make the ensemble more interesting and the costume more varied, and are welcome after several seasons of unimaginative monotones."[6] A 1935 article in Vogue described these new trends in accessorizing:

Gloves: You might even build your outfit around your gloves, cart before the horse fashion. That's how important they are . . .

Shoes: Small jodhpur boots, only a fraction higher than an ordinary Oxford are what Schiaparelli sprang at her collection . . . New, too, are buckled Oxfords mounting high over the instep and square-toed Bunting shoes with the toes slanting downward . . . fairly flat heels everywhere . . . narrow gold leather frogs over the instep of military shoes . . . double breasted buttons over the instep . . . gold and silver Greek evening sandals . . . and . . . heel-less sneakers of lame' or pearl-embroidered velvet.

Belts: Wide crusader belts of embossed or cut-out gold and silver leather, worked bronze stomachers, thonged belts, jewelled belts, studded with multicoloured cathedral-window stones . . .

Jewelry: Decidedly barbaric, big lumps of it in bright colours . . . wide gold bracelets with blobs of semi-precious stones. No modest little diamond on your decolletage, but handfuls of them in something large and impressive. Diamonds in your hat and as many as you can buy."[7]

From the Hamilton Watch Company, here are *Hamilton Classics Authentic Reproductions from America's Past*. Still hand-assembled in Lancaster Pennsylvania, they are, left to right: the Wilshire City Edition (1939); the Ardmore (1934); the Cabot (1935)—all reflecting the beauty of the Art Deco influence; and the Ventura (1957), with its classic modernism. During the years following their introduction of timepieces for both sexes, the name *Hamilton* became an almost generic term for the wristwatch, and the ultimate gift for many occasions, especially graduations. Young ladies and gentleman were proud to receive their first "Hamilton" after earning that high school or college degree. It was, in some respects, part of a rite of passage to adulthood. Photo courtesy of James Marsh, President, Hamilton Award and Incentive Division.

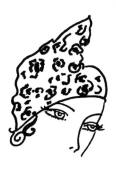

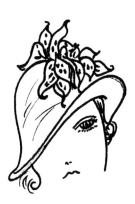

Hats were tiny in the early years of the 1930s, becoming broader brimmed in the latter half of the decade. The final years of the Thirties heralded the return of chapeaus that looked like "things"—from flower pots to crowns—which were plunked on the head with hapless abandon. The epitome of daring was, not unsurprisingly, to be found in Schiaparelli's designs, for her creations carried innovation to the brink—and toppled it gleefully over the edge. Among her more daring millinery masterpieces was one that emulated a lamb chop complete with ruffled "panties," and another in the shape of an inverted shoe.

Open-toed shoes "opened" new fashion doors when they came into vogue around 1937, along with colorful, strapped sandals for evening wear. And to complement the new footwear, gossamer silk chiffon hosiery was preferred by the women who could afford it. By mid-decade skirts were timidly rising once again, and when the decade came to an end, they had lifted to a more interesting, and acceptable, 15"-17" from the floor.

It's not surprising that the beauty shop of the 1930's became an even more essential component to good grooming, and just the right cosmetic, coupled with scrupulous care of skin and hair, was supremely important. Beautician's services were available at a reasonable cost, so that even those of modest means could treat themselves to an occasional trip to the palace of beauty.

In 1937 another name that has more than weathered the "test of time" was first offered to the public. It was the luxurious Hermes silk scarf, which usually depicted intricate "horsey" designs, reflecting the company's beginnings in 1837 in the harness-making trade. The popularity of these unique creations has never wavered and, both old and new, they continue to dominate the fashion accessorizing scene as a status symbol and valuable collector's item.

The beginnings of a drastic turnaround in swimwear took place in the 1930s, when swimming was no longer the principal purpose for wearing a bathing suit. Instead, spawned by Chanel's suntanned look of the 1920s, *sunbathing* was the overriding obsession, and thus swimwear became less intrusive as women strove to expose more and more of their bodies to the sun's tanning rays. Sports clothes followed suit. Tennis, especially when played on the professional circuit, demanded shorter costumes, and the shorts that were eventually worn by female "pros" made their way into everyday fashions.

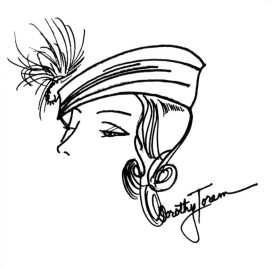

The pall over Europe severely impeded the creativity of the major Parisienne fashion houses as the decade drew to a close. With the advent of World War II, haute couture suffered a mighty blow. There was little possibility of generating "electricity" at a fashion showing when the spark had been extinguished from daily life. Paris—at that time still acknowledged as the fashion capital of the world—was, by the beginning of the next decade, occupied by Nazi forces. Many designers, anticipating the inevitable, had fled. Some took their talents across the Channel . . . with mixed results, for the British were also suffering the cruel restrictions of war and a wartime economy. Others simply bided their time. And for still others there was no recovery at all. One thing was certain: the world could no longer look exclusively to Europe for its inspiration in fashion. Yet circumstances never totally snuffed out the message of *couture*. Undaunted, she continued to make herself known and, among the monied classes, fashion remained glamorous and innovative.

Although fashion "ins" and "outs" remained under the influence of haute couture and the media, in the United States the "homespun look" also captured the public's imagination throughout much of the decade. Cecil Beaton commented on this surprising phenomenon in a 1932 *Vogue* article by observing that, "In America's 'West' blue canvas dungarees, leather jerkins, large sombreros and windbreakers . . . are piled to the ceiling in the local store and can be had for small coin."[8] The trend was not short-lived, for a March 1936 *Harper's Bazaar* feature titled "Dress America" made reference to the fun and treasures to be found in country general stores and the ". . . vast and hysterical selection of 'Heavy Duty' (89 cents) suspenders . . ." The mail-order catalogues of Sear's & Roebuck and Montgomery Ward offered plain and fancy clothing at bargain prices . . . like leather gloves for 57 cents a pair and a moleskin vest lined with sheepskin for $2.65!

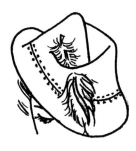

Much admired for their brilliant colors, native American Indian clothing enjoyed a resurgence of popularity too. Buckskin and beaded boots and boleros, silvered and decorated belts that became pieces of prized jewelry in their own right, and of course, the always dependable moccasin were much in demand. The Western look was but one that was fostered at least in part, by films—with more than a little help from fashion magazines, like *Harpers* and *Vogue*—which brought the very latest from the fashion world to women in all walks of life. The movies, however, were bound to reach a larger, more diversified audience, and consequently much of what is now viewed as the "look" of the Thirties is, in great degree, a reflection of what people saw on the *silver screen*. This costuming was influenced by the glamorous designs of fashion's creative geniuses, as well as a new breed—the costume designers, many of whom worked almost exclusively for the film studios.

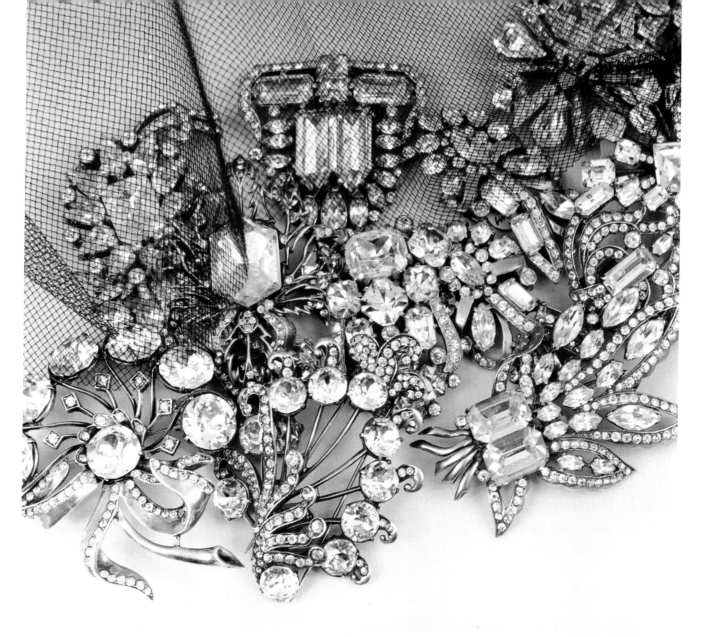

A scrolled ''E'' for Eisenberg...and Exciting! These brooches and clips are all early pieces in Sterling and base metal. Each a masterpiece. Collection of Joanne Ball.

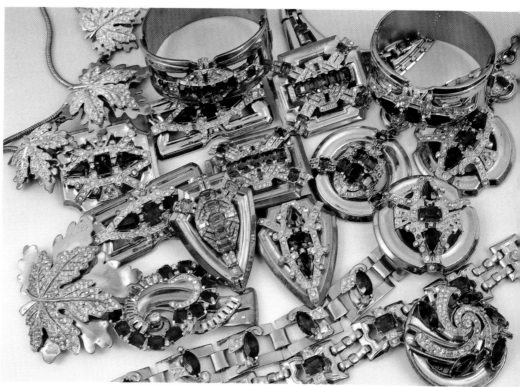

The Deco splendor of McClelland Barclay is captured in this grouping of colorful brooches, bracelets, and necklaces. Each reflects the ''artist's eye'' of this renowned illustrator, who lost his life during World War II. Collection of Joanne Ball.

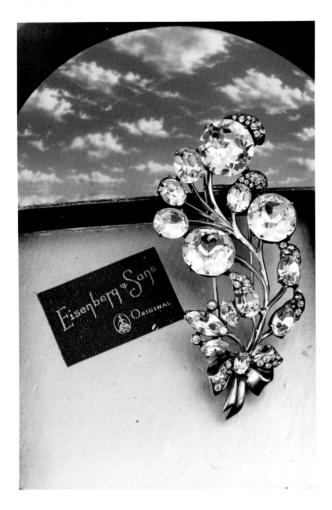

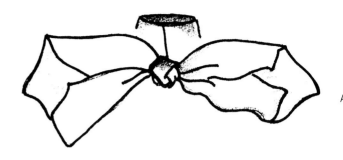

A.

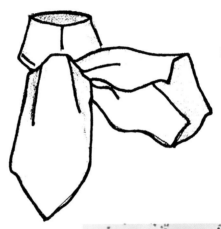

B.   Puff tie in the making.

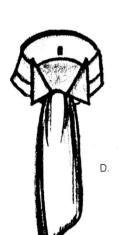

D.   Completed tie.

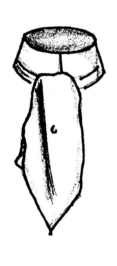

C.

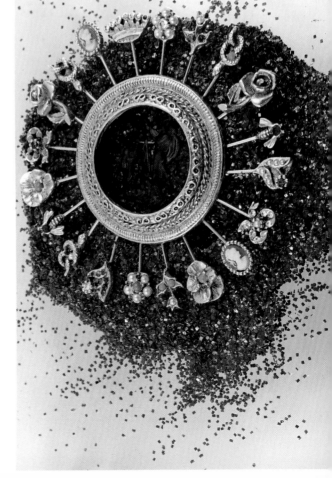

Movies and radio had become the solace of a population eager for a glimpse of the "better life" that hopefully lay ahead. Even the best was not beyond imitation—that was the "silver lining" in the 1930's fashion story. Hollywood gambled and won, for by giving the public what they instinctively sensed it needed, the scions of the industry created a heyday for films. Although screenwriters pumped out popular tales of hope and survival, the drawing room comedies and flamboyant musicals also succeeded in capturing the audience's imagination. It transported them out of the Depression doldrums and provided glimpses of worlds they probably would never see and glamorous lives they could only dream about.

Films helped to institutionalize the distinctive look of the 1930s by developing the promise of glamour-made-affordable. A few hours in a dimly-lit movie theatre could tease the audience with Jean Harlow in satin lingerie and feathered boas, Ginger Rogers in swirling gowns and glittering jewels, and Fred Astaire and Adolph Menjou in tails and spats. Carole Lombard might appear the epitome of glamour as she swept confidently across the screen in a simple felt hat with upturned brim, but the average 1930's woman could have one of those, too. Feather boas may not be practical for a mother with growing children and a low-paid, laboring husband, but she could occasionally treat herself to a pair of rhinestone clips from the dime store to fasten on that simple crepe dress. Women were perhaps most susceptible to "movie images," but even the conservative male of the 1930s wasn't immune. He flung a scarf flamboyantly over his shoulder, just as gentlemen had during the Twenties when scarves epitomized the bon vivant of the movies.

Thus, three important elements combined during this period to create a *core of fashion* that penetrated all layers of the social and economic strata: designers of fashion for film, the established couturiers worldwide, and the enormous impact of fashion magazines. Women eagerly pored over the "latest," like the colorful description in a 1936 issue of *Harpers*, describing flowered berets, black enamel bracelets, and ". . . Darwin tulips looped through the belt of your black day dress. Molyneaux does this sometimes with yellow tulips, sometimes with white, and they're artificial though they look fresh as the dew." Hats that year included those of chiffon and straw like ". . . Suzy's latest pill-boxes made of several layers of stitched chiffon with a chou tied high on one side. Or a pillbox in peacock colored chiffons swathed around the head and tied center back like a kerchief with the ends flipped out."[9]

The public's fascination with America's own Wallis Warfield Simpson made her a "star player" in the saga of the 1930s. Her romance and eventual marriage to England's king, who relinquished his crown for "the woman I love," became the bittersweet love story of the decade, if not the century. The Duchess's opulent jewelry and accessories transfixed lovers of luxury and beauty everywhere. Commissioned mainly during the 1930s and Forties, they stand as a brilliant beacon of splendor in a world where the lights were slowly dimming. Not only were there breathtaking necklaces, bracelets and rings of diamonds, sapphires, rubies, and emeralds, but a magnificent array of other accessories, like eighteen carat gold lipstick cases and compacts embedded with gigantic precious gems. One enamel, ruby and diamond evening bag, circa 1930, is described thus, "The front of the frame decorated with black enamel dart and scroll motifs, pave set throughout with brilliant cut diamonds and with diamond-tipped ruby beads at intervals, the wedge-shaped pull similarly set, the reverse decorated with star-set rubies and diamonds, the pink and gold bag embroidered in a design of foliate and stylised flowerhead motifs on an ivory coloured ground . . ."[10] The Duke, on the other hand, had his own impressive accessories . . . officer's swords, Scottish dress dirks and Skean Dhus of silver and ivory, badges and belt clasps, highly-detailed silver tobacco boxes, cuff links of 18-carat gold, and ornate snuff boxes, many items going back through hundreds of years of British history. They were all, nonetheless, overshadowed by the opulence of the Duchess's magnificent jewels--timeless and awe-inspiring.

Another "jeweled look" that surfaced during this time had a tremendous impact on the future of jewelry design. In 1927 a young man from Sicily—Fulco Santostefano della Cerda, duke of Verdura—started his career as a textile designer for Chanel. With her growing focus on the importance of jewelry to complement her fashions, Chanel quickly recognized his talents and appointed him chief jewelry designer. Many fine and costume pieces that became popular mid-century and beyond are a direct result of designs by Fulco—from coins and coats-of-arms to ropes culled from drawings of seafaring knots. He was responsible for popularizing figural pieces like jewel-encrusted chessmen, Chinese horsemen, and fluttering hummingbirds, then in a stroke of genius, reviving the art of baked enamel over a gold base, resulting in a soft, lustrous sheen. One of Fulco's flagship designs was the wide enamel bracelet centered with a Maltese Cross of various hues that Chanel always wore in duplicate, one on each wrist. All promoted a look that was destined to endure.

Prior to this, most of the century's fine jewelry consisted of precious stones set in platinum, with gold rarely used in adornment of this type. Fulco, however, mixed precious and semi-precious stones and then pressed them into gold, much as one would press a

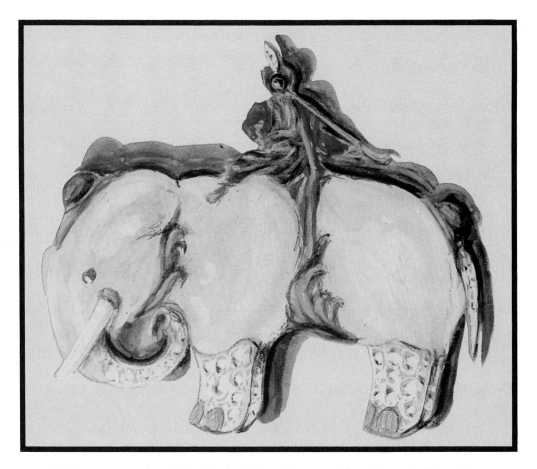

stone into wax, creating a look of stained glass. As reported by a former fashion editor many years later, "'It was costume jewelry in real. People wore it like bunches of flowers—outside, on a suit, at lunch. . .nobody had done that kind of thing until Fulco came along."[11] Decades later, costume jewelry mavens like Kenneth Jay Lane would happily acknowledge their debt to Verdura when they offered similar designs in costume pieces to eager customers who otherwise could not have enjoyed them.

In 1937 Fulco arrived in New York to collaborate with New York jeweller Paul Flato, founding his own business there two years later and adding another shop in Paris in 1947. For two decades thereafter his creations appeared repeatedly on the covers of *Harper's Bazaar* and *Vogue*. The grande dame of fashion, Diana Vreeland, reflected on his contributions years later when, as fashion editor at *Harper's*, she mused, "Everything he did was wonderful. He was great artist, like someone from the Renaissance. No one ever made gold things like he did. If he's forgotten, it's because people don't really remember anything except diamonds."[12] In truth, the Duke di Verdura had pioneered new frontiers and redirected jewelry design from the beaten path, opening breathtaking vistas from extraordinary new heights.

High on the list of the 1930's contribution to the world of jewelry was the use of Bakelite and similar synthetics, which reached the masses as gemstones and gold obviously could not. Fashioned into pieces that have enchanted consumers and collectors ever since, this medium allowed designers to explore new areas and carry their imaginations into delightful flights of fancy. From fruits and vegetables to elaborate figures and flowers, the possibilities were endless. Designers worldwide contributed to the renderings so prized today, and the magic of these synthetic materials continues to provide present-day artists with a medium the public still finds intriguing.

The 1930s gave us a panoramic view of real characters as diverse as the likes of Bonnie and Clyde, Al Capone, and Bugsy Siegel were to society mavens like Brenda Frazier and Barbara Hutton ("the poor little rich girl"). It was a view that encompassed the depths of poverty and the playgrounds of the rich. From the tragic exodus of Oklahoma farmers driven westward by dust storms, to Shirley Temple look-alike contests with little girls curled, ruffled and be-ribboned—and mothers hoping for a pot of gold somewhere over that tarnished rainbow—it was a decade of *hope* in the face of seemingly insurmountable odds.

On that cheery note, brimming with a vast assortment of whimsical delights, another decade passed into history. It too painted a broad spectrum of society, reflecting both its ills and a steadfast determination to overcome them. In entertainment—and fashion—the world was trying to create some semblance of normalcy when everything else seemed to be spinning out of control.

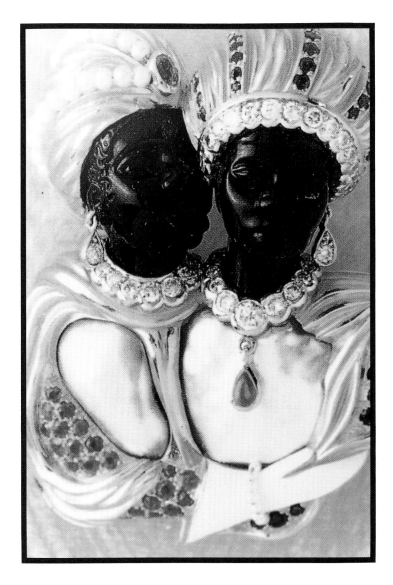

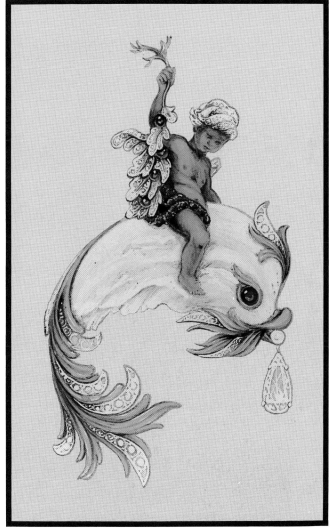

Sheer artistry. Three original drawings
for jewels by Verdura. Verdura's
recognition of the symbolism and artistic
possibilities in "decoration" jewels
created a revival for heraldic pieces that
depicted the crests and symbolic icons
of military and social orders, as witness
this elephant inspired by the Royal
Danish Order of the Elephant. And
returning to the Renaissance, "His
blackamoors might have stepped out of
a Venetian banquet scene painted by
Veronese. Their dusky skins contrast
with their Baroque pearl chests,
aigrettes sparkle in their turbans, and
their necks are encircled with pearl
chokers." (*Country Life,* June 7, 1990,
Diana Scarisbrick.)

1930-1940
[1] "Beaton in Vogue" p. 156
[2] "Beaton in Vogue" p. 156
[3] "Fashion, the Mirror of History," p. 231
[4] "Vertes", p. 19
[5] "Fashion, the Mirror of History"
[6] "Vogue," October 1, 1935 p. 135
[7] "Vogue," October 1, 1935, p. 132
[8] "Beaton in Vogue" p. 156
[9] Harpers Bazaar, March 1936, p. 109
[10] Jewels of the Duchess of Windsor, The, p. 132

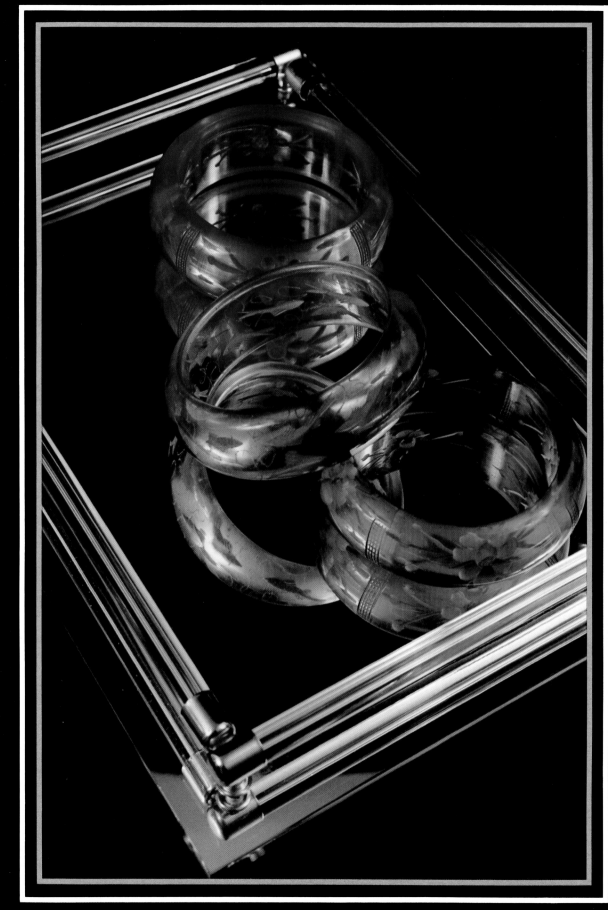

Lucite bangle bracelets carved with fish

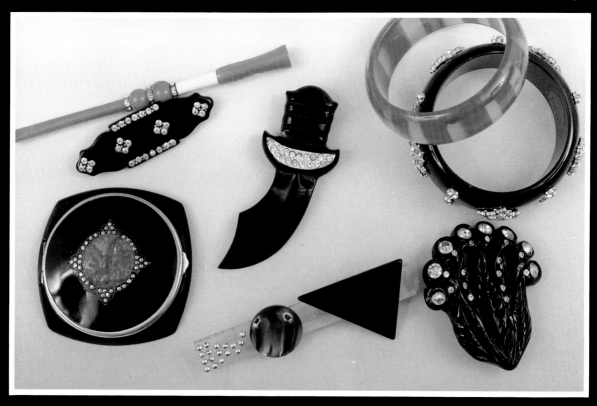

An array of bakelite and synthetics,
including a black compact with cut steel
and celluloid decorating the top, a
rhinestone-studded cigarette holder, and
a modernistic brooch inspired by the
1939 World's Fair.

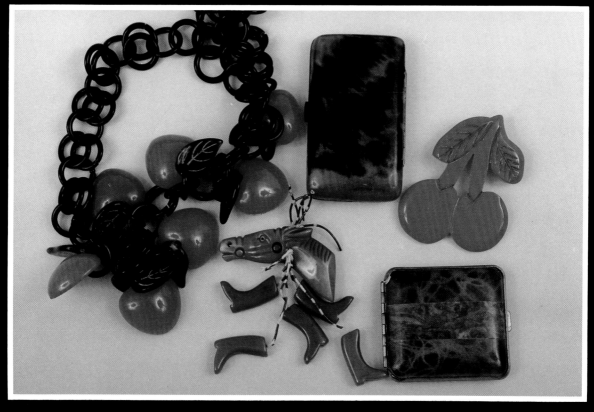

Synthetics from luscious cherries to
equestrian delights, flanked by faux
tortoise compact and cigarette case.

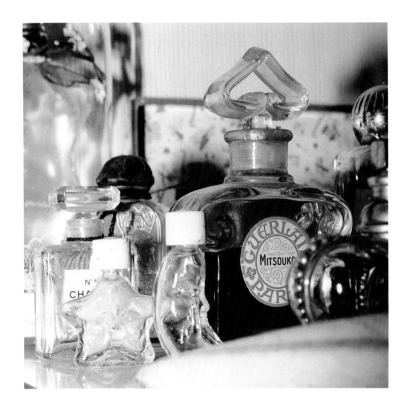

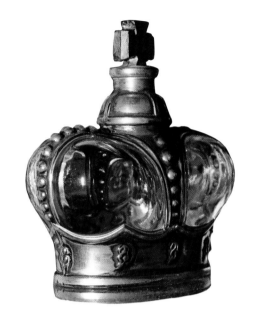

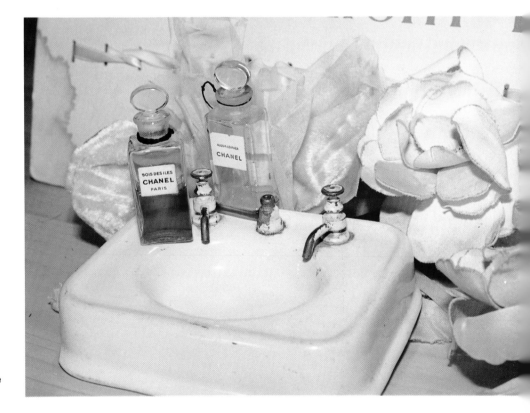

Madame's toilette...from
dime store perfumes to Mitsouko by
Guerlain, the "royal crown" of Prince
Matchiabelli, timeless Chanel, Art Deco
floral scents in a charming carrying
case, the inimitable Schiaparelli...and the
mysterious Golliwog.

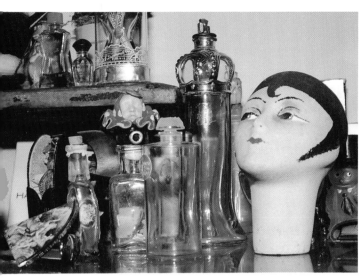

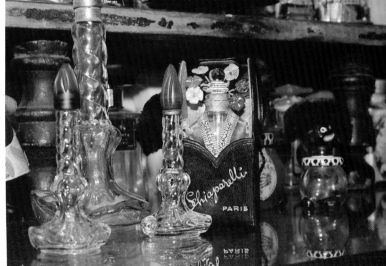

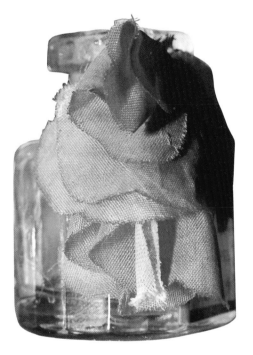

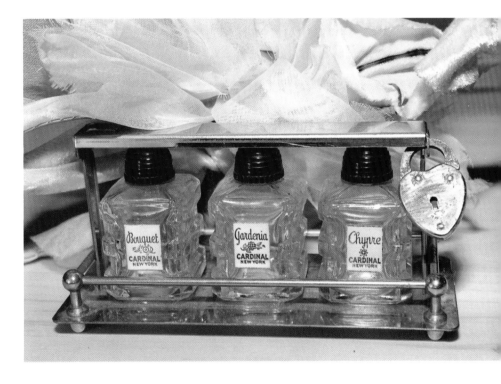

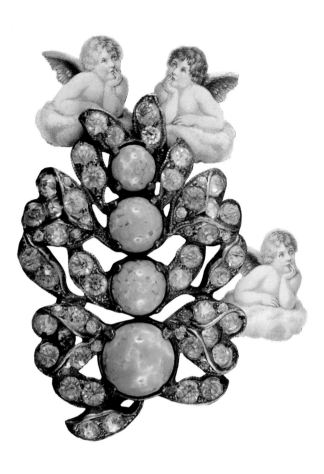

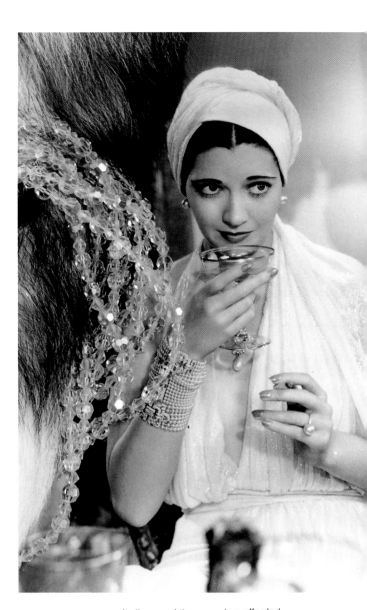

Eisenberg sterling fur clips, one ablaze with faux turquoise, the other with faux turquoise, rubies and diamonds.

A glimpse of the escapism afforded audiences in 1930s Hollywood. Surrounded by wealth, wide-eyed glamorous Kay Francis sips champagne wearing a pearlized turban and an armful of Joseff of Hollywood matching bracelets with glittering Deco clasps. Photo courtesy of Joan Castle Joseff.

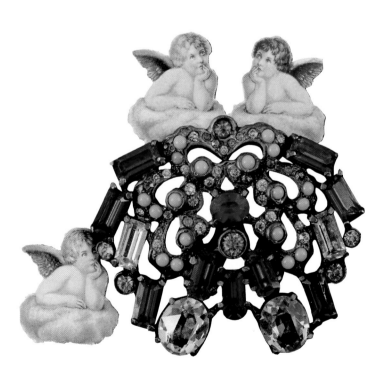

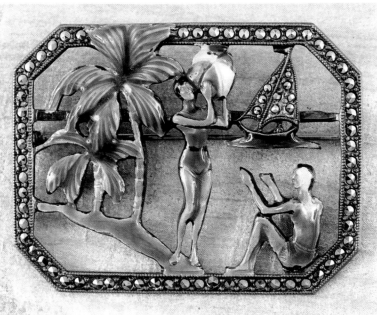

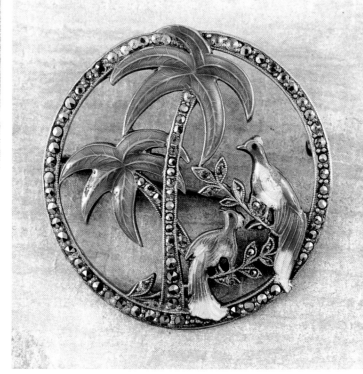

Two sterling marcasite, hard enamel pins. Havana..."at play on the beach"...and Cuba..."birds in the trees," and below, a giant marcasite flower.

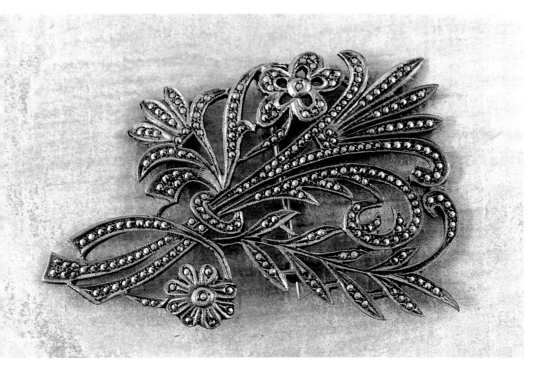

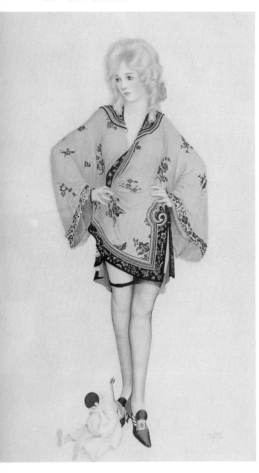

"Sleepy Time Gal."

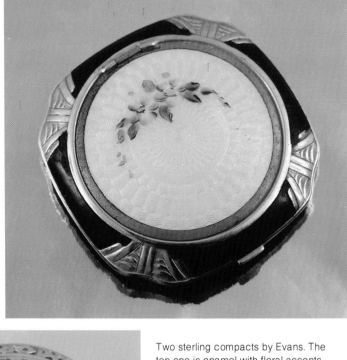

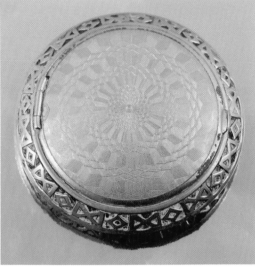

Two sterling compacts by Evans. The top one is enamel with floral accents, the bottom has intricate designs and a top of champleve peach enamel.

The rare beauty of two sterling and enamel champleve brooches, studded with marcasites.

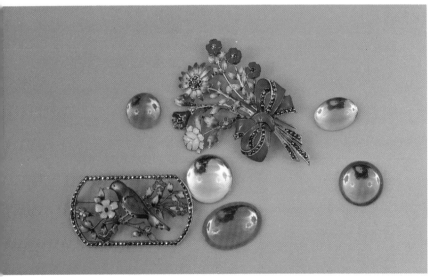

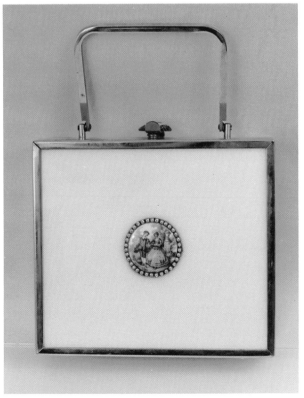

A white synthetic bag with gold frame and Limoges insert.

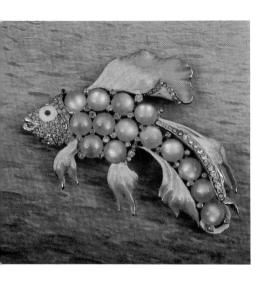

With an early Coro marking, a huge "pearl-bellied" fish enameled in shades of pink and studded with pave rhinestones.

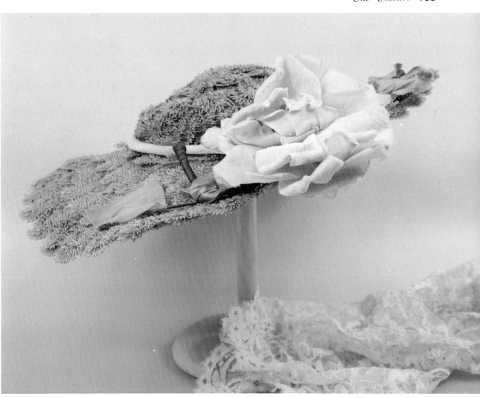

This is femininity! Courtesy of Clar-Mar.

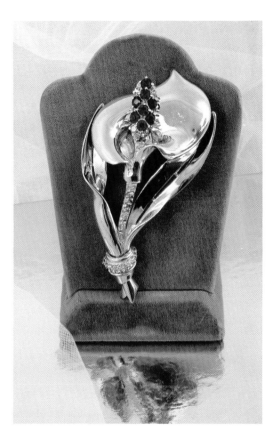

A majestic 5″ CoroCraft calla lily that's been plated again and again to give it exceptional weight and sheen. The ruby-studded stamen is moveable.

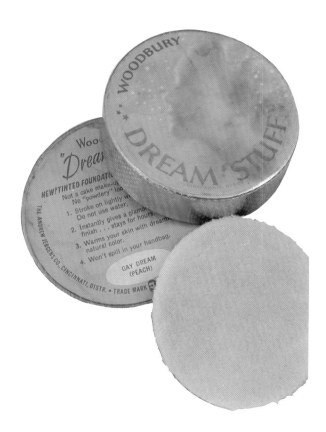

Gay dreams and champagne bubbles. Woodbury "Dream Stuff" powder.

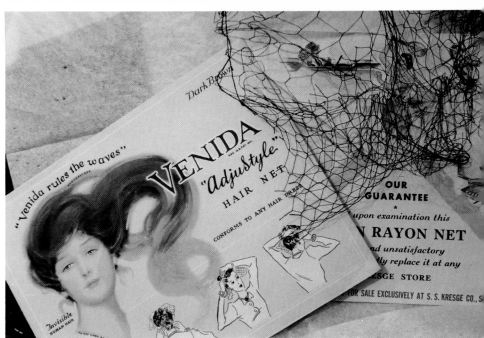

It can't be all glamour! A human hair net, circa 1930.

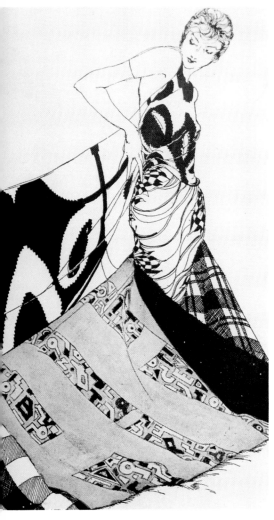

The scarf-wrap technique. *Harper's Bazaar*, 1939.

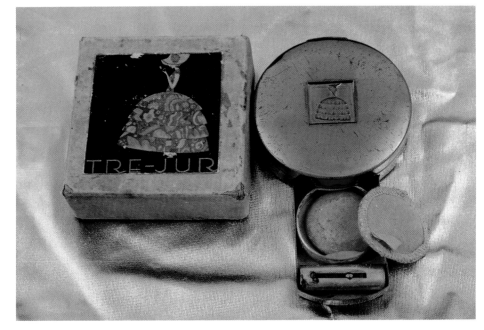

Powder, rouge and lipstick combo from Tre-Jur, in original box.

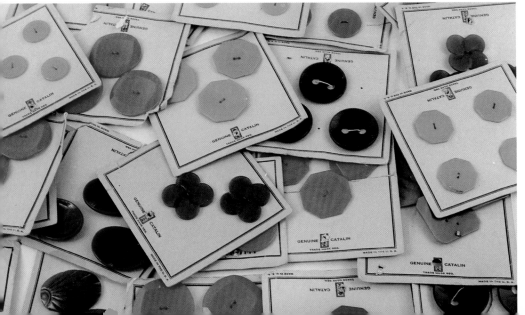

Deco Catalin buttons, on original card.

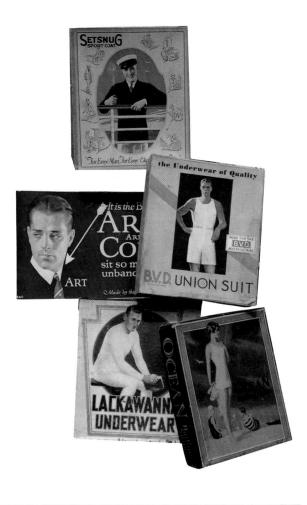

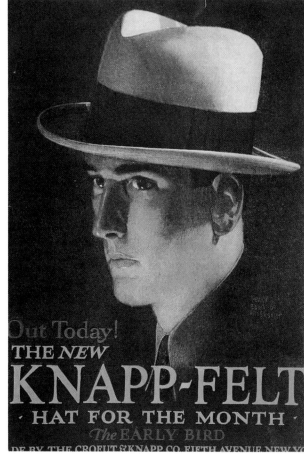

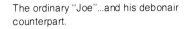

The ordinary "Joe"...and his debonair counterpart.

Pearlized tops with enamel designs add a look of Deco beauty to amber glass dressing table containers. A whalebone walking stick (circa 19th century) nestles between.

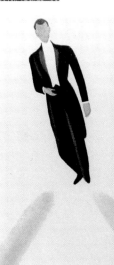

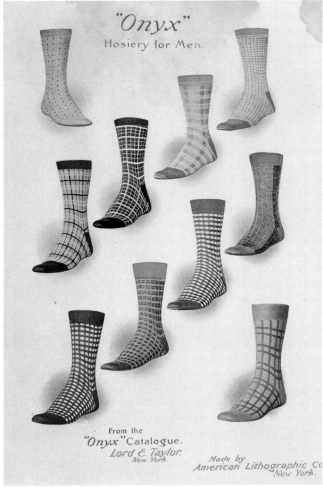

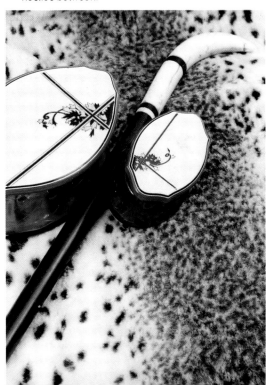

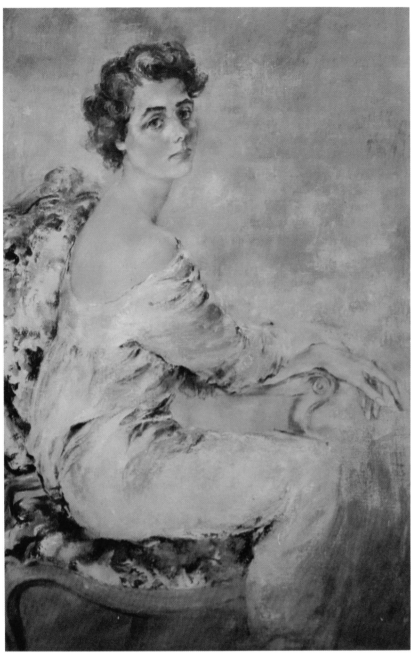

"Lady in Green," 1935. Howard Chandler Christy (1873-1952). Oil on canvas, 44-¾" x 29-½". Courtesy of Alan M. Goffman, The Fine Art of Illustration, New York.

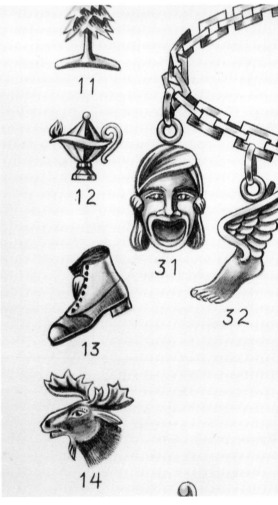

Moveable overlays of pavé rhinestones on golden leaves from the graceful layers of this McClelland Barclay necklace and matching brooch.

Stylized charms of the 1930s. Designer: John F. Dubbs.

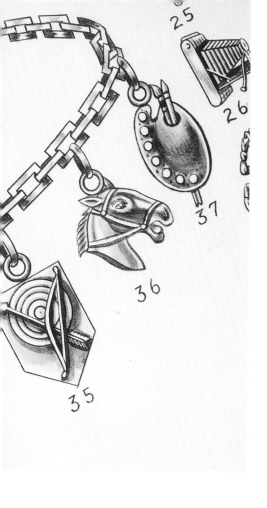

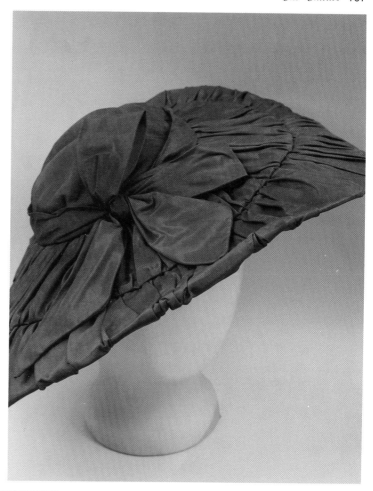

Pouffed, pleated, and "cocksure."
Courtesy of Clar-Mar.

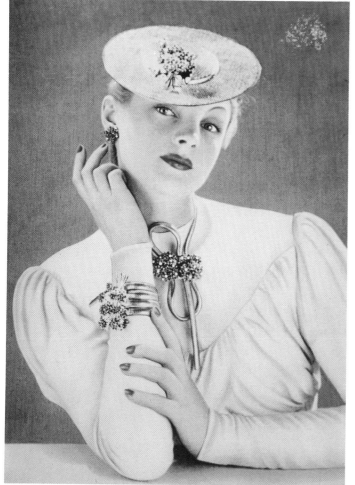

Plasiar de France, July 1939.
Mauboussin.

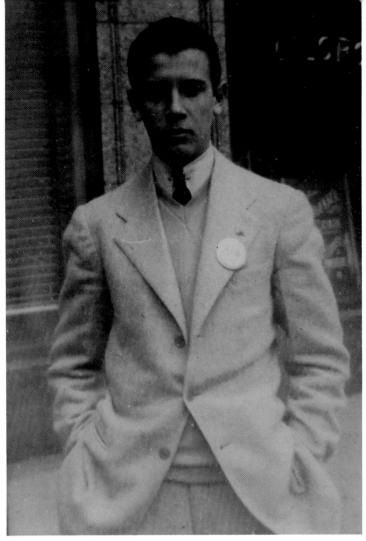

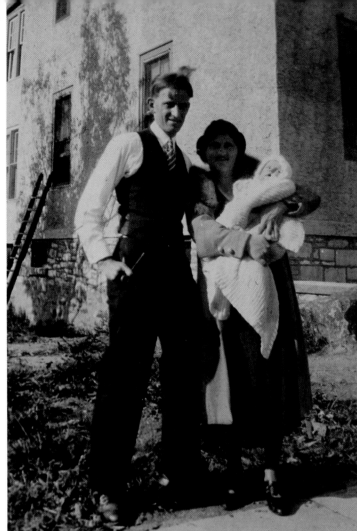

Faces and Places

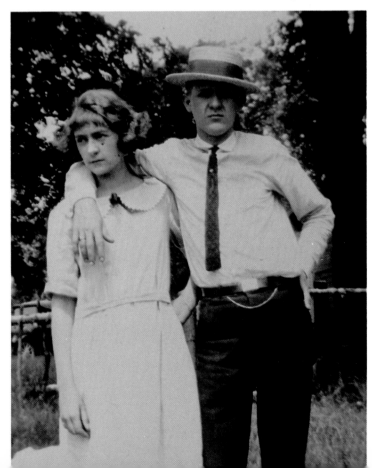

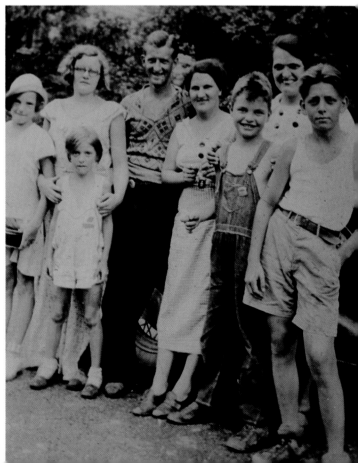

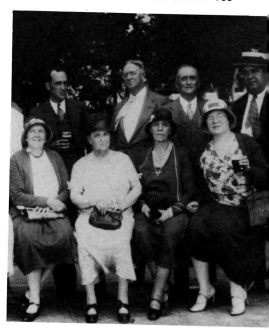

Vogue, November, 1931:

"This year the anatomy of the debutante has changed. The typical young girl of to-day is a creature of curves. She knows her waistline well, and when she dances, she unconsciously flaunts her little behind . . . She loves the big puffed sleeves of evening and the square padded shoulders of day. Her hair is often parted in the middle and always in curls . . . She pulls her hat over one eye more like a rake than an Empress Eugenie. She takes like a duck to water to the new removeable furs . . . and finishes her costume with a new school of accessory . . ."

"Muffs are back and smarter than ever this season. And a short fox cape that just covers the shoulders is among the sensations of the winter."

"Here . . . is Schiaparelli's wooden soldier (coat) . . . done in deep, bright blue corduroy with an enormous rib. It fastens first horizontally at the waist-line, then vertically, with silver curtain-ring clips.

Vogue, November 1, 1931 ("Tips on the Shop Market")

"Twenty or thirty bracelets on the arm—more if you insist-. . . They don't look too barbaric either, for they're very thin gold or silver bangles—not much heftier than a stout picture wire . . . The imports are twisted in pleasant variations; the made-in-America ones are of plain silver or washed gold. You mix the two together and you have one of the smartest medleys that ever weighted down a wrist."

"From darkest Africa via the French Colonial Exposition, come two nifty notions for enlightened America. One, baptized 'Congo,' is a broad scarf necklace of braided silk strips, primitive yes, but extraordinarily smart to wear with your wool dress. 'Dakar' is a two-inch wide belt of braided silk strips in various colours and edged with fringe meant to gird your wool sports dress . . . Also very nice to wear with wool dresses are the new scarfs of 'Chelita'—a thin wool, crepe-like fabric. Most of these are of the Ascot type and have strips joined together in geometrical designs."

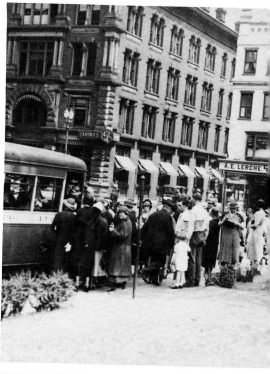

Vogue, October 1, 1935:

"Chanel is doing things with shawls. Not the cashmere shawls of our grandmothers or the riotously botanical pieces that are known as Spanish, but elegant, extravagant shawls entirely of paillettes, or of heavy, coal-black crepe, with miles of fringe . . ."

"Bergdorf Goodman has gone royalist. Their new vanity case for irrepressible young things is a gold metal sceptre, almost a foot long, hung by gold cords and glittering with pomp and majesty. Inside this rod of empire are a purse for keys and change, room for cigarettes, a handkerchief, powder and rouge, and all the rest, down to a lipstick in the very bottom of the gadget."

"Don't cry 'too theatrical!' when you see the pearl-studded, gold braid headbands at Saks Fifth Avenue. In the hand, they do look prima donna but, on the head, they're charming and a change from the usual flora and fauna of hair-dos."

Vogue, June 15, 1938:

"Luxuriously correct is this cleverly designed companion bag with accessible outside zipper pocket that carries a 7 piece dresser set of cloissone enamel. Silk lined with ample space in the body of bag for personal accessories . . $20.00 as illustrated in brown lizard cowhide."

"Always a little nonsense in accessories. Beetles or strawberries embroidered on Schiaparelli's reverse. Quite a bit of embroidery. Buttons like leaves, caterpillars, stag heads, tree-trunks, gold acorns . . . White celluloid belts on Balenciaga's nice day dresses. LeLong's gold metal bracelet from which dangle three chains with rings—one each for three fingers . . . Chanel's necklace of glass globules you'd swear were soap bubbles."

Vogue, May, 1, 1939:

"In days of old when knights were bold this luxurious hand-shirred, satin-lined muffbag would stir romantic fancies. Sinuously curved to fit under your arm . . . or like your heart, wear it on your sleeves, if you wish. Black transparent velvet—a yard of it—or Black Antelope—8 feet of it . . $18.50."

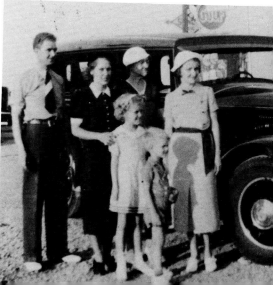

"These irreverent pants and petticoats are the direct descendants of Grandma's underpinnings, worn when she was young. But, where hers were prim and quaint, our 1939 scalawags are impudent . . ." (R.H. Macy advertisement)

"You'll go to the theatre, much as queenly beauties went in the 1900's . . . See the lorgnette, the beige fox muff, the dog-collar, the square neckline of the beige lace dress."

And, in celebration of the 1939 World's Fair:

"See the Liberty Bell, made with 11,600 Mikimoto pearls and 366 diamonds . . . at the New York World's Fair."

"This big Glentex pure-silk scarf shows George Washington calmly surveying the Panorama of the Fair . . . you may buy in any number of colour combinations, calm or riotous. You'll find it at Altman, and it's your very own scarf for just about $2."

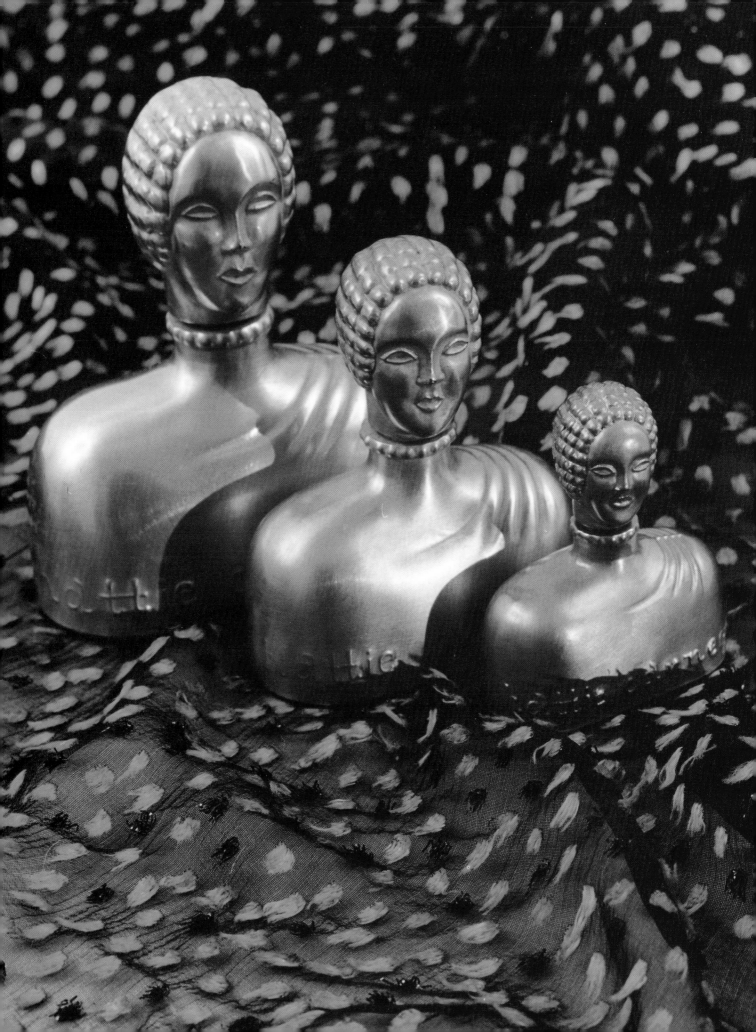

The Forties

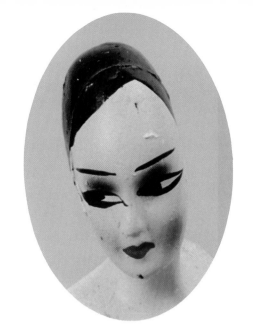

"FASHION TODAY IS SIMPLIFIED AND STRIPPED OF ALL THAT IS SUPERFLUOUS. IN RETROSPECT—IN TWENTY OR THIRTY YEARS—WILL SHE CALL FORTH JEERS AND LAUGHTER? WE PREFER, OF COURSE, THAT SHE WILL NOT. Marcel Verte

The celebration welcoming the birth of the 1940s found the United States seemingly impervious to the disastrous conditions existing a mere ocean away, as the ravages of war cast their pall over much of Europe. The "nothing can touch us" attitude was short-lived, for two short years of peace were followed by four harrowing ones of war. Few individuals were spared as its impact left far-reaching and indelible marks on everyone. Some were devastating and irreversible. Others were light and even frivolous.

In the United States, the decade started on a cheerful note. Bright colors, in daring combinations, were "in" for 1940. As *Vogue* reported in its September, 1940 issue, "Black is all very well for evening. But this year more than ever you'll love colour too. Hypnotic-red, for example . . . Strange muted combinations of colour—like plum colour and violet, mustard yellow and pale blue. Benedictine brown and black . . . Pink and black—for the young. Dark purple gloves with a red dress; royal blue or bright red gloves with a pale blue dress. Over a pale pink or bright orange dress, wear a short-sleeved brown fur jacket; long brown gloves that meet the fur sleeves, and match them exactly." But, all that was "bright and gay," like the word from those lyrics in the melancholy 1940's song, "I'll Be Seeing You," became muted. December 7, 1941 turned life in the U.S. "inside out," just as September 1, 1939 had transformed the face of Europe.

The attack on Pearl Harbor marked the beginning of a radical turning point for women. She served in the Armed Forces and was also called upon to work in defense plants, taking the place of men who had left jobs and family to answer their country's call. This created an entirely new set of "needs" when the average woman of the Forties opened her closet to start a new day. "Rosie the Riveter" couldn't rivet in a cotton housedress. And thus, slacks and shorts finally gained more than marginal acceptance. This wasn't a mere trend of the moment, devised of necessity and later relegated to "has been" status. It was another corner that couture turned—one that would be built upon and refined throughout the ensuing years. Movie stars like Katherine Hepburn and Marlene Dietrich had introduced this "look" during the late 1930s and early Forties. But it took the circumstances of World War II to make fashion designers and the buying public comfortable with it.

Once socio-economic conditions of this magnitude occur, accessories must also adapt to changing times. Bandannas wound their way around previously unprotected heads, turbans became not only practical but glamorous, and sandals and open shoes accommodated the more relaxed ambiance women were able to finally achieve in their everyday life.

Scarves continued to cast a spell when viewed on the movie screen, ". . . by the classical way in which Katharine Hepburn was able to turn a white silk scarf into something approaching a commandingly regal headdress."[2] And Lana Turner projected a girlish innocence in those famous "sweater-girl" photos by tying a demure little scarf around her neck. With role models like these, wearing a scarf for protection while working in a defense plant became a glamorous way to wrap and tie one's hair. It was simply an extension of the influence of movies on fashion, an influence that began from the moment the *silver screen* captured the imaginations of viewers decades before. The simple scarf had, in fact, taken on a new allure as early as 1937 when ". . . the kerchief industry got an unexpected sales bonanza because Joan Crawford tied one around her head in *The Bride Wore Red*.[2]" Two years later, ". . . sales of chenille robes skyrocketed when Deanna Durbin wore one in 1939's Three Smart Girls Grow Up.[3] Both trends continued into the 1940s and were joined by many others that were "movie inspired."

The strange "utility" clothing of the World War I years had an updated revival during World War II. Not considered necessary in the U.S., they became "standard issue" in Great Britain due to massive shortages of just about everything. Their design was controlled by the government, which took pains to employ the services of major designers to produce fashions that would be palatable to its citizenry. Of course, this regimented look made accessorizing even more important. Hats, scarves, and jewelry all added that individual touch so necessary for morale.

In the United States meanwhile, shortages of wool, cotton, silk and synthetic fabrics forced the government to place restrictions on the amount of material manufacturers could use in women's wear. Silk stockings became a precious commodity. Women hoarded the few precious pairs they might be fortunate enough to own, and resorted to leg makeup instead, even ingeniously "painting" seams up the back. To cope with all these shortages, "Designers used whatever unrestricted materials were at hand. Furs, wings, feathers, beads, sequins, veils, felt and velvet were included in the materials for winter; laces and straws were used for spring and summer. 'Hats' appeared in the forms of snoods and scarfs, tied into knots at the front of the head while draping over long bobbed hair at the back."[4]

Golden triplets inspired by civilizations past. Hattie Carnegie bottles with 14K overlay for her "49" perfume rest on a 1980's Paco Rabanne scarf.

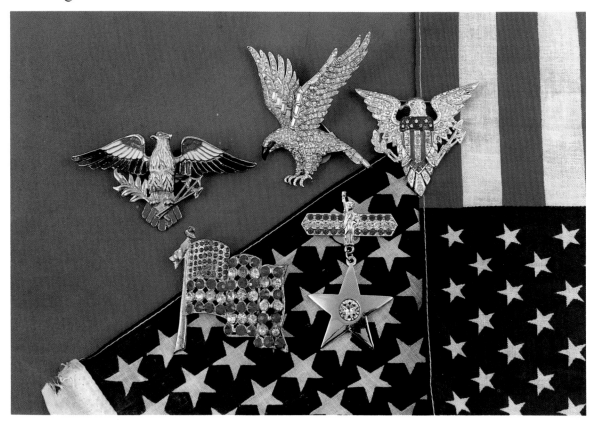

Patriotic pins for civilians.

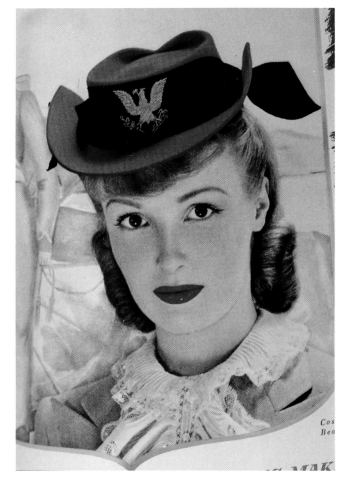

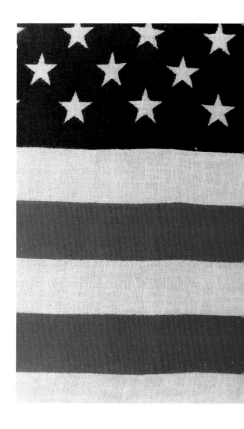

A DuBarry cosmetic ad from *Harper's Bazaar*, April 1941 features a saucy felt hat with a patriotic American eagle.

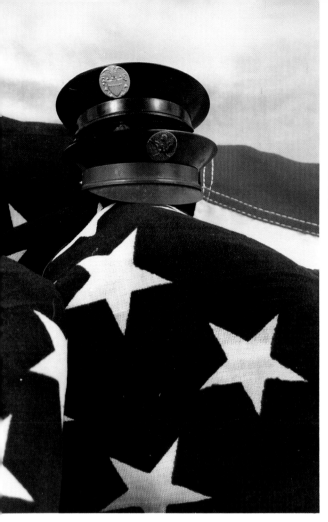

Patriotism as we powder our noses!
Clever service hat compacts by
Henriette. Courtesy of Joan Orlen.

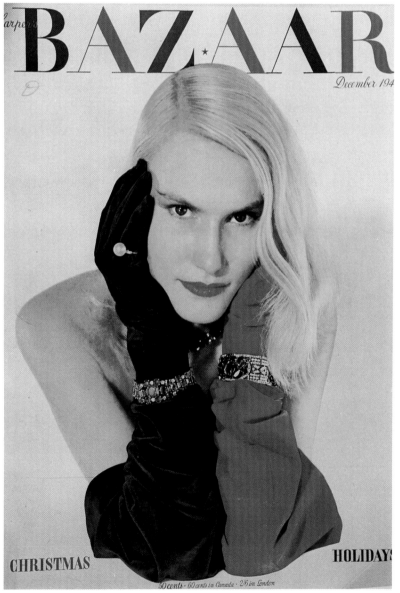

The 1940's woman unfolds before our
eyes. With her Veronica Lake hairdo,
she appeared on the December 1941
cover of Harper's Bazaar.

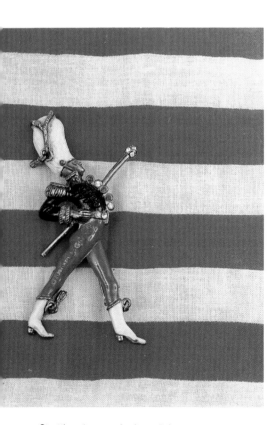

Strutting drum major brooch in gay,
patriotic colors.

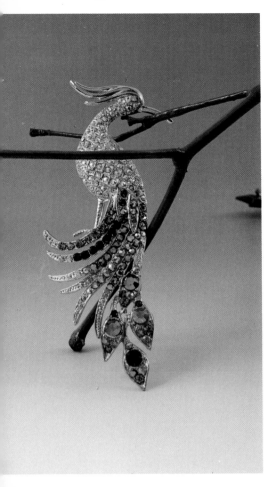

"Real" hats, however, refused to be relegated to the back of a shelf, and maintained a very prominent place in fashion of the 1940s. As described in an article in the January 1944 issue of *Vogue* titled "This Spring . . . Hats Sit Tight":[1]

"If you are interested in a new spring hat . . . you must look first to your hair. The ideal head is small, smoothly rounded, well-tended . . . either with a shingle or with long hair dressed close and sleek. With the small defined head achieved, All is Yours: the Cloche, the Bowler, the Chaplet, the flexible Beret, the little hat you pin over your ear, the miniature hat that sits forward, or crouched between two upswept curls . . . consider the cloche. The cloche 'Twenty Years After' is no 1926 bathing-cap. It is much softer, much more gentle. It starts a little further back. Shows a little hair. There are some sailors about . . . with the narrowest brims you've ever seen . . . Berets are the all-engagement hat . . . They are 'good' worn any way that's most becoming; straight on the head; pulled back off the forehead, and flattened out as though heading into a ninety-mile gale; . . . Many a beret enobled with a brilliant jewel and a tiny nose veil goes out, with great elegance, to dinner."

This popularity of hats that sat back on the head, exposing the forehead—which had gained prominence, so to speak—came about mainly because one of the most popular hairdos of the time was the turned-back, soft pompadour effect. This, along with the youthful pageboy, or a combination of both, was considered the hairdo of the 1940s. Indeed the simple, swept-under pageboy, usually brushing the shoulders, contributed to the look of the "All American" girl, whose image came to the fore in the same decade. She wore bobby socks and saddle shoes or loafers, emanated wholesome innocence, and was a cross between a Norman Rockwell painting and the photo servicemen carried in their wallet or displayed inside footlockers as a reminder of the "girl back home."

In Paris, meanwhile, Schiaparelli's wit and style, so evident in her 1930's millinery designs, had served to inspire designers during the war years and, above all, to elevate spirits. As Karl Lagerfeld noted in an interview with "W" in 1978, "People who make clothes should avoid at all cost the idea that because Paris is in a difficult mood, fashion must be severe and serious. During the war, fashion in Paris was unbelievably amusing . . women often wore hats that looked like wedding cakes.[4]

Costume jewelry maintained its hold on the accessorizing business—and the consumer's imagination. From funky to elegant, the American woman had a treasure trove to choose from. Giants like Trifari, with its master designer Alfred Phillipe, and Coro, with the genius of Adolph Katz, gave her more costume jewelry choices than had ever been seen anywhere before. Elite, family operations like Eisenberg, Hobe, and Panetta, and the husband and wife team of Marcel and Sandra Boucher, honed glitz and glitter to a fine edge, with remarkable designs that emulated the real thing in a manner rarely seen before.

The saga of the Eisenberg family is a entrepreneurial success story. Starting in the dress business early in the century, they recognized the marketing possibilities in costume jewelry in the 1920s, when the pieces they had added to their garments as decorative accents—and as an extra incentive toward purchase—began disappearing. Putting two and two together, only one conclusion seemed logical—or cost effective. Obviously, women loved these jeweled creations, so why not market the product separately? It was a revolutionary idea that gave birth to sections in department and specialty stores devoted exclusively to the sale of costume jewelry.

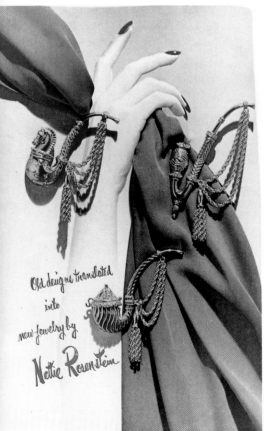

Old designs translated into new jewelry by Nettie Rosenstein

During the 1940s, jewelry by fashion designers like Coco Chanel, Nettie Rosenstein, Elsa Schiaparelli, and Hattie Carnegie were carried in only the finest emporiums, along with boutique designs created by Miriam Haskell, Nadja Buckley, and the inimitable Joseff of Hollywood, who carried the art of merchandising and promotion to new heights. By this time, the industry had grown to such an extent that hundreds of companies were manufacturing costume pieces, with the best of these still treasured by eager collectors. They ran the gamut from glamorous and glitzy to whimsical and funky. Jewelry became even more playful, and "obviously fake" was at last an acceptable alternative to the more staid, formal—and sometimes prohibitively expensive—look of the "real thing."

Movies, like those starring Carmen Miranda, the wild and comedic Latin bombshell, ignited a trend toward "fruity" accessories. Cherries, bananas, oranges, strawberries, pears and peaches no longer grew on trees and bushes—instead they sprouted from the brims of jaunty hats, perched on lapels, and dangling from wrists. There were also vegetables, animals, bugs, and mythical creatures, characters resembling those from the pages of a comic strip—sailor boys and drum majors, animals on seesaws, bird baths, frogs playing saxophones . . . a seemingly endless array to delight the child in everyone. Many of these were fashioned after the ever popular synthetics of the 1930s. From the most expensive "real gems" by Cartier and Tiffany to the bunch of Coro plastic bananas attached to a card in the dime store, there was something for everyone—and everyone was happy.

Continuing a trend that had started in the 1920s, even female accoutrements became pieces of jewelry in and of themselves, and it was important for women to have attractive compacts, cigarette cases, pill boxes, and boudoir items. Dressing tables were adorned with perfume bottles of etched glass and vibrant colors, and matching brushes, mirrors and combs in materials ranging from glistening sterling silver to plastics and celluloids (another carry-over from the 1930s).

During the war, patriotic jewelry was, of course, extremely popular. Flags waved not only from flagpoles—they were placed proudly on men's and ladies' lapels, coats and scarves. The pea jackets of Navy seamen, and Eisenhower jackets named after the hero general who wore them, enjoyed popularity with the younger crowd. Shoulder bags, copied from the style of women in uniform, became popular. Drawstring purses gained favor at the close of the war, and small clutch styles also vied for the attention of the 1940's woman. Due to wartime shortages, plastics and synthetics frequently replaced the leather formerly used in handbags and shoes, and these materials have never relinquished their importance in these categories. Even the hatboxes that were the trademark of New York models were carried by the average woman on the street when B. Altman converted this idea into the "hat-box" handbag made of shiny patent leather.

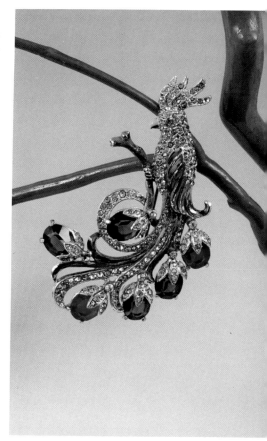

Although a good portion of the male population spent much of their time in uniform—at least during the early years of the decade—and had absolutely nothing to say about what they'd wear, or when, there were fashion favorites for men both then and after the war ended. Among these were wide ties made even bolder by overpowering prints, pleated pants, and lightweight straw hats with colorful bands—although most men of the Thirties and Forties still preferred the felt hat with "standard" brim made popular by movie tough guys like Humphrey Bogart and James Cagney. Regardless of their choice, hats were considered an absolute necessity by most men, and businessmen and blue collar workers alike were rarely seen on the street without one.

Some young males found a unique way to express themselves that widened eyes and brought groans of disbelief. The zoot suit—a by-product of the jitterbug craze—seemed to meet a vicarious need for expression during the mid-1940s but, as might be expected, was viewed with considerable disdain, at least by the older generation. In the extreme, these outfits consisted of broad-brimmed hats, below-hip-length outer coats with gigantic shoulder pads, and full, peg-bottomed trousers. To complete this rather amusing ensemble, from the belt of these ballooning pants hung a long "zoot" chain that the wearer could nonchalantly twirl. All in all, the complete "zoot suit" package gave the term "angular fashions" a whole new meaning. After all, if Joan Crawford could sport "shoulders out to here," surely young males could also affect a wedge-shaped appearance. If these "hooligans" proceeded to the dance floor in this get-up, what took place was labeled "dirty dancing," although certainly tame when compared to many of the dance crazes that would follow. Many of these young men went on to become captains of industry, scientists and teachers, and pillars of their communities. They simply put their youthful excesses behind them, and said a silent prayer that no embarrassing photographs would be unearthed for their children or grandchildren to find years later.

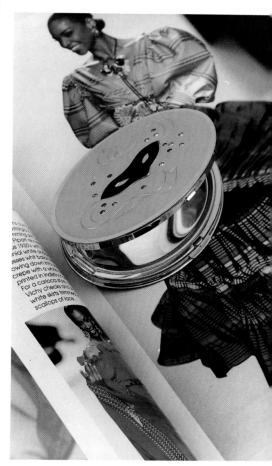

During much of the 1940s, shoe purchases were at the mercy of ration cards. Consequently, each pair was precious and chosen with care, not only with practicality in mind but to boost morale through the lean times. Along with sky-high heels and ankle straps, platform soles and "wedgies" were the shoes of choice. In footwear, as in just about everything else, wartime conditions created fashion ingenuity and a modicum of fun. Nothing could take away the personal fears and tragedies, but the simple pleasures of day-to-day living created an exterior brimming with hope—and even good cheer!

August 14, 1945 brought about an enormous metamorphosis. Fashion, especially for men, was drastically affected. For many, the uniform had been their "outward covering," and one over which they had no control. Needless to say, the men's clothing industry boomed when these servicemen finally returned home. Many started or continued their college educations, and as a group they were generally older and understandably more mature than the young men before them or those that would follow. Most World War II veterans—as well as countless others who were drafted near the end of the conflict but had to complete their service obligation—were still matriculating four years after the war's end. This "different breed" of collegian is reflected in an *Esquire* "Big 4 for Fall" September 1949 feature that listed, among others, the following somewhat questionable "necessities" for the returning collegian:

For Town and Travel... striped rep, foulard knit, narrow four-in-hand ties; bold stripe or solid color braces, garters to match; pigskin wallet; foulard or cashmere mufflers; leather travel slipper; *For Prom and Party* ... midnight blue and white dinner jacket; patent leather plain tip shoes; smoked pearl, maroon stone, white pearl studs and links; money clip, key chain, cigarette case, wallet; white plain or monogrammed handkerchiefs; grey mocha or white kid gloves; *For Campus and Classroom* ... strapped back tweed cap; striped rep, crocheted, wool, foulard, ribbon bow ties; tooled Western belt; tie holder, collar pin or bar; tennis, squash, swimwear; *For Club and Country*... khaki color snap brim hat; tan polo coat; cashmere sweater; chukka boots; golf, riding and ski wear.

A "masquerade" compact by Dorothy Grey.

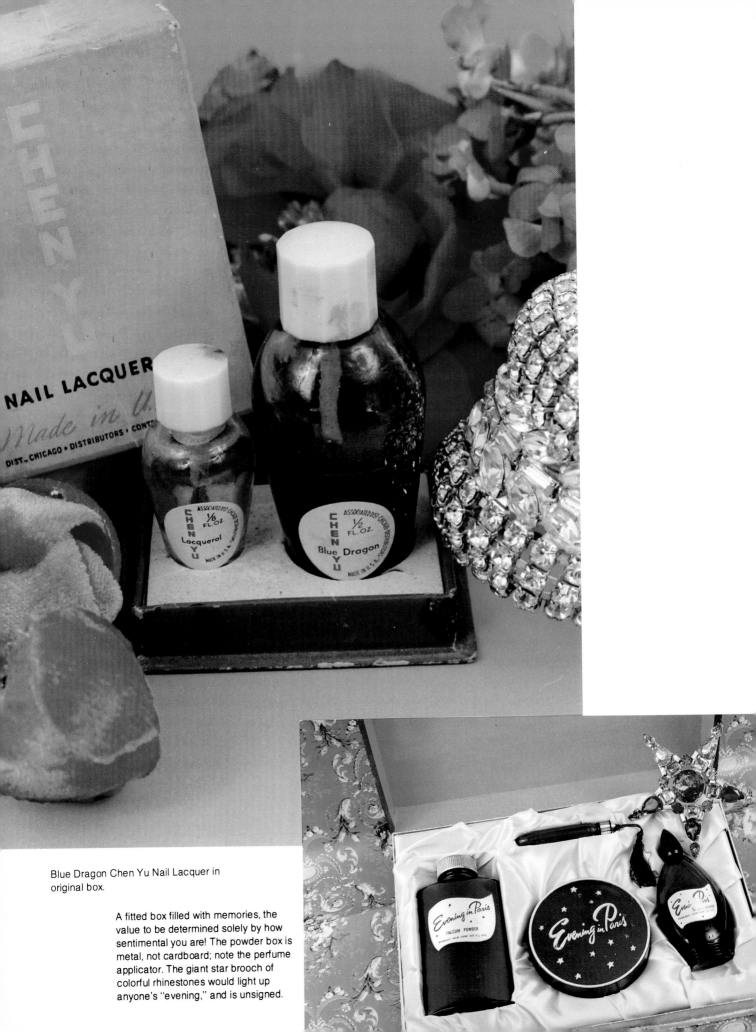

Blue Dragon Chen Yu Nail Lacquer in
original box.

A fitted box filled with memories, the
value to be determined solely by how
sentimental you are! The powder box is
metal, not cardboard; note the perfume
applicator. The giant star brooch of
colorful rhinestones would light up
anyone's "evening," and is unsigned.

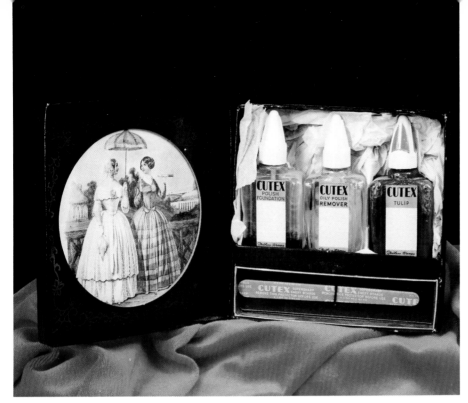

The Cutex "Tulip" collection, with case.
Courtesy of Magi.

Ferocious! This plush bulldog wears
miniature hat from salesman's sample
box.

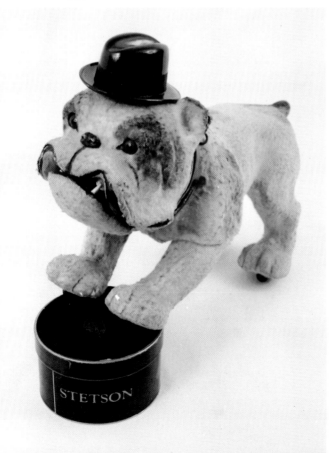

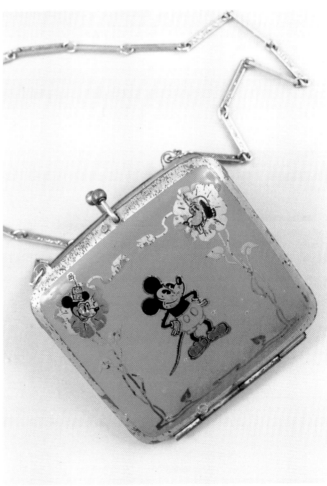

Blowing bubbles on a Mickey and
Minnie Mouse change purse. Minnie on
one side, Mickey on the other. A
priceless treasure!

Hats of the Forties. Left to right, a bizarre little turban; pleated cloche with a Parisienne look; a navy straw confection with peach chiffon and an English-made, burgundy felt with taffeta bow to cock at any angle, marked Frenchie.

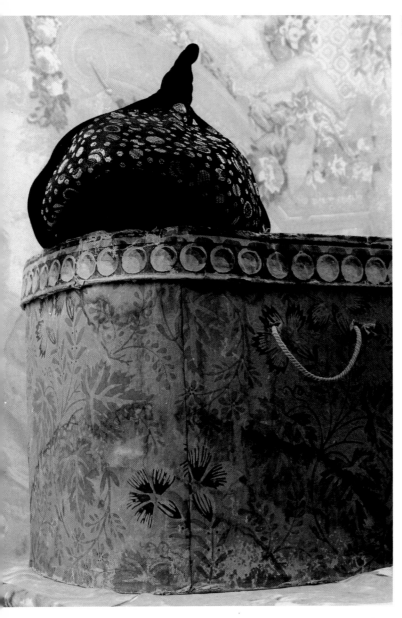
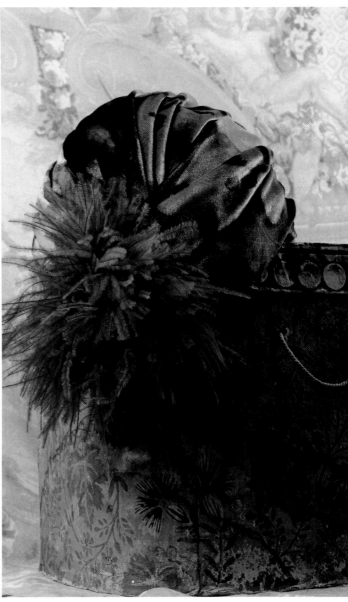

This awesome list may have reflected the needs of a wealthy Ivy Leaguer but, although it does provide an interesting look at male accessorizing, it's unlikely many of those returning G.I.s, some with wives and children, were particularly concerned with—or able to afford—a wardrobe of this magnitude. Nevertheless, with modification, some of this look crept into items that most males could hang in their closets or pile neatly in dresser drawers—and it does serve to highlight what was "in" for men during the latter years of the decade. For more mature men, a somewhat sophisticated Edwardian look was in vogue, with longer waistcoats, slim trousers, and even bowler hats. It signified a return to safer more comfortable times, and men, especially those in Great Britain, embraced it.

The war's end also brought drastic changes in women's fashions. Clothing lines had been somewhat angular, with shoulder pads and peplum effects that accentuated tiny waists. Although the 1940s at long last gave American designers the recognition they deserved, they were overpowered in 1947 when this wedge-shaped look came to an end, and a young Frenchman returned French couture to its pre-war eminence. This time it was Christian Dior who created another fashion revolution, loosely based on the styles of

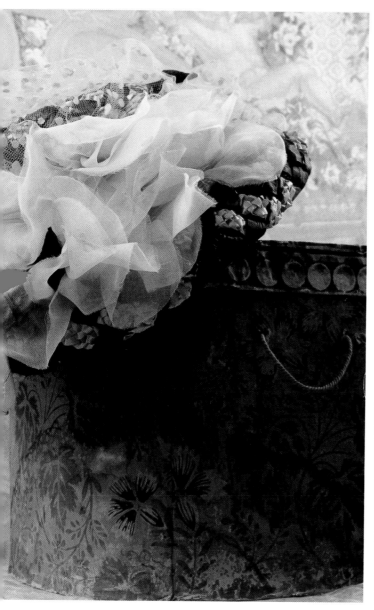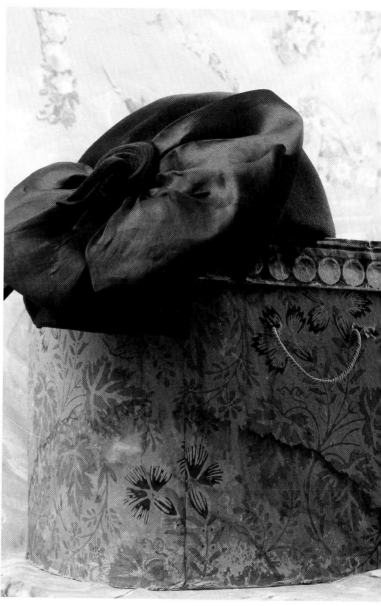

the 1860s, and "...it was largely left to Dior, in the post-war era, to recapture many of the crinolined effects recorded by the Empress Eugenie's pet artist..."[6] Aptly called the "New Look," his designs were graceful, with nipped in waists and longer, fuller skirts, some nearly brushing the ankles, and coat lengths frequently hitting the tops of shoes.

As described in the April 1947 issue of *Harper's Bazaar,* "The big news in the Paris spring collection is the shift in silhouette. The agent provocateur and hero of the day is the couturier, Dior. He is revolutionizing daytime fashions as Poiret did in his day and Chanel in hers." With shortages a continuing problem in Great Britain and rationing still in effect, this extravagant departure, with its yards and yards of fabric, was viewed with alarm by the British Board of Trade. As might be expected, women were not to be denied. After years of wartime deprivation, they needed a change—and with the "New Look" they surely got it.

The decade had been launched by the frightening "bang" of war, but in the world of fashion it made a steady and highly-popular three-year exit with an astounding barrage of another kind—the "New Look" of Christian Dior.

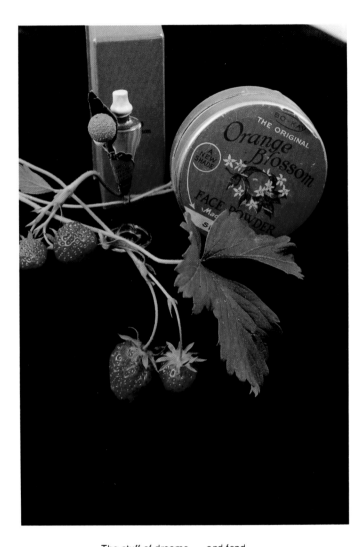

The stuff of dreams . . . and fond
memories. Orange Blossom face
powder and cologne.

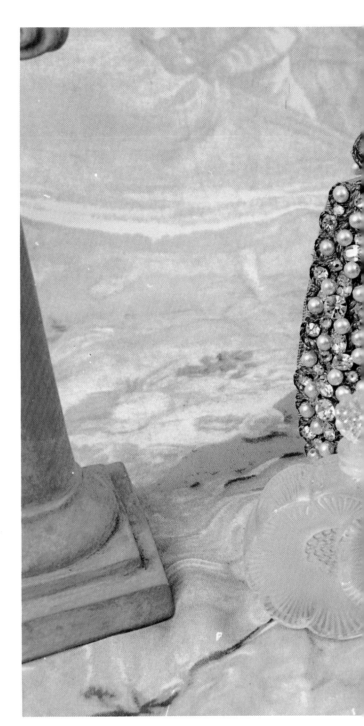

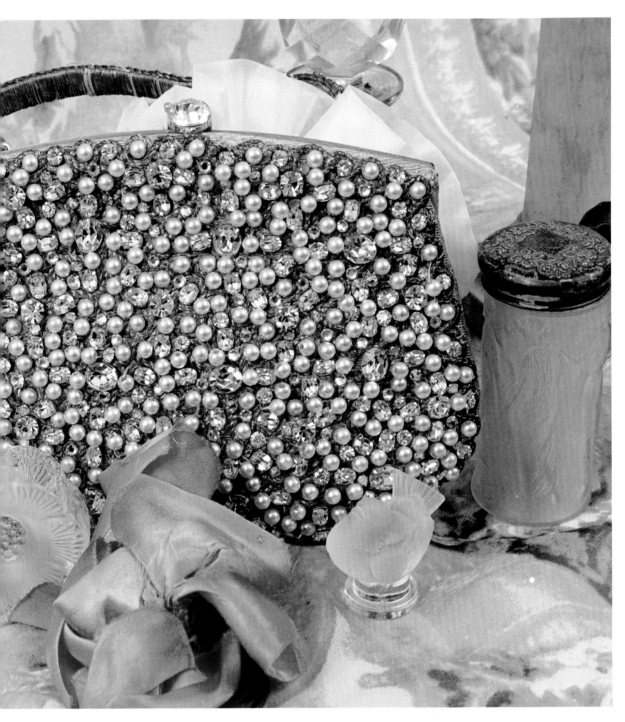

A Nettie Rosenstein masterpiece. With a base of braided gold, this pristine 9″ x 6″ evening bag is studded with faux citrines and pearls (a weighty handful!).

1940-1950
[1] Scarves, p. 34
[2] Jewelry of the Stars, Creations from Joseff of Hollywood, p. 123
[3] Jewelry of the Stars, Creations from Joseff of Hollywood, p. 123
[4] "Historic Costume" p. 259
[5] "W", March 31-April 7, 1978
[6] "Fashionable Mind, The" p. 88

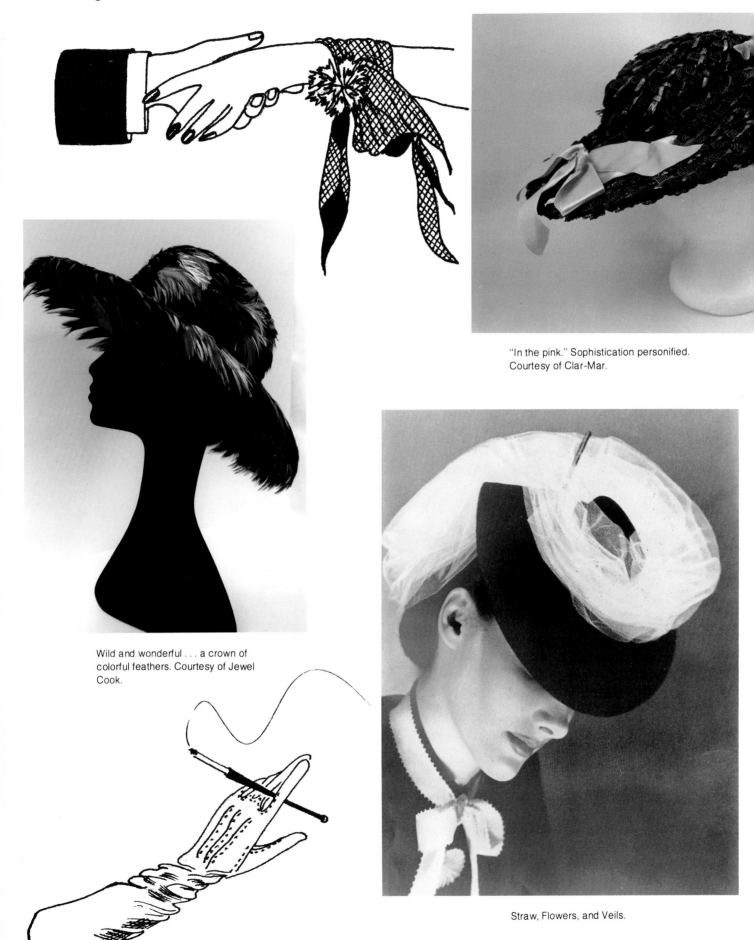

"In the pink." Sophistication personified. Courtesy of Clar-Mar.

Wild and wonderful . . . a crown of colorful feathers. Courtesy of Jewel Cook.

Straw, Flowers, and Veils.

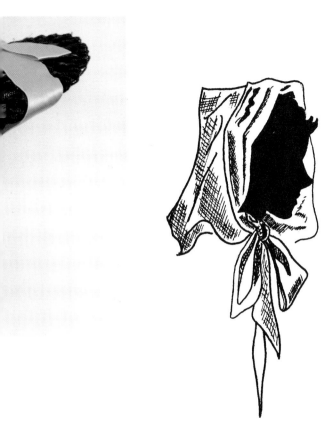

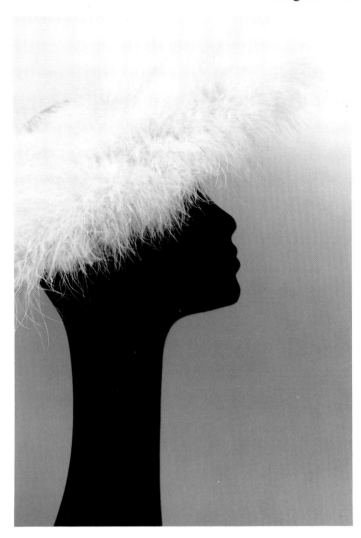

A strikingly feminine silhouette . . . this
pale blue hat, like a giant fluffy boa.
Courtesy of Jewel Cook.

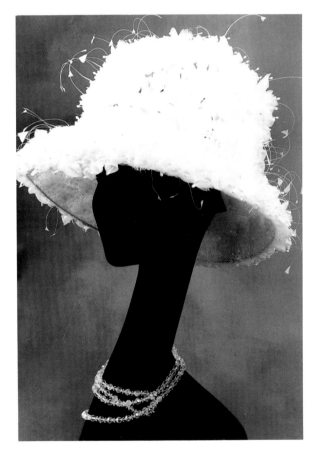

A hat like a giant, gossamer beehive.
Courtesy of Jewel Cook.

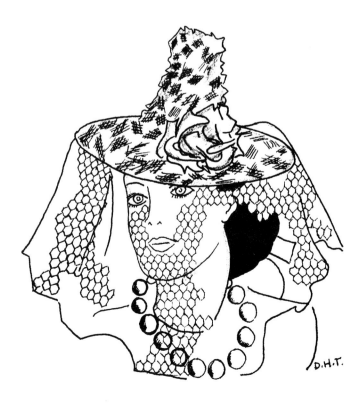

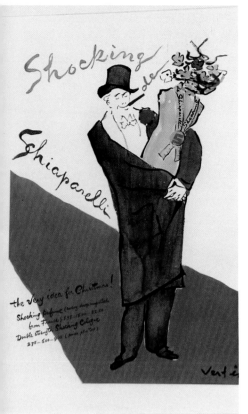

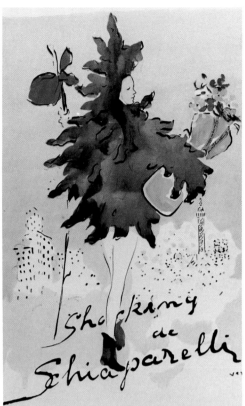

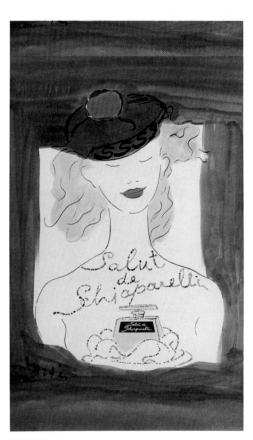

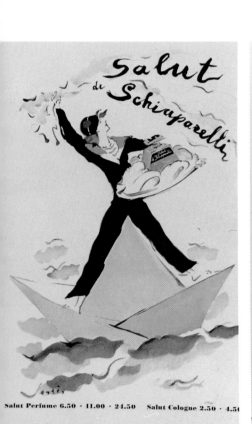

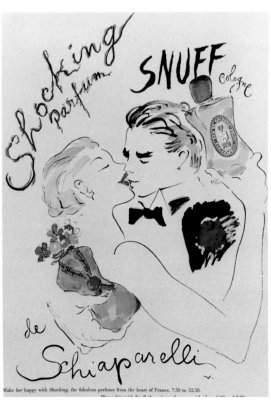

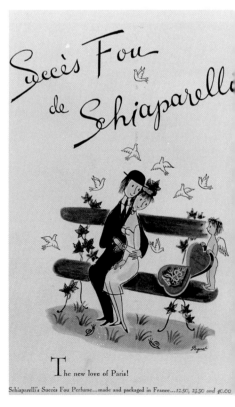

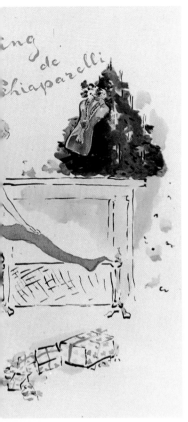

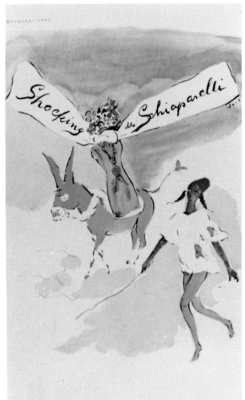

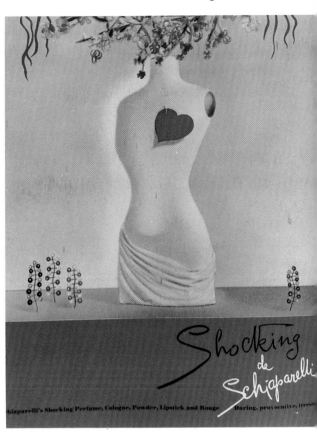

Schiaparelli's Shocking Perfume, Cologne, Powder, Lipstick and Rouge ... Daring, provocative, irresi

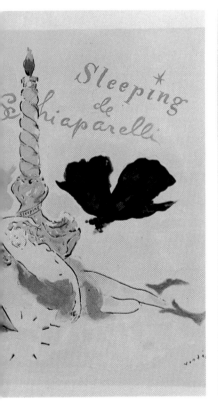

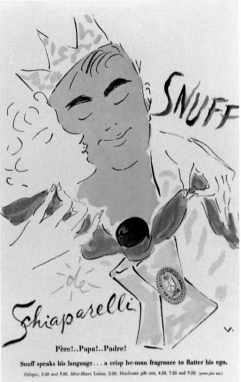

Père!..Papa!..Padre!

Snuff speaks his language . . . a crisp he-man fragrance to flatter his ego.

Cologne, 5.00 and 9.00. After-Shave Lotion, 2.50. Handsome gift sets, 4.50, 7.50 and 9.50. (prices plus tax)

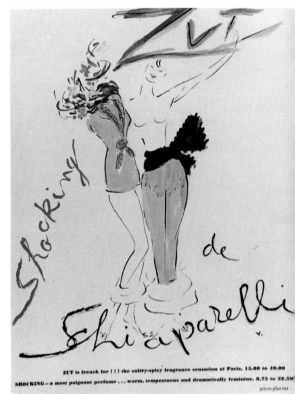

ZUT is french for ! ! ! the sultry-spicy fragrance sensation of Paris, 15.00 to 40.00

SHOCKING—a most poignant perfume . . . warm, tempestuous and dramatically feminine, 8.75 to 32.50

prices plus tax

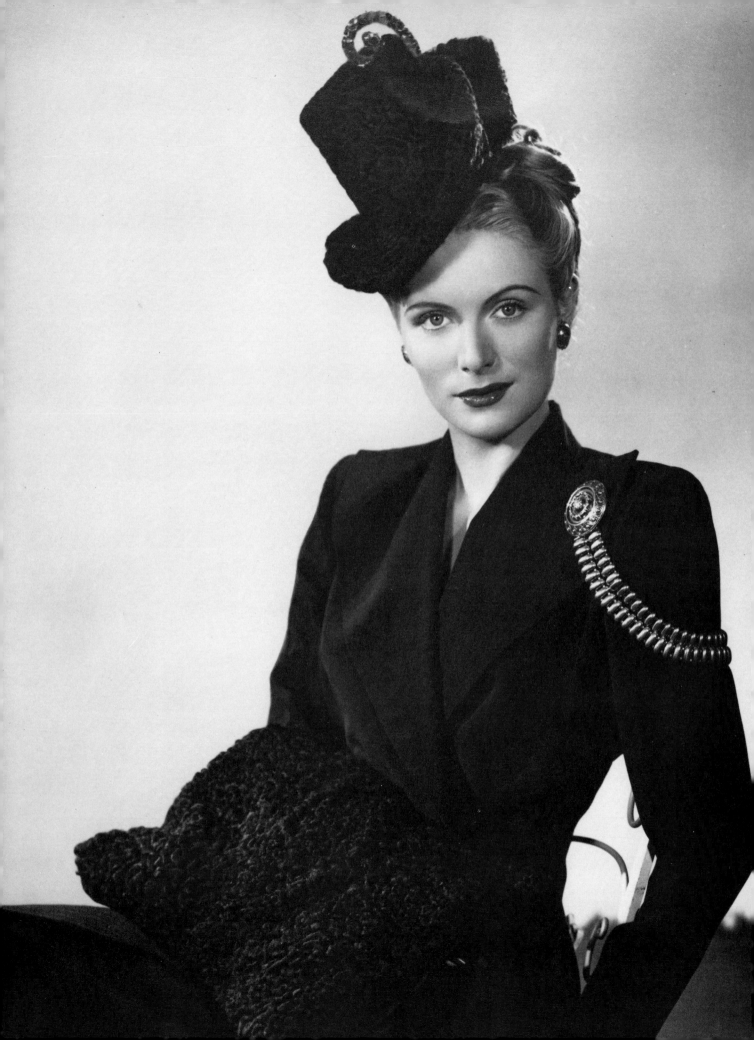

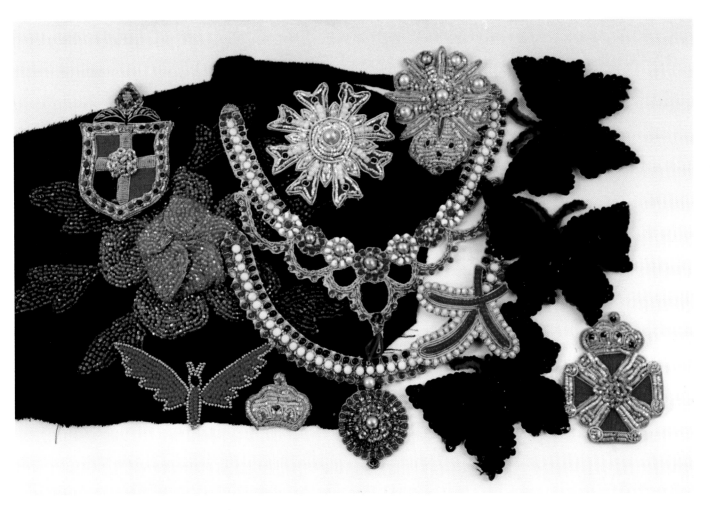

The "necklaces" are Lesage-style, with
jewel-studded embroidery, as are the
patches featuring embroidery and
vintage Indian beading.

Starlet Virginia Huston, pictured here in
a 1946 photo, is the epitome of 1940's
glamour with her upswept hairdo and
Persian lamb hat and matching muff,
with an over-the-shoulder, cartouche-
type brooch by Joseff of Hollywood
completing the outfit. Photograph
courtesy of Joan Castle Joseff.

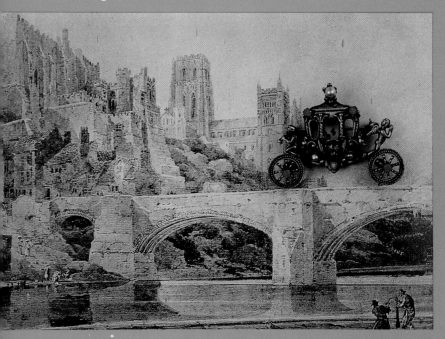

This Coro coach pin travels a medieval byway to the castle above.

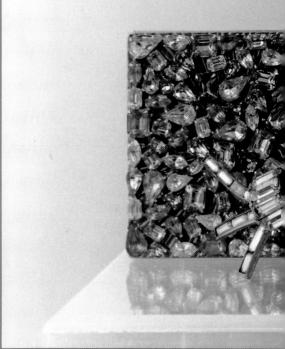

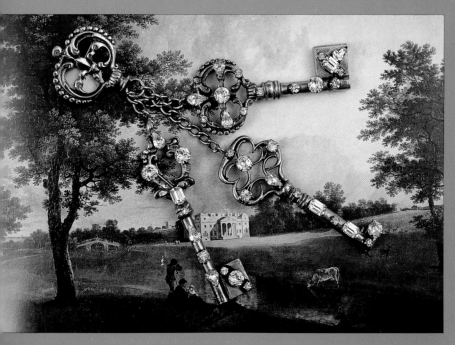

And here are the keys to that castle -an unsigned lapel "show-stopper"; each key is 3″ long.

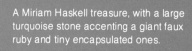

A Miriam Haskell treasure, with a large turquoise stone accenting a giant faux ruby and tiny encapsulated ones.

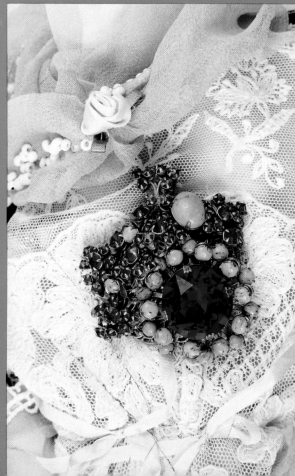

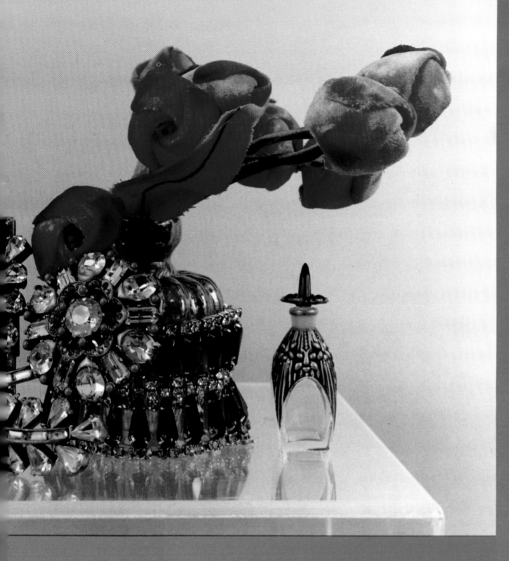

Timeless beauty knows no decade. The silk poppies and perfume bottle are from the 1920s. The giant rhinestone flower is a theatre piece from the 1930s, the jewel studded Evans compact lit up the 1940s, and the bracelet with giant keystones is an unsigned beauty from the 1950s.

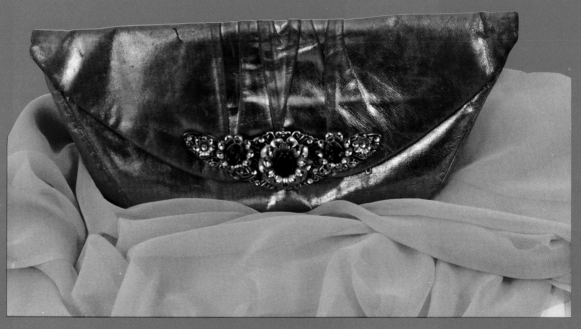

A buttersolf, oversized evening bag with jeweled clasp. Courtesy of Jan Schtavino, *Ragtime*.

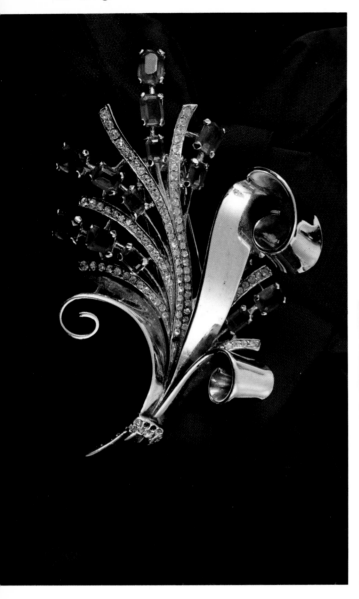

Classic beauty of line and form—a majestic sterling (vermeil) Trifari brooch.

Brilliant in its composition, color and diverse stones, this 5-piece parure by an unknown maker is a magnificent testimony to the artistry found in many unsigned pieces.

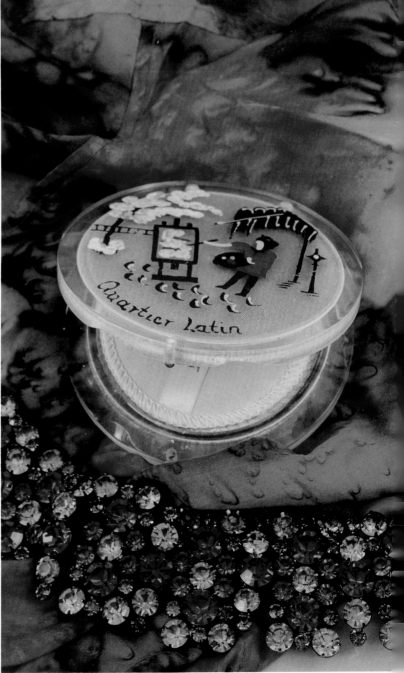

A lucite compact decorated with a painted scene of artist and easel, and a brilliant KJL 1960's amber choker with gunmetal backing. Compact courtesy of Joan Orlen.

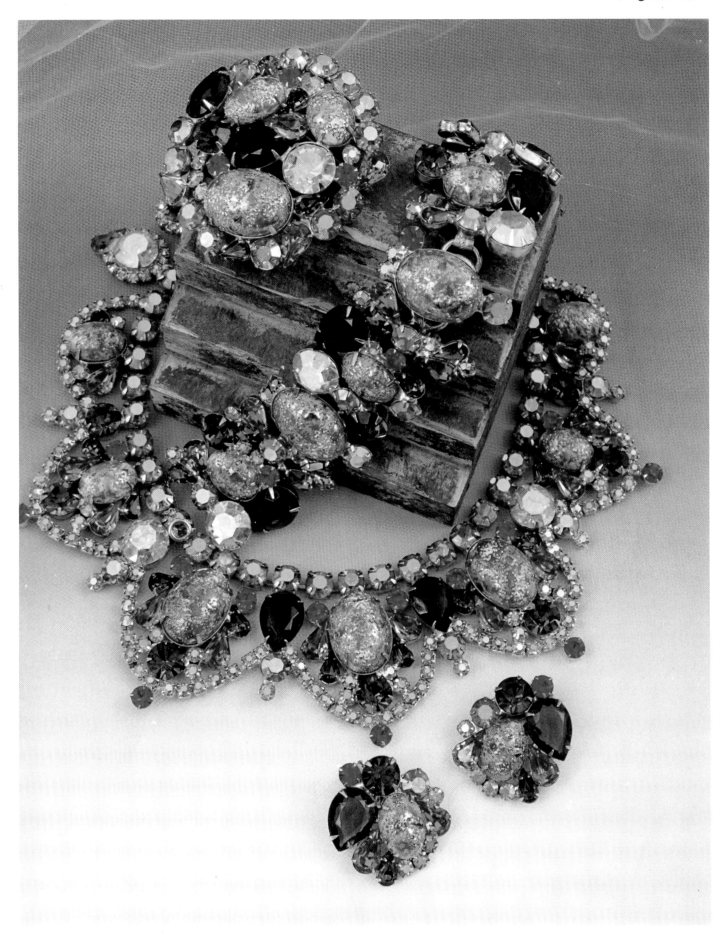

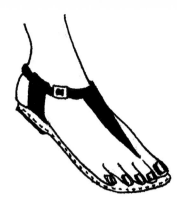

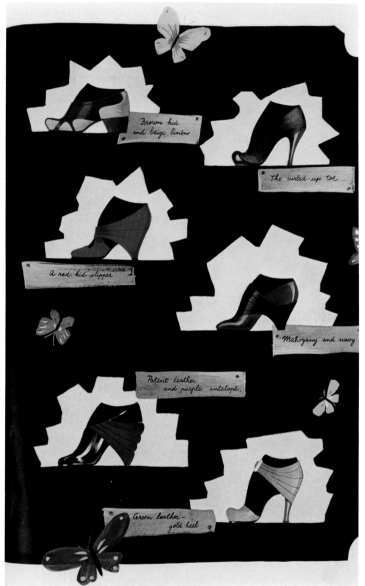

Brown kid and beige linen

The curled-up toe

A red kid slipper

Mahogany and navy

Patent leather and purple antelope

Green leather— gold heel

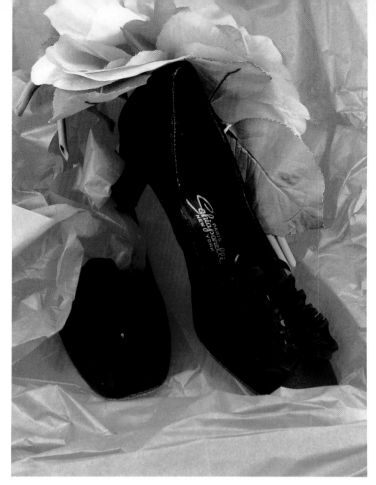

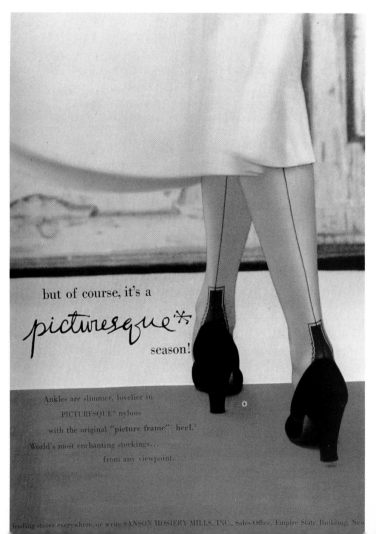

The walk of Schiaparelli.

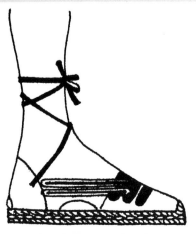

but of course, it's a

*picturesque** season!

Ankles are slimmer, lovelier in PICTURESQUE* nylons with the original "picture frame" heel. World's most enchanting stockings... from any viewpoint.

leading stores everywhere, or write SANSON HOSIERY MILLS, INC., Sales Office, Empire State Building, Ne

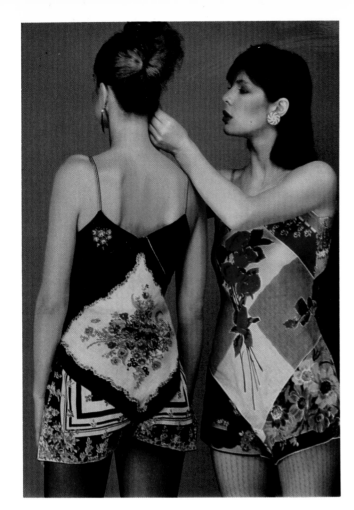

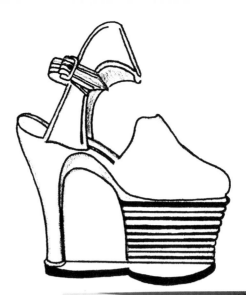

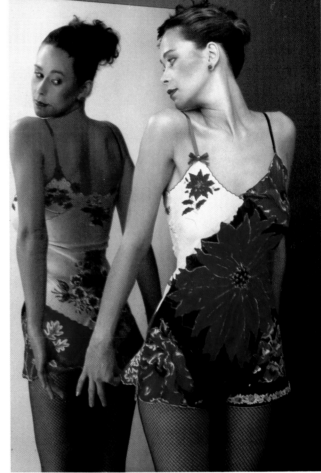

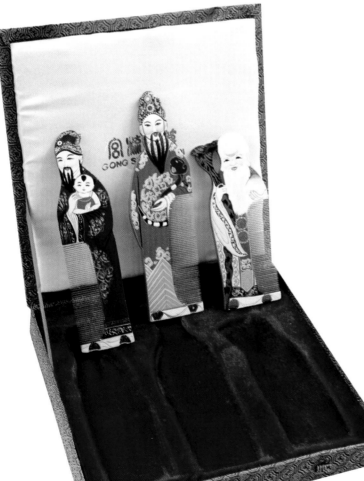

A boutique delight! These one-of-a-kind teddies, made from 1940's hankies, were a New York boutique "hit" in the 1970s. Courtesy of their designer Michelle Stoneman.

Oriental combs...a fortune for your hair. Courtesy of Golden Heart Antiques.

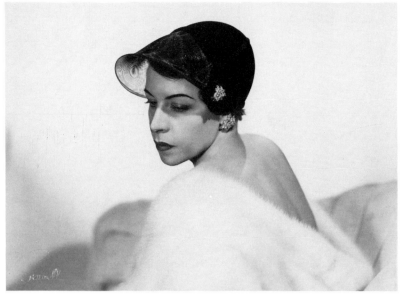

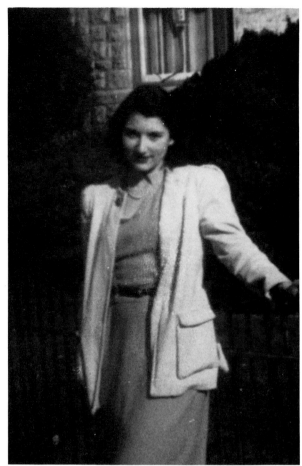

Joan Castle Joseff is pictured here in a 1940's photo by Seawell. Her velvet visored cap is lined in moire and accented by a glittering pin and matching earrings. Courtesy of Joan Castle Joseff.

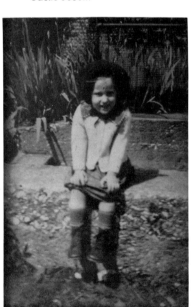

Faces and Places

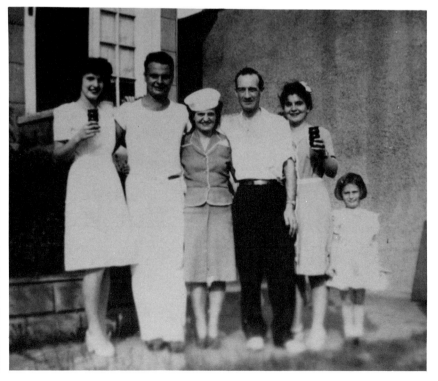

From Periodicals of the Time

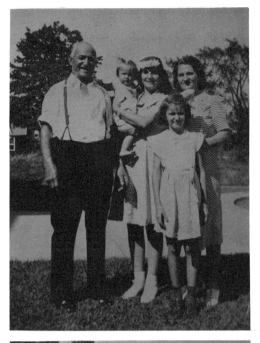

Harper's Bazaar, March 15, 1942:

"You won't be sorry if you always have two or three daffodils pinned with a jeweled clip or brooch to your navy blue coat . . . or a single tulip . . ."

"As far as we're concerned, this bracelet is one of the niftiest gadgets in town. It's two-tone gilt with a big detachable curly bow on the front. Wear it with the bow when you want to be dressy; without the bow it's just right for tweeds and you can pull off the bow, which is fastened on with two clips, and pin it on your dress. $14.75, Ciro of Bond Street."

Harper's Bazaar, October 1942:

"To fill in the V of a suit jacket, to make a plain wool dress something special, to wear instead of a fur piece, Lord and Taylor presents a triangular rayon knit scarf. Tying around the neck on its own string, it has a ruffle threaded with gold that makes a little high collar. You can also wear it tied over the head like a prosperous *babuska.* At $3.50 it does a lot for any autumn's day. Black and colors."

Harper's Bazaar, June 1943:

"Drop Tested Swimsuits . . . Not literally dropped from the sky as are the Cole parachutes for the Army Air Force—but constructed with the same painstaking workmanship." (Cole of California advertisement)

"You can now indulge all those hidden desires to beg, borrow, or even steal the red pompom cap off a French sailor's head, for the American-French War Relief . . . sells the exact copy for $5 in all sizes . . ."

Harper's Bazaar, November, 1945:

"Something round . . . A disk of gold to hang from a bracelet or a neck chain or even to pin on a lapel. Nadja Buckley of Bonwit Teller has designed this one, engraved with a medieval-looking guardian angel who wears rubies on her wings, holds a diamond-tipped wand, and flits through a diamond-studded sky. $395 plus tax."

"Something silk . . . A big square of scarf called "You and I are one"—it proceeds to prove this to you by multiplication, subtraction, addition, and division. In each corner is a fat, bright red heart to give a romantic touch to the modern version of a schoolroom blackboard. The scarf is, of course, pure silk, hand-rolled, hand-screened, and completely washable. In white, splashed wildly with numbers of gold, royal, scarlet, and bright green. $18.50. Bergdorf Goodman."

Harper's Bazaar, October 1947:

"A handbag in golden alligator, polished to a depth of brilliance and standing as slim as a reed—although it is fully lined with cross-grained morocco leather and contains a zipped central pocket and five side pockets. The slender handle is twisted about a shining, ring-jointed bamboo bar. $290, including tax. At Cartiers.

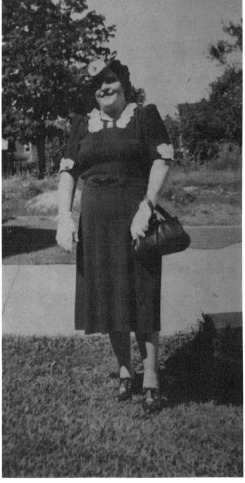

"A typical Dior afternoon decollete—as low and as wide as the law permits, and always with sleeves. Huge yellow or white solitaire diamonds twined round the throat, often tied in back with black velvet ribbon. Sometimes there are dog collars, or, more becoming, two rows of big stones."

"Take a furled umbrella. That's one silhouette in fashion. Open it part way. There's another. Blow it out full and you have a third. The Paris collections divide the honors. Young women seem to take naturally to the full skirts; older women look elegant furled . . . on the other hand, you may be a half-closed umbrella in a suit with a pleated skirt or in a black chiffon dress pleated from top to hem . . . Full-blown . . . are all the big skirted evening dresses, often cut to clear the ankles, sometimes with deep flounces at the hem, like ruffled parasols."

Motion Picture Magazine, "Broadway Fashions," February 1948:

"Four miniature bottles of Dana Perfume—20 Carats, Platine, Emir and Tabu—fitted in a slim gold kid envelope. $10.50."

"Ask Paris what makes the peplum so popular. It's out-and-out feminine flattery, of course! Here—for you in this wonderful new two-piece dress. Rich contrast in the front panel, bow-back peplum and little cuffs . . . only $6.98."

Harper's Bazaar, May 1948:

"The basic line of fashion is set, but now things are beginning to happen on heads and feet. The newest of the new hats do not shoot out at angles. Instead they sit level on the brow, determined but naive."

"Balenciaga creates an evening dress of beige and white striped satin, extremely tight at the waist, cuffed at the decolletage with folded white chiffon—and equips it with separate sleeves that are merely circles of chiffon mounted on black velvet garters."

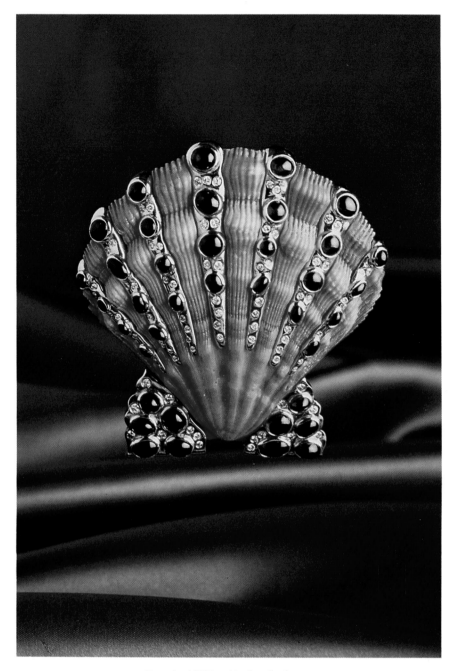

From the 1950's, a Verdura lion's paw
shell with cabochon sapphires and
diamonds rises majestically above a
swelling sea of royal blue. Verdura
transformed such "natural" objects into
bountiful treasures by draping them with
gems and emerald "seaweed," or
heaping them, upturned, with precious
and semi-precious stones. Courtesy E.J.
Landrigan, Inc./Verdura. Photographer
David Behl.

The Fifties

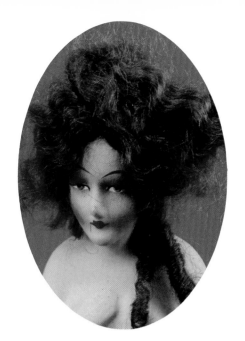

IT IS ONLY SHALLOW PEOPLE WHO DO NOT JUDGE BY APPEARANCE.
Oscar Wilde

In many respects, the 1950s were a panacea . . . and a puzzle. In 1950 another war, the Korean conflict, disrupted the short-lived peace—and the lives of more of its young men, including seasoned veterans from World War II. Most of the latter had long since returned home and established themselves in the communities with career-track jobs and growing families. Added to this unexpected disruption, a cloud of another kind appeared in 1953. This time it was "McCarthyism," and throughout much of the decade this accusatory witch hunt spawned a country looking right and left with a suspicious eye. Neither war nor distrust was an auspicious way to start the decade.

From a sociological standpoint, change was taking place that would eventually reshape the business and economic climate in a manner that would have seemed unthinkable a few decades before. The die was cast when all those returning veterans from both World War II and Korea initiated a virtual stampede for housing, causing a boom of gigantic proportions. Real estate developments spread like ink blots on a once pristine blotter as they expanded ever outward from the core of established cities and towns. Most homes were on small lots covering huge tracts of land sub-divided by eager entrepreneurs. The implications were vast, marking the beginning of an exodus to the suburbs, away from the urban areas and much that they represented. A new breed of American emerged, one that was destined to live a life different from that of parents and grandparents. The baby boom that followed World War II was well underway as the 1950s began, and it continued throughout much of the decade. The conditions brought about by the conversion from a wartime to peacetime economy introduced a plethora of goods and services to meet the needs of newlyweds and new parents—and slowly but surely changed the face of American culture.

The enormity of providing "essentials" and "non-essentials" for these growing families that sprouted up side by side, like rows of Nebraska corn, had to be met. This included furniture and appliances for new homes and cars to transport dad to work and mom to the city for shopping or to school with the children. Garments and accessories to complement the tidy package presented by this "picture perfect" life were an important part of the scenario. Suburbia was *safe*; home and family were *safe*; everything was compartmentalized into a tidy, non-threatening package. It was only natural that fashion would reflect the attitude of cautious optimism and conservatism that permeated the culture. Accessories did not fall victim to caution, however, as the prim fashions of the time demanded more of them. That fact was made abundantly clear in a 1951 article in *Glamour* titled "Accessories . . . the difference between clothes and fashion," when one dark green suit with nipped in jacket, modified peplum waist, and full, mid-calf skirt was given a host of different accessory looks: ". . . pearl and rhinestone jewelry, a red handbag, bright brown shoes and gloves," or ". . . a gold jersey velveteen turban with a pointed crown, gold and pearl beads . . . masses of gold bracelets, chamois gloves, and black calf bag and shoes," or ". . . a turquoise knit hat worn on the side . . . a green turtleneck sweater," or ". . . a black jersey blouse, low cut, with pearls and sparkle at the throat, a black satin cummerbund," and finally ". . . a little black satin beret, white gloves, black suede bag and shoes."[1]

The same article goes on to emphasize a credo for the well-placed accessory that applies at any time, in any decade, although the conservative 1950s seemed to desperately need the "jolt" they could provide. "But whether it's this suit or another, whether it's new or something you've had, remember that the final trick lies in the addenda . . . the little things that have so big an importance. The *additions*. Because it's really these that can make you look like a million dollars.[2]

Since jewelry was an important part of that accessorizing addenda, the popularity of costume jewelry gained momentum. When the War ended, manufacturers were able to return to pre-World War II production, free from the material restrictions that had hindered them during much of the 1940s. Hundreds of new manufacturers tossed their hats into the jewelry "ring." Glitz and glitter gained a foothold on the imaginations of top designers—and the public. Jewelry became bolder and more ornate. The smaller, somewhat dainty pieces of the 1940s were replaced by larger, more showy designs, many elaborately detailed and replete with imported Austrian stones. It was the beginning of yet another trend in the jewelry industry—one that would create a boom of its own for nearly 20 years. But, of course, there was much more to the "jewelry story" than the popularity of costume pieces. Fine jewelry design kept pace with the ever-changing whims of the public, and upscale retailers like Tiffany, Harry Winston, Black Starr & Frost, and Van Cleef & Arpels more than held their own amid the stiff competition.

The 1950s saw the rise of a phenomenon in the jewelry world. In 1948, when he was only seventeen years old, David Webb met Nina Silberstein, a certified public accountant. Webb was already a brilliant designer, but at such a young age he, of course, had a limited knowledge of the business world. Together, Webb and Silberstein were a well balanced combination, their skills and personalities perfectly complementing each other. Webb's rise was meteoric. Less than a decade after showcasing his jewelry at Bergdorf Goodman he moved to an exclusive East 57th Street location. Tragically, Webb died while still in his prime. The business had always been a group effort, and to the credit of Nina's son Stanley and a loyal staff, Webb's legacy is lovingly carried forward in the glorious pieces bearing his name in shops in New York, Houston, and Beverly Hills. That name—*David Webb*-inspires awe in the Nineties just as his raw talent did in the Fifties. The look remains distinctively Webb's—fine, classic jewelry that carries the jeweler's art to another dimension.

Men of the Fifties became more conscious of unusual items with a "jewelry" look, like belt buckles, tie clasps, and cuff links. Their clothing styles remained conservative, especially in the office, where businessmen gave credence to the theme of "the men in the grey flannel suits," one a seeming carbon copy of the other. While conservative prints will always be in style, these same gentlemen remained loyal to the sometimes loud and always wide 1940's necktie and the standard felt hat.

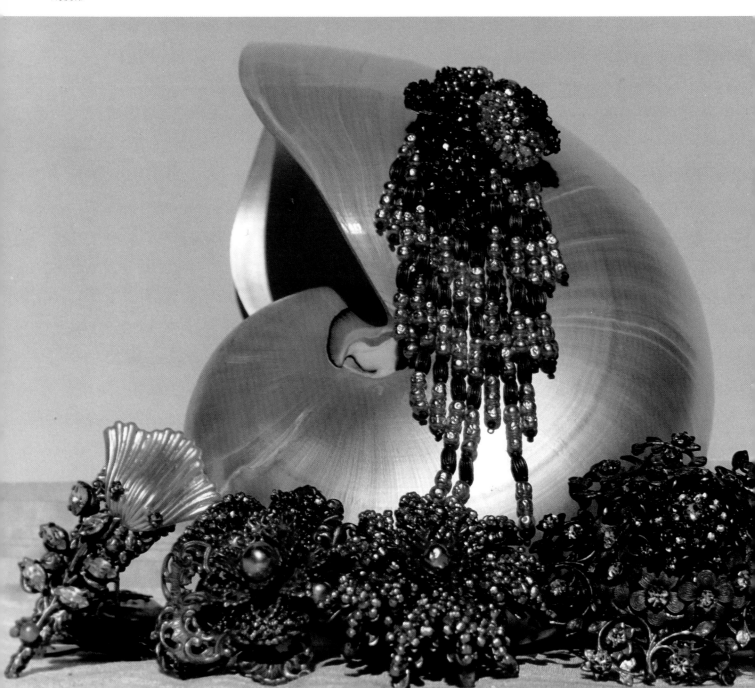

"A la mer." A giant shell drips with jewelry treasures by Miriam Haskell and Robert.

Women's hats were basically "unobtrusive." They were, with few exceptions, close to the head to complement *the* hairstyle of the 1950s—the "poodle cut" with minor decorative appeal, like tiny face veils or a single feather. Shoes were, to a great extent, boxy looking, with rounded toes, but there were, thankfully, some glamorous exceptions. Seamed stockings with "heels" that rose partially up the back of the ankle remained popular and, once again, women struggled to keep those seams straight.

The bouffant skirt of the late 1940s continued its hold on the public's imagination and was frequently accessorized with flat ballet slippers to complement the "ballerina look." Teenagers of the 1950s took the look a step further with poodle skirts (appropriately decorated with felt cutouts of dogs, balloons, or whatever) that brushed their bobby-soxed ankles, with penny loafers or saddle shoes barely showing below. These young people also favored tight, ankle-length trousers. For the more daring, the beatnik look—an offshoot of the zoot-suited guy of the Forties—had its tentative beginnings in the late 1950s. The needs of the young were being addressed with more vigor, a precursor of the decade to follow.

For those of a more staid bent, a new interest was added to gloves, involving a replacement of the three top-stitched seams that covered their backs. The basic design of gloves had changed little in fifty years, and it was time for something different. Buttons, buckles, stripes and embroidery brought renewed attention to the old favorite. Driving gloves with non-slip palms were not only popular but necessary for the careful motorist, and "little white gloves" remained *de rigueur* for the proper young lady to wear to the office, and in most social situations. In fact, as in the 1940s, no job interview was complete without them. Gloves were so important, in fact, that some handbag designs featured an attached "glove holder."

The 1950's fashion theme was a familiar one, for the overall refrain was one of conformity. The public was reticent to venture too far into unknown territory, and the results were what one might expect—generally uninspired. Sociologists could undoubtedly provide in-depth theories, but to the layman it seems only logical that after two wars "playing it safe" was the least threatening way to go. Most folks revered home, family, friends, and career—and they wanted nothing to disrupt any of them. As in any time, under any circumstances, creativity could not be stifled, and there were interesting tidbits here and there. The public always yearns for at least a glimpse of "something different." This time, however, the timid voice of the 1950s seemed to be pleading, "But not too different"! The result was an air of restrained sophistication. More and more women were entering the job market—if only until they married or established families—and suburban lifestyles and entry by husbands into the world of free enterprise involved many changes, including business travel and at-home entertaining. Once again, women could indulge in items like furs and cashmere sweaters, the latter updated into chic, tight-fitting, beaded styles.

Designers tried mightily to capture the public's attention with titillating styles, but the average woman of average means was in no mood for it—and in many instances these new designs totally missed the mark. For instance, the early 1950s saw a modification of Poiret's harem pants. This time it was the harem skirt. Its questionable popularity was of short duration, and with good reason. "The harem skirt of the early 1950s qualifies . . . as one of the most extraordinary fashions of all time. How did one sit in these bloomer-hemmed balloons, which look like giant puff balls that have settled around the legs?"[3] Adventuresome women, of course, managed, but this was not the decade to experiment with sweeping changes. On a lesser scale of discomfort was the 1959 Yves Saint Laurent line that introduced garments daringly hobbled at the knee (at least the hobble had moved up the leg from its beginnings at the calf early in the century) but, like its predecessor, its popularity was fleeting.

Dior, the fashion genius who had changed everything so dramatically the decade before with a look that had carried over into the 1950s but with much of its electricity drained, continued to wield influence on fashion until his untimely death in 1957. His designs—and those of his predecessors—were eagerly awaited at the approach of each new season. Certainly Dior must be credited with the foresight to give women what they craved. As described in a 1957 issue of *Vogue*, "In this new collection, Mr. Dior presents both facets of his brilliant talent: one his painter-architect mastery of abstract design; the other his gift for making women look completely feminine (the basis of his great success in 1947)."[4] Dior was astute enough to recognize this need of the 1950's woman, since women were still drawn to tried and true variations on the "New Look," which had long since become an "old" one. Chanel's design philosophy was much the same. "It is Chanel's premise that respect for the individual should dominate design; that clothes must be more important on the woman than on the designer's drawing board."[5] In any event, circumstances seem to have conspired not only against those women who longed for a burst of fashion excitement instead of being mired in fashion quicksand, but against the designers themselves.

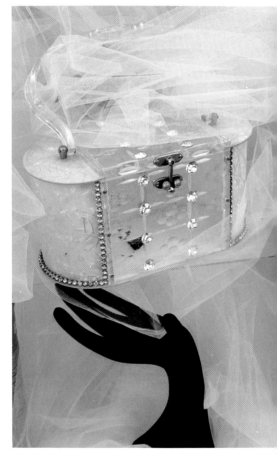

Early plastic bag...Oh, so fine! Courtesy of Magi.

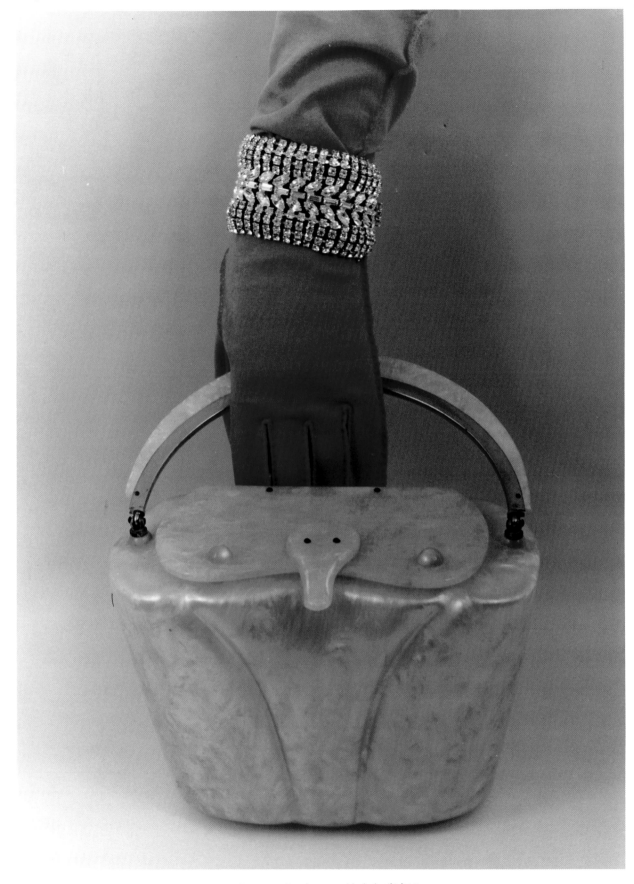

An unusual and rare molded plastic bag,
rose colored glove and rhinestone cuff
bracelet. Courtesy of Magi.

Couture finally succeeded in gaining a "seal of approval" for one new fashion look. It dealt the ordinary woman of ordinary means a "triple whammy," and is probably the look for which the Fifties will be remembered. Introduced first as the sack dress (a simple, loose-fitting, unbelted sheath), it was transformed into the A-line in 1958, and shortly thereafter the trapeze—an exaggerated A-line that begged for a very broad-brimmed hat to give the look some semblance of proportion. The A-line was exactly what the name signified—narrow shoulders evolving downward to a wide, wide hem. Although the silhouette was not a new one, it would continue to reassert itself in the ensuing years.

There was, however, another look that rightly belongs to the 1950s. It started in Europe, just as it had under Chanel's influence in the 1920s, but this time the trend reached beyond the beaches of St. Tropez and the playgrounds of the wealthy. Sunbathing, and the outwardly "healthy" results, became a benchmark of the times, and ". . .It was the Italians who gave to the men and women of the 1950s the look of people who live 'in the sun.'. . . now Italian sandals and sunglasses characterized fashionable summer dress for the decade."[6] This casual look of sun and sandals widened the demands and endless possibilities to be found in simple, easy clothes to fit the suburban lifestyle of so many. And then there was plastic and lucite—shoes and handbags in see-through styles were all the rage. An enchanting phenomenon, they created a look that remains distinctly Fifties . . . and highly collectible.

Despite its foibles, the decade was deserving of the posthumous title, *The Fabulous Fifties*. But little did anyone envision to what ends the youth of the next decade would take it!

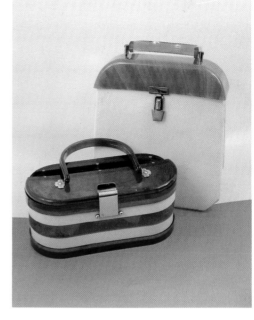

Toffee and creme! Two plastic beauties. Courtesy of Magi.

1950-1960
[1] *Glamour*, October 1, 1951, p. 173
[2] *Glamour*, October 1, 1951, p. 173
[3] "Fashionable Mind, The" p. 86
[4] *Vogue*, September 1, 1957, p. 216
[5] *Vogue*, September 1, 1957, p. 220
[6] "Fashion: The Mirror of History", p. 365

As timeless in the fifties as it is today...the window of Didier Ludot, Paris, 1991.

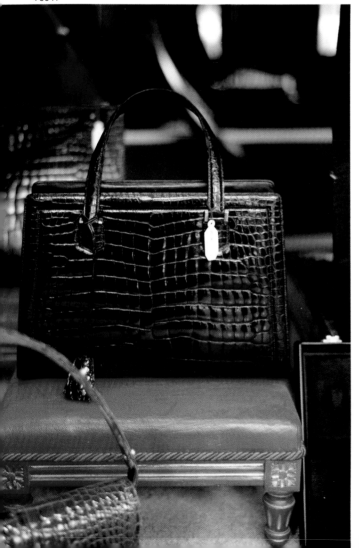

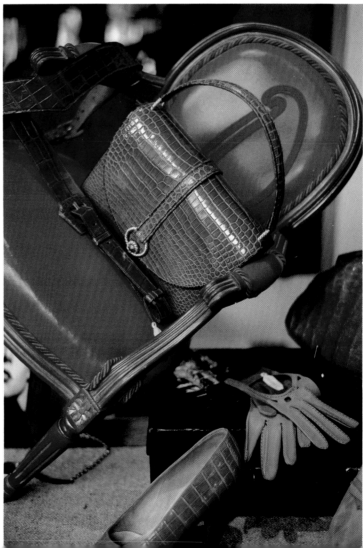

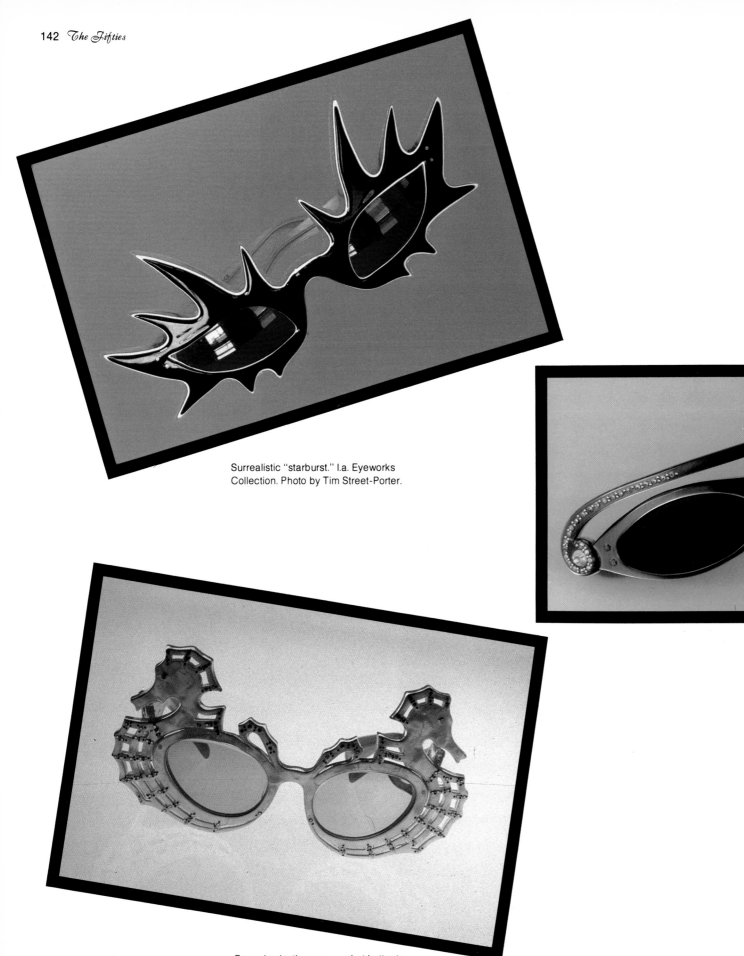

Surrealistic "starburst." l.a. Eyeworks
Collection. Photo by Tim Street-Porter.

For a day by the sea . . . what better to
wear than these Seahorses? Courtesy
l.a. Eyeworks Collection. Photo by Tim
Street-Porter.

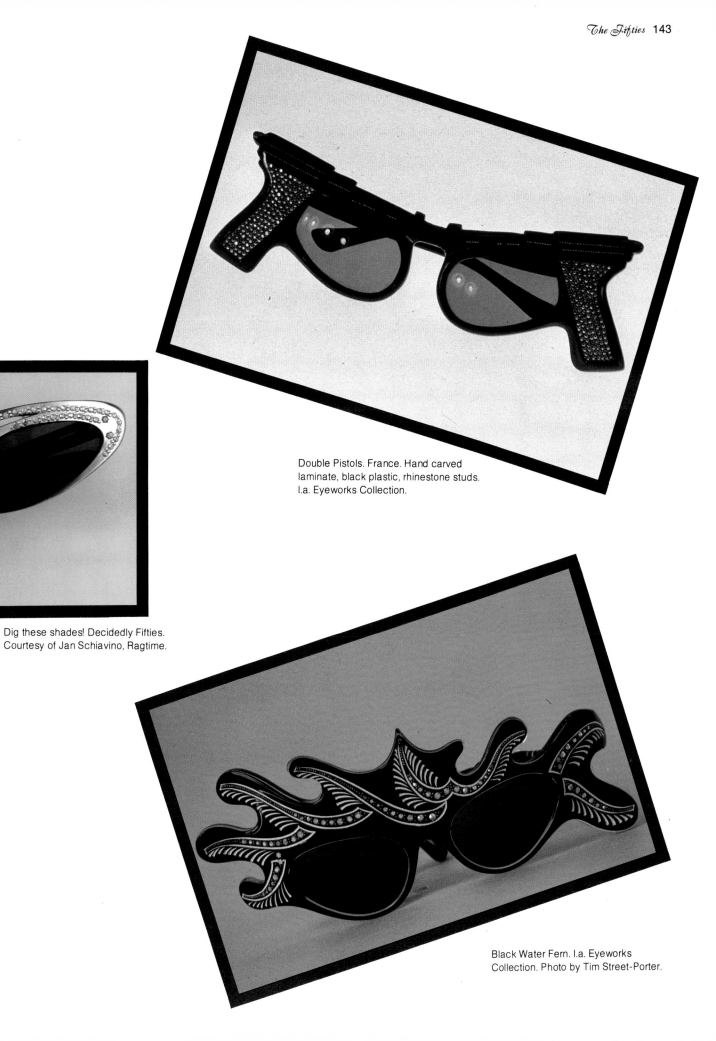

Double Pistols. France. Hand carved
laminate, black plastic, rhinestone studs.
l.a. Eyeworks Collection.

Dig these shades! Decidedly Fifties.
Courtesy of Jan Schiavino, Ragtime.

Black Water Fern. l.a. Eyeworks
Collection. Photo by Tim Street-Porter.

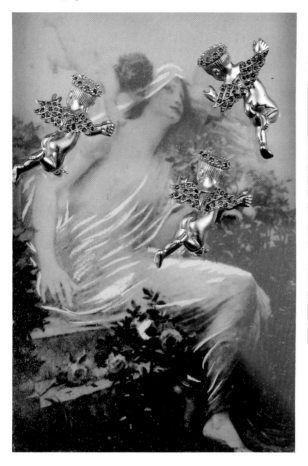

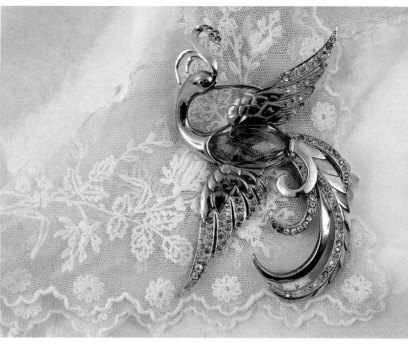

Grace in motion and design. This unmarked costume piece in tones of gold and silver with giant faceted center stone measures 4″ by 4½″.

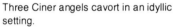

Three Ciner angels cavort in an idyllic setting.

Who else but Miriam Haskell? Fifteen strands of gossamer crystal beads and tiny pearls, with matching 3″ earrings. Smashing!

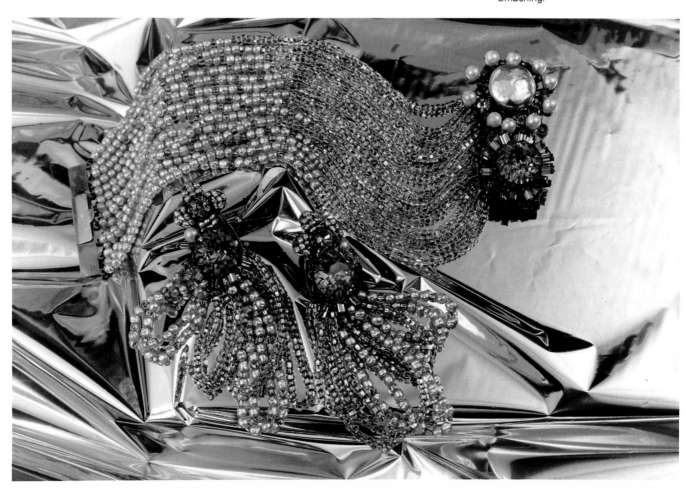

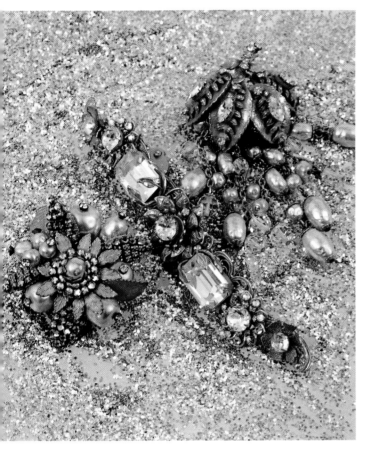

A gigantic 5¼" Miriam Haskell brooch nestles between two Robert pieces of similar design.

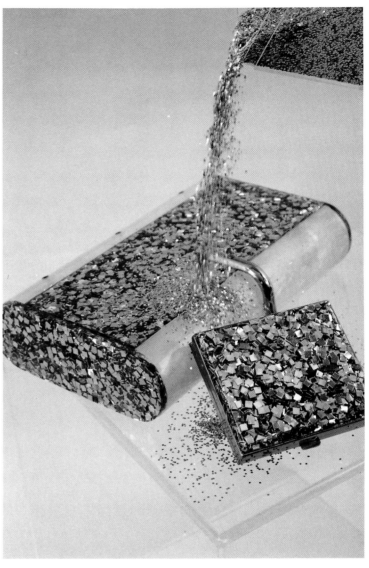

"All that glitters." Clutch bag with matching compact. Courtesy Magi.

"Floundering" around with a wild and crazy Miami fish bag...to make it even more interesting, the head opens and so does the mouth!

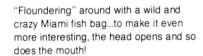

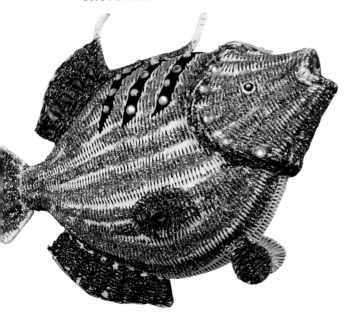

Good things in small packages! Orlane perfumes in charming drawstring pouches.

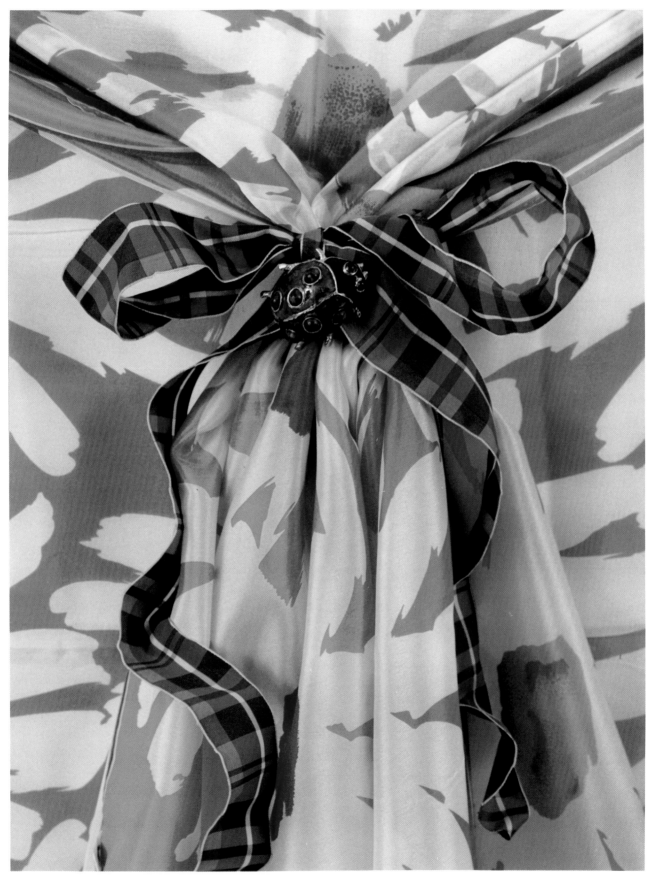

A Beetle (KJL), a bow, and the vibrant
beauty of a 1950's Vera scarf (reissued
in 1990), courtesy of Vera.

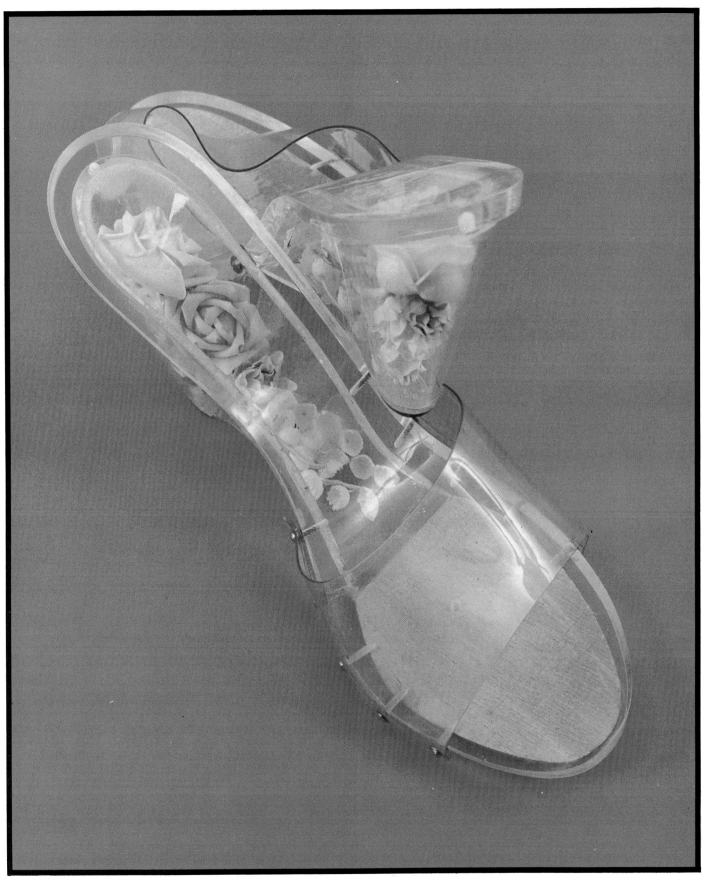

Walking is no bed of roses! See-through
plastic "wedgie" shoes with flowers
blooming everywhere.

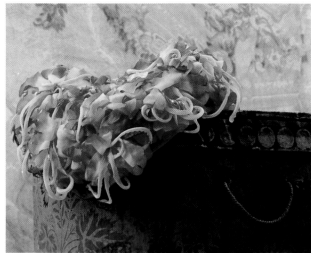

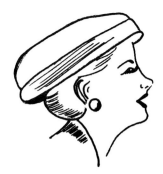

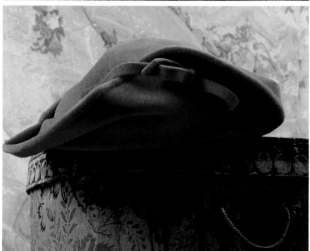

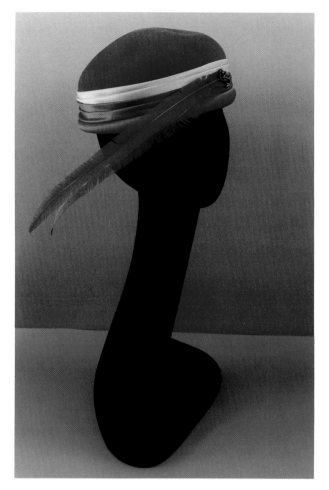

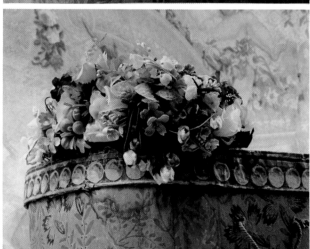

This hat of double-banded satin was worn with the 1950's "topper" coat. Courtesy of Gloria Malloy.

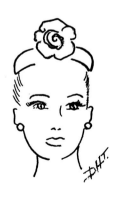

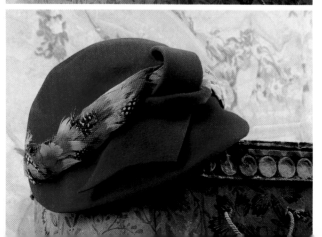

Hats of the Fifties . . . close to the head! The rose felt was made in Italy by Bursalino, the red felt and florals were custom designed by Anne Sary, Hartford, Conn.

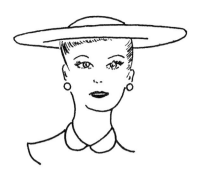

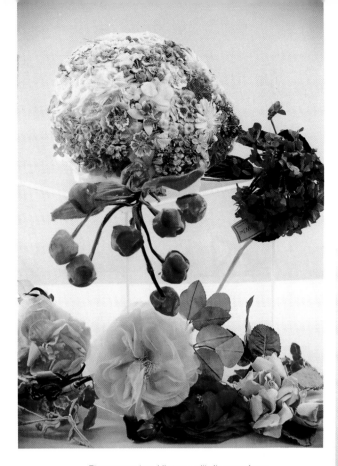

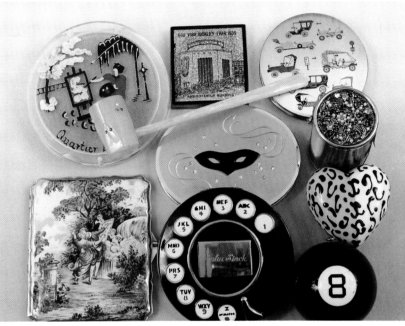

Flower garden. Vintage silk flowers from the '20s, '30s and '40s...and a precious Schiaparelli hat.

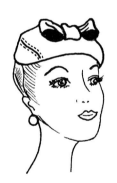

From the Forties and Fifties—compacts galore! Left, top to bottom: Lucite Latin Quarter compact by Bell DeLuxe; Stratton cigarette case. Center, top to bottom: Zell World's Fair Administration Building compact; Dorothy Grey compact with black enamel mask; telephone dial compact. Right, top to bottom: Stratton automobile compact; Dorset cylindrical compact with colored rhinestones; Illinois Watch Case Co. enamel compact from the 1930s; black plastic 8 ball compact. Courtesy of Joan Orlen.

And here are more. Bottom, left to right: Italian goldtone and plastic, hand-painted portrait, enclosed in glass; large square Rex fifth Avenue compact in red lucite with Sterling overlay; Parisienne souvenir compact with plastic dome, by Daniel; Bakelite rhinestone poodle compact; unusual K & K bracelet/compact with red and clear rhinestones; Evans elongated cigarette case with goldtone scrollwork and beige applied repousse; Bakelite tortoiseshell compact with rhinestone top and matching comb; center: Volupte brushed gold hand compact. Courtesy of Joan Orlen.

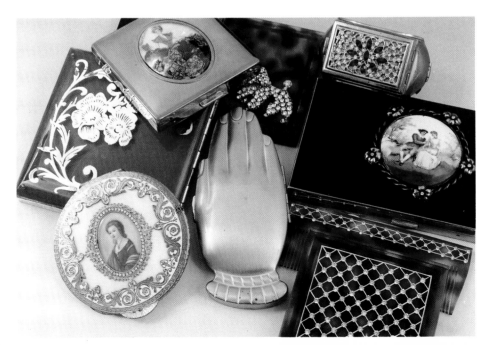

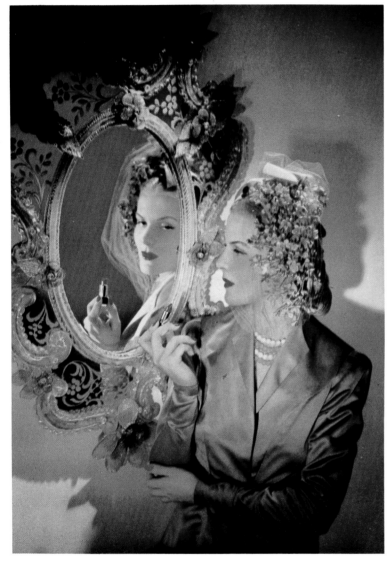

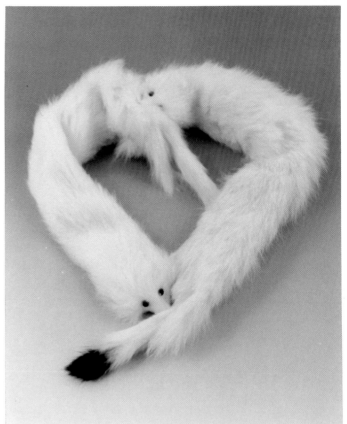

Just friends! An ermine collar for coat or suit.

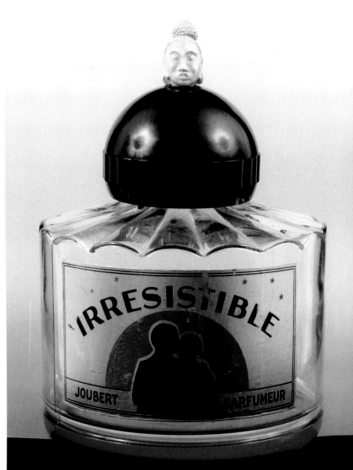

Call me irresistible. Courtesy of Magi.

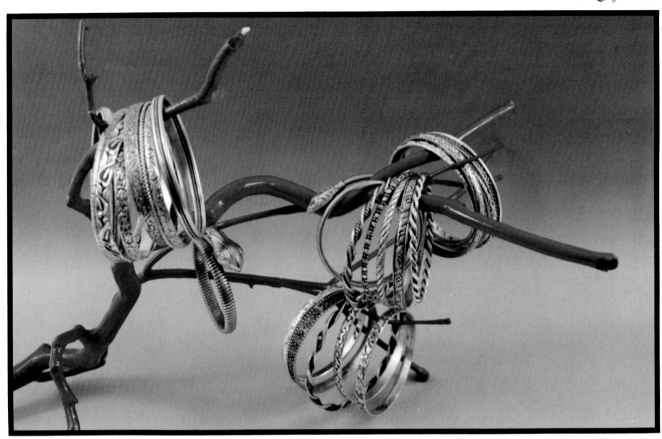

Out on a limb! A mass of sterling
bangles . . . with a few "snakes in the
branches."

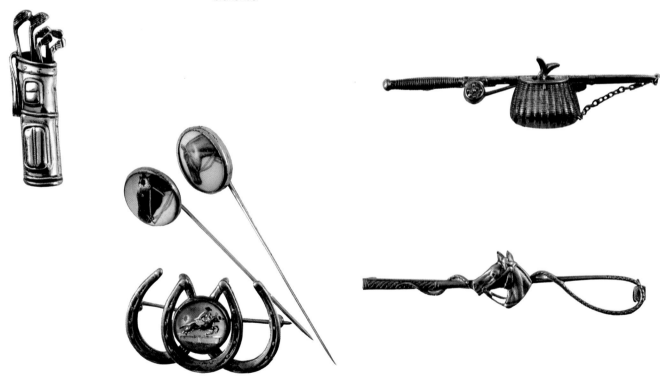

"Something for the golfer and angler (all
in sterling) and also the "horsey" set.

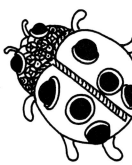

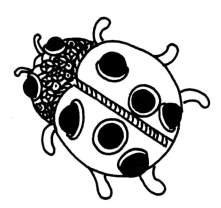

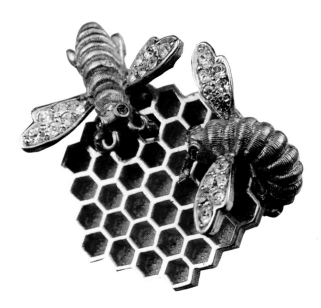

A "honey" of a brooch . . . Boucher bees
cavort on the "comb."

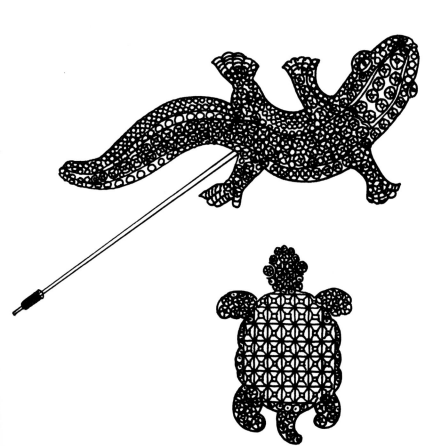

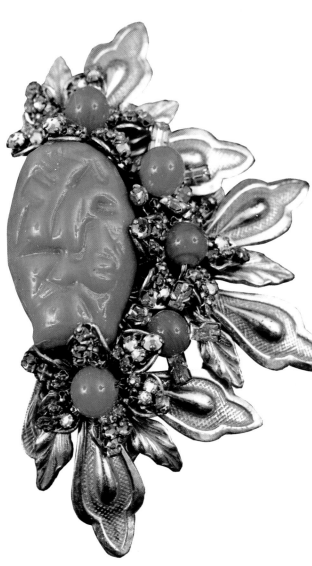

A 3½" Miriam Haskell brooch, magnified
to show detail.

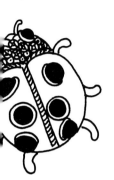

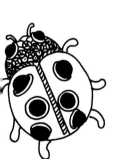

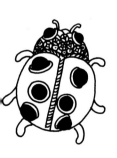

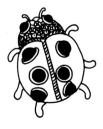

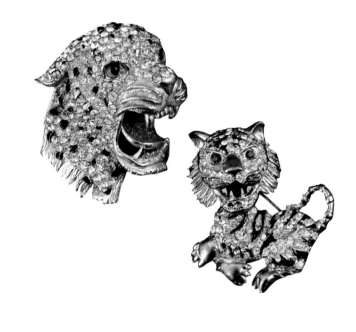

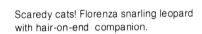

Scaredy cats! Florenza snarling leopard with hair-on-end companion.

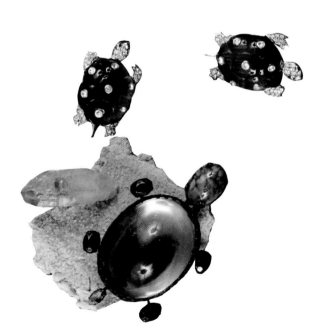

"On the rocks." A 1950's Schreiner turtle with giant lucite "shell" and trembler head watches over her "babies"—amber, rhinestone-studded earrings by Kenneth Jay Lane, circa 1980s.

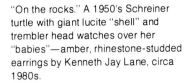

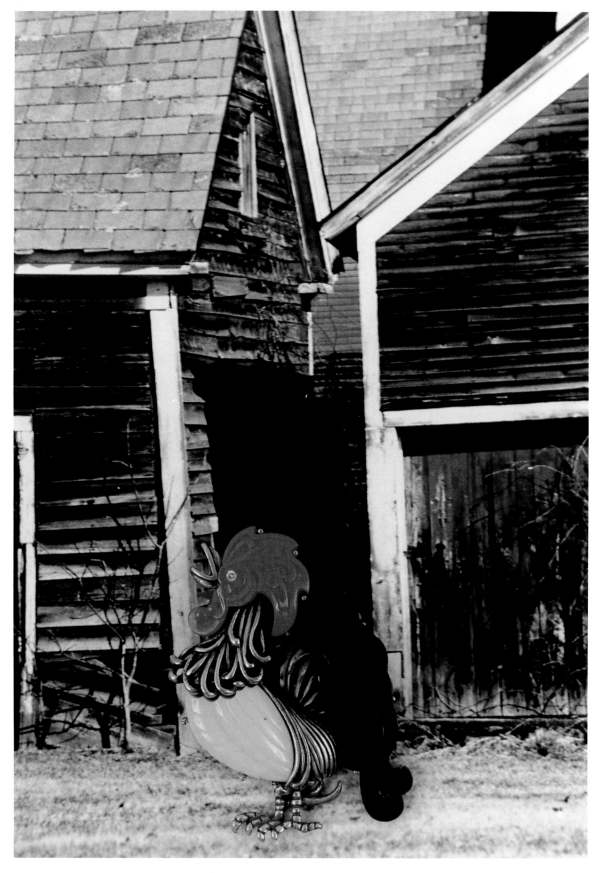

Surveying his domain...A majestic
Bakelite "king of the barnyard" by Hattie
Carnegie.

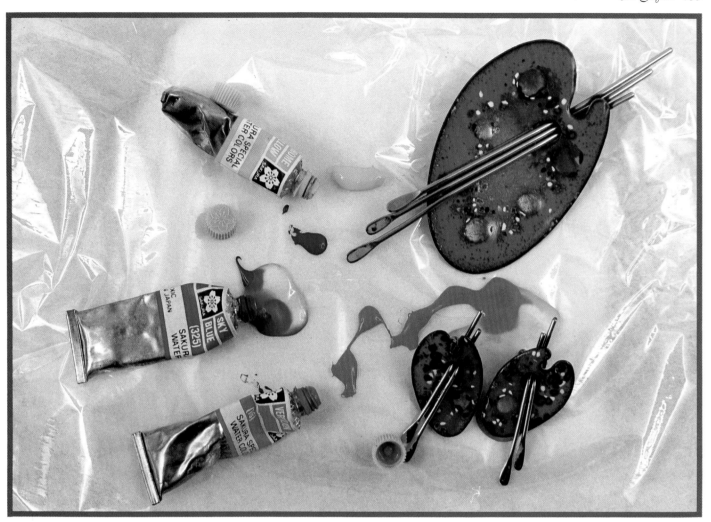

What better subject for copper jewelry by Matisse than an artist's palette? With matching earrings.

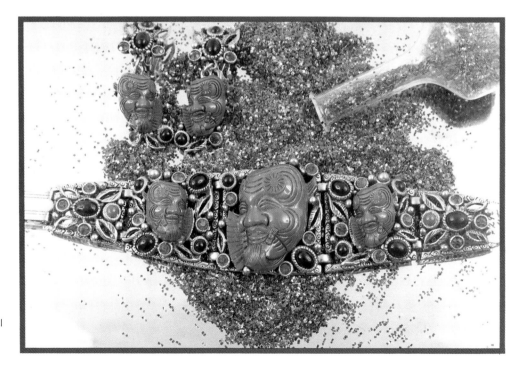

Smiling Japanese gods are the focal point of this bracelet with matching earrings by Selro.

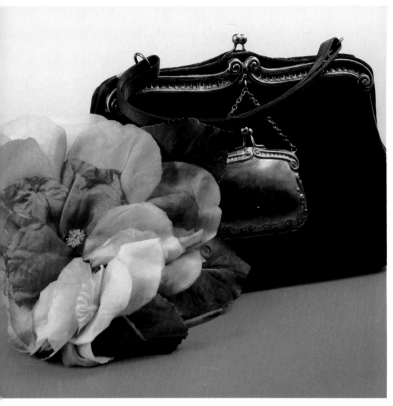

Victorian elegance revisited in this red velvet Italian bag with antiqued brass trim and an attached change purse, by Roberta Camarino.

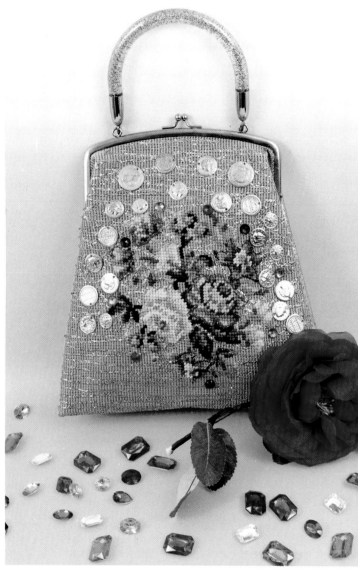

Just rewards! This bag has everything-a plastic handle, embroidered flowers . . . and gold coins. Courtesy of Magi.

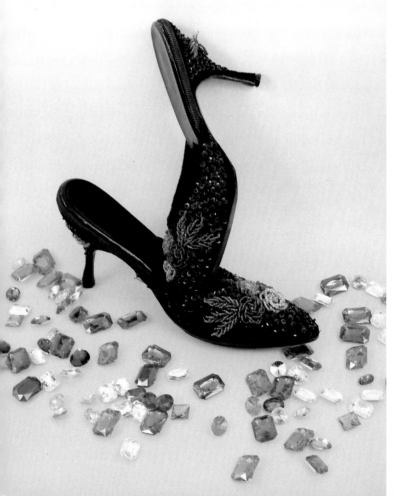

Great expectations shoes...with beading from heel to toe! Courtesy of Magi.

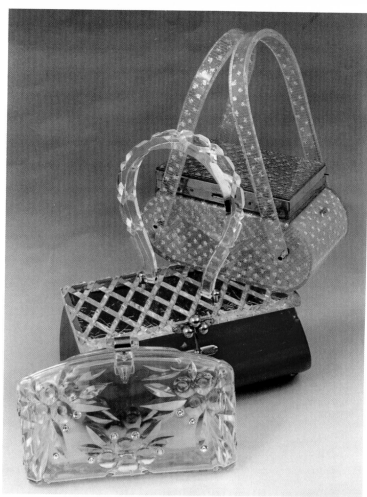

Lucite bags . . . Rhapsody in Three!
Courtesy of Magi.

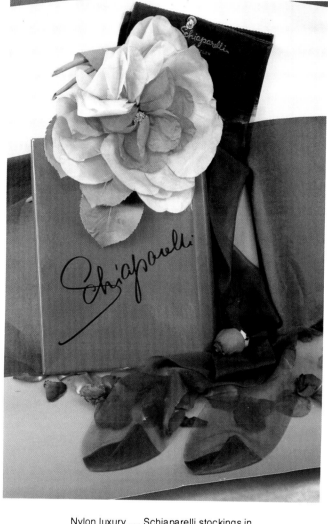

Nylon luxury . . . Schiaparelli stockings in
the original box. Courtesy of Irma.

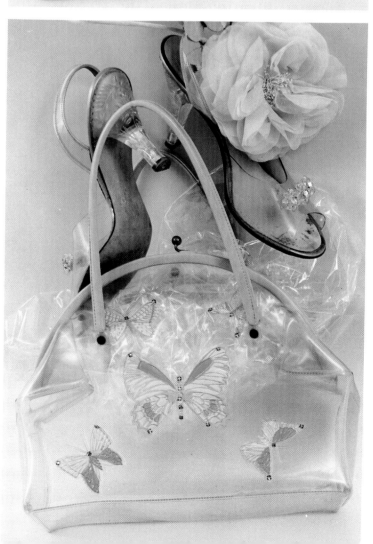

Butterflies R Us! Courtesy of Magi.

This Leo Glass necklace could hang proudly from any Yuletide tree . . . or better yet, provide a charming accent for madame's decolletage!

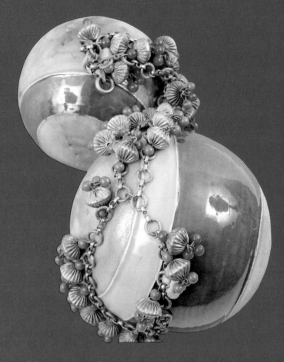

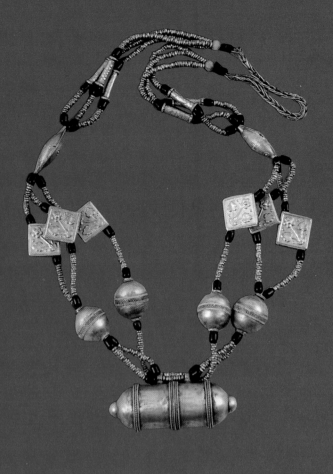

A Berber silver tribal necklace.

"Bingo, Bango, Bongo." A cotton Chipie warrior scarf, Paris, 1990, is surrounded by African necklaces and trade beads.

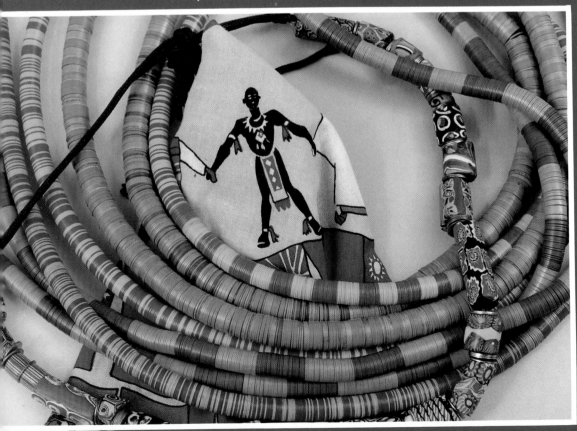

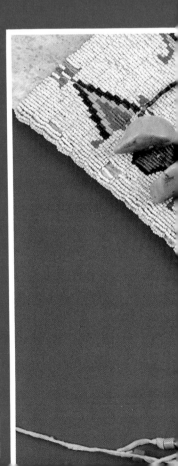

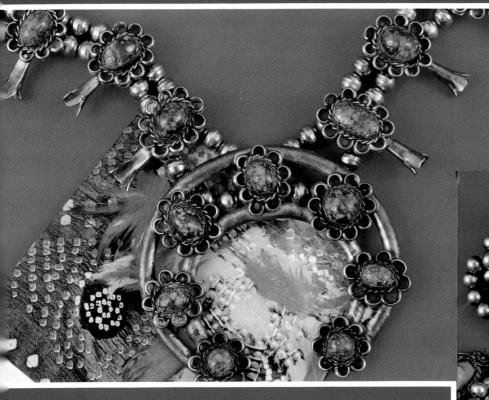

Squash Blossom...silver beads...and fine old cuff.

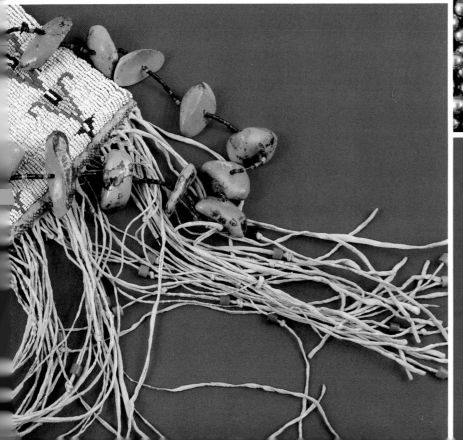

A 1950's Heishe bead and turquoise necklace rests on a Plains Indian pipe bag from the 1930s.

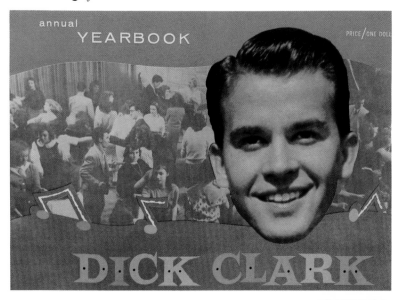

"I give it an 85—it has a good beat and it's easy to dance to!" From the American Bandstand Yearbook, 1957.

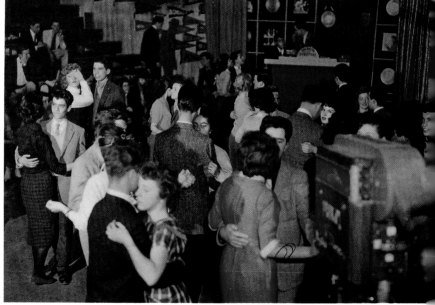

Woven wicker bag with felt insets of a girl...a dog...and glitz! The ceramic poodle was a popular accent. Courtesy of Magi.

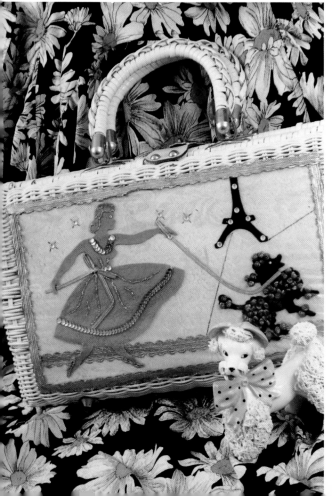

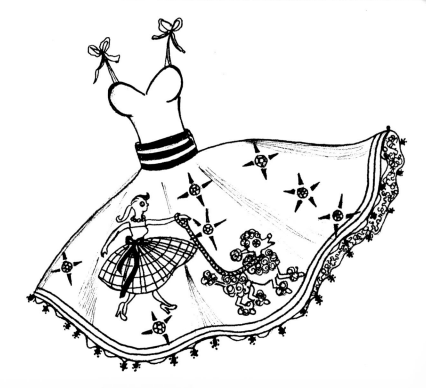

Harper's Bazaar, February 1950:

"Hat, white straw. A John Frederics charmer . . . $5.00.
Earrings, rhinestone buttons. By Kramer . . . $1.00.
Stockings, 20 denier nylon . . . $1.50.
Shoes, black calf pumps. By DeLiso Debs . . . $12.95.
Brassiere, black satin and lace. By Exquisite Form . . . $2.00.
Handbag, shiny black plastic . . . $4.95.
Gloves. Stitched black cotton . . . $2.00.
Bracelet of gilt and not-real carnelians. By Reja. $7.50.
$12.75 for a small clutch bag of cobra, ready to move in the best circles. By Josef."

"$2.50 for red cotton gloves with a zippered pocket in one palm for those exasperating bus fares."

"The bound wrist—bound in chiffon or metallic mesh to catch the eye and hold it when you lift a glass or light a cigarette. Silk chiffon squares in pink and gasoline green. $1 each. By Sally Gee . . . with the yellow square and the green, Castlecliff pins. With the pink, Trifari bracelets."

Harper's Bazaar, October 1950:

"Sable lipstick brush in sterling silver. $8.50. Silver-plated bobby pins with rhinestone drops. $1.00. Wadsworth gold-finished compact with jeweled chevrons $49.75."

". . . black velvet hat with a border of cock feathers that ends in a swishing tail."

Glamour, October 1951:

"For the ladies, $2.25. Cigarette holder from the Continent. Chromium with red or black mouthpiece that ejects the cigarette when you press it with your thumb. A smart four inches long . . ."

"New earrings flow forward to meet the cheek or upward to outline the ear."

"Cuddly cloche of just about perfect proportions for practically anyone. In divine hues of Bloomsburg satin—blue, smoke, absinthe, faced with velveteen. Wear it anywhere, anytime. From the master designer, John Frederics . . . $14.95.

". . . a gold jersey velveteen turban with a pointed crown, gold and pearl beads, tight at the neck, masses of gold bracelets, chamois gloves and black calf bag and shoes."

Harper's Bazaar, May 1954:

"Van Cleef & Arpels will soon dismount the fabulous Marie-Louise tiara which Napoleon I gave to his second wife on the birth of their son, the King of Rome (circa 1811). Before dismounting this famous heirloom, Van Cleef & Arpels invites you to select one or several emeralds from this tiara to be fashioned into a special jewel for you . . . Each purchaser of the Napoleon emeralds will receive a special parchment illustrated with a reproduction of the tiara showing where his emeralds were originally set." (Van Cleef & Arpels advertisement)

Harper's Bazaar, November 1954:

"Cartridge cuff links . . . The perfect gift for that sportsman. Genuine 32 calibre cartridge (with charge removed of course) and loaded with a silver bullet. $4.95 pair."

Vogue, September 1, 1957:

"For a woman whose fur hat is temporarily in the hat box, there's the fur bag, biggish, possibly yellow-dyed Persian lamb, or red fox . . ."

"Bronze shoes, attenuated and certainly pointy, reappear and add to the possible choice in late-day or little dinner shoes."

"Tiny crystal beads are strung and massed together in jewelry as unweighty as chiffon; some with pearls in shimmery, waterfall necklaces . . . alternate for pearls: grey stones, grey-crystal, grey jet beads, worn in a melange, especially good with grey flannel."

"In this new collection (1957), Mr. Dior presents both facets of his brilliant talent; one, his painter-architect mastery of abstract design; the other, his gift for making women look completely feminine (the basis of his great success in 1947)."

"It is Chanel's premise that respect for the individual should dominate design; that clothes must be more important on the woman than on the designer's drawing board."

"Incidental table intelligence: a ruby-eyed gold poodle cigarette lighter . . . a latticed gold shell pocket watch, a reed-slim gold cigarette holder, a fish shaped gold key chain."

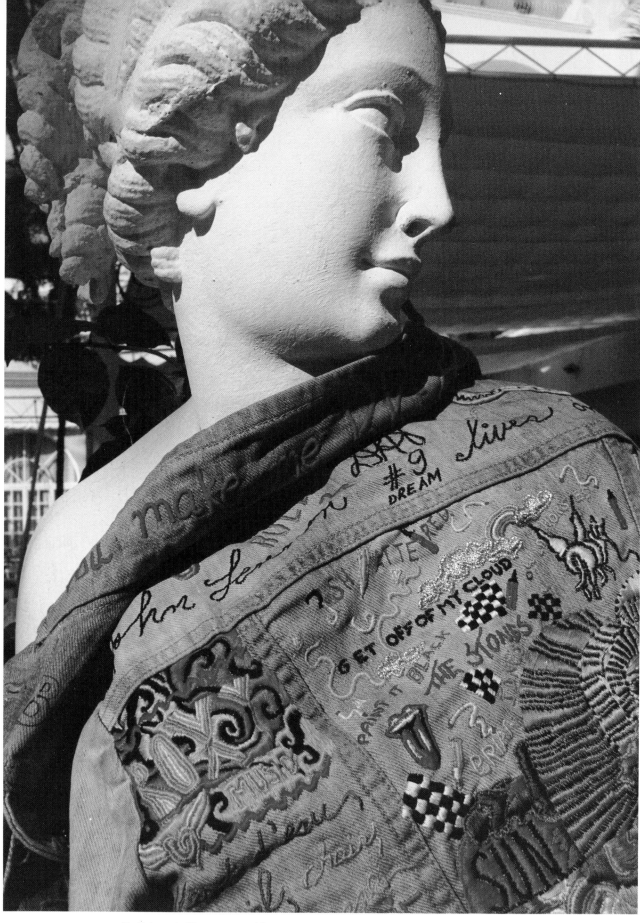

Emblazoned with messages of the Sixties, a lovingly hand-drawn and needlepointed denim jacket by Dorothy Torem unites with the classical when draped over this statue on the sun-drenched isle of Capri.

The Sixties

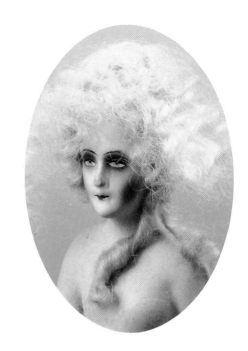

UNCONTROLLABLE LAUGHTER AROSE AMONG THE BLESSED GODS.
Homer, *The Iliad*

A "youthquake." That name, perhaps more than any other, most clearly describes the 1960s. Rejection of old mores—triggered in part by political questioning and anger over the Vietnam War—became a vehicle for self-affirmation. And what better way for those who felt politically powerless to express their feelings of frustration than in attitudes and clothing?

Skirts ran the gamut from short-short minis—which had their beginnings in England—to lengths coming to the ankles and below. Either legs didn't show at all, or they were covered by fishnet or metallic stockings. There were wild prints, mismatched outfits, jeans of all styles and shapes, pants riding low on the hips, and flaring bell-bottom trousers, and the end result may have seemed little more than a conglomeration of bemusing items of apparel to some.

In their hip-hugger jeans and baggy shirts, the new "unisex" fashions made distinguishing the sex of the young and "mod" well nigh impossible. Adding to the puzzle were males with long flowing locks, just like their counterparts, and females sans makeup. The "message" was not uncommon to decades past. "Androgyny returns each decade in different variations: the twenties flat-chested flapper with bobbed hair and without waistline, thirties tailored ensembles even for tennis, hunting and golf, forties utilitarian wartime outfits, fifties chemise and oversize men's white shirts for teens, sixties unisex denims and army clothes . . ."[1]

Rock 'n roll supplanted the movies as the primary influence on the clothing styles of teenagers. The United States did not have a corner on this trend, since many of that era's stars were British—and the rest of the world listened, and watched, just as intently. London and France were the centers for many clothing styles and "pop" music sounds that never quite caught on in the United States. San Francisco and a few other "hippie havens" were another story altogether, and they became the site of "flower power," with its own standards of dress and behavior. Nevertheless, the message was clear. On both sides of the Atlantic, youth was influencing fashion as never before.

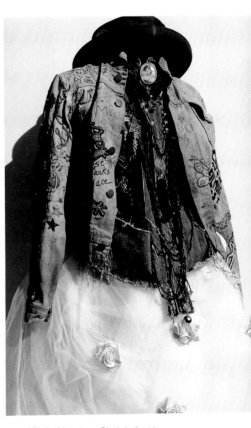

Dresses, referred to as "granny" dresses, were ankle length and shapeless, and looked like something even pioneer women would have rejected. Clunky shoes and boots, jewelry with leather thongs and the ambiance of handmade crafts, or strands of "love beads," completed the outfit. As Kennedy Fraser wrote in a *New Yorker* article about the youth of the Sixties, "It has all been done more tumultuously, more authentically, by people who are barely their seniors in life span, let alone in history."[2] The power of this grass-roots movement was not lost on designers of high fashion. Trendsetters like Andre Courreges—generally acknowledged, along with Londoner Mary Quant, to have started the mini-skirt trend—made the indispensable flat, white boots his trademark. But that was not the extent of Courreges' influence or ability. An article on Paris fashions in *Vogue*'s September 1963 issue heaped praise on his abilities: "Courreges has perfected the straight line, bringing everything close to the body. His tailoring is without peer, subtle, correct, and modern. Many coats on the narrow side with easy shoulders, small stand-up collars, leather-ribbon belts that tie in a flat bow at the waist . . . and winter white leather will be the niftiest thing on two feet this year—after boots, shoes; then gloves, exciting domed caps . . ."[3]

Just as Cape Canaveral launched our first astronauts into space, Pierre Cardin catapulted space-inspired, avant garde fashions to the fore, while Rudi Gernreich shocked even the usually "unshockable" with his daring topless and see-through dresses and teeny, weeny bikinis. "Cat-suits" clung to the bodies of the lean—and not so lean—and were worn with a mini-skirt and Courreges-style boots. Paco Rabanne introduced daring chain mail clothing and others made solely of plastic discs. This fueled a trend for huge synthetic disc earrings—veritable flying saucers dangling from the ears.

All or most of these designer creations were incorporated into fashions that clothes-conscious yet trendy individuals would find acceptable. They were often complemented by enormous pieces of "body jewelry," which covered the wearer's chest like elaborate medieval armor. Other jewelry was almost as dramatic, and long, long ropes of pearls became a favorite. More and more women recognized the accessorizing possibilities in earrings, and they were popular in all sizes and styles. Paris haute couture reflected the trend to "jeweled" accessories. ". . . Jewels with everything; lustrous pearls the size of mothballs, jeweled buttons . . . flat medallions, stones bursting with light mounted in huge squared Byzantine pins in the Empress Theodora manner." [4]

The "tried and true" designers, like Yves Saint Laurent, must not be dismissed when one looks at those wielding fashion influence in the 1960s. Elegance and verve commanded the attention of sophisticated women everywhere, and we are able to

Mix 'n Match...a Sixtie's fashion statement...denim jacket, tulle and...roses!

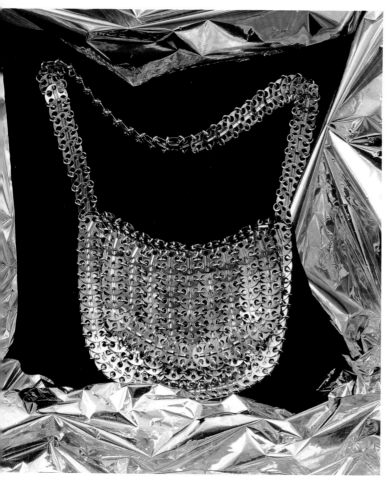

High theatre! Paco Rabanne . . . on stage! Collection of Mark Walsh.

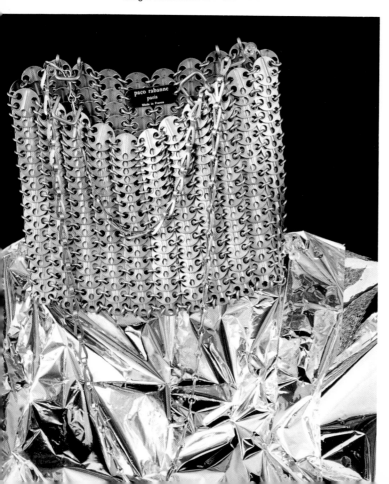

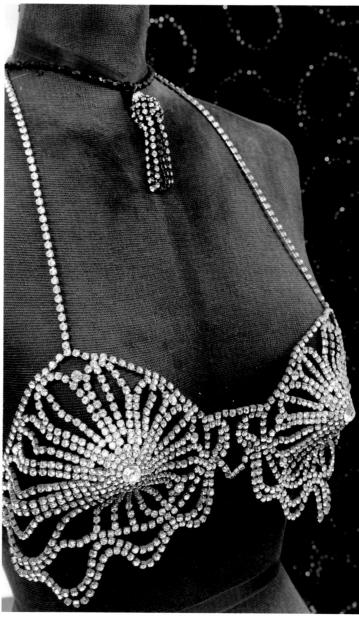

"Topsy 'n Turvy." The bra to end all bras. Courtesy of Joan Schiavino, Ragtime.

Meet you at the Peppermint Lounge!

Paco on ice . . . an imposing Paco Rabanne bag. Collection of Mark Walsh.

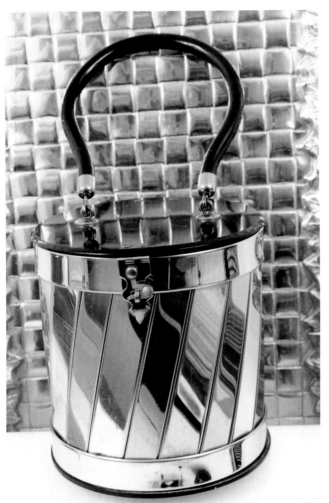

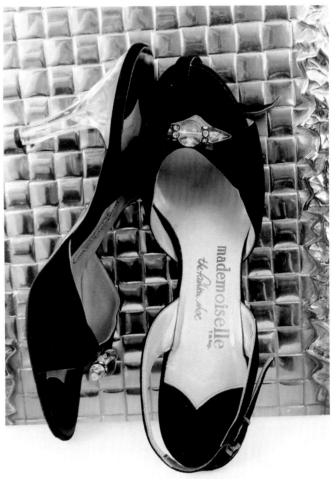

These black suede beauties with carved lucite heels and trim are by Mademoiselle. Courtesy of Magi.

"Beat the drum" for the ultimate in bags. This evening beauty has metallic bias stripes. Courtesy of Magi.

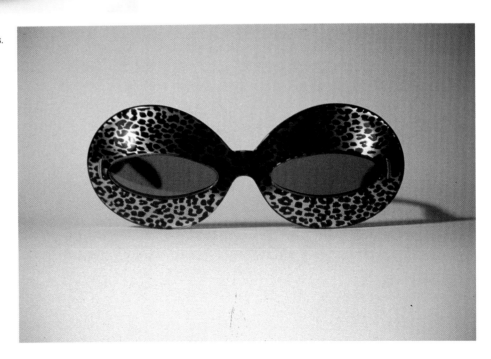

Queen of the Jungle . . . leopard sunglasses. l.a. Eyeworks Collection.

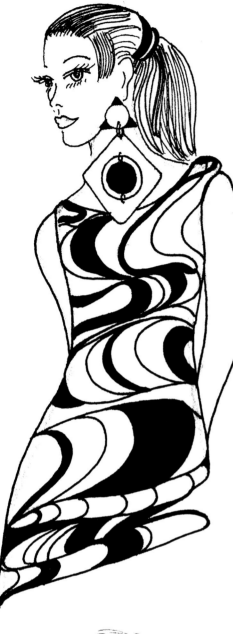

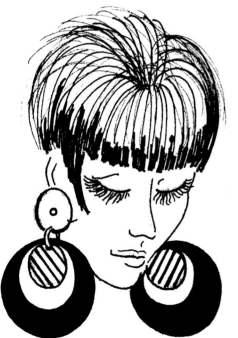

glimpse the magic of these fashion mavens via *Vogue's* reaction to the Paris showings in their September 1963 issue. "The air was charged with pinpoint bubbles of anticipated success as we entered the door at St. Laurent. Shining copper beeches stood ceiling high in the corners of the double salon . . . on and on they came like a rush of trippers from Mars, wearing jerkins and overblouses of checked wool and suede and mink with slack gold chains circling their waists, under their collars; chains rimmed jaunty porkpie hats . . ." [5]

Shawls, like those wound around "granny" dresses, became a decorative accessorizing item for the more sophisticated when made of dressier fabrics, sometimes decorated with fringe, embroidery, and glitter. Emilio Pucci was one designer who brought colorful, modernistic prints in luscious color combinations to a kaleidoscopic array of silky lingerie. These and other romantic yet upbeat designs were enormously popular with that powerful army of more mature women who were unwilling to sacrifice their fashion sense on the altar of the "hippie" culture.   Fake furs were a sensation— and many were almost impossible to tell from the genuine article. Simple suits and dresses were given a feminine touch with the addition of lace collars and jabots. As in the Fifties, the early 1960s saw handbags trimmed with flowers and other ornamentations and covered with see-through plastic. The end of the decade revitalized a short-lived interest in the midi-skirt, a more upscale and fashionable alternative to "granny" fashions. Frequently decorated with fringe, they were complemented with boots that grazed their hems. However, the midi probably arrived too soon on the heels of the mini to seriously capture the attention of women who were already more than a little confused by fluctuating skirt lengths and mixed fashion messages.

Turban-style hats, many of real and "fun" fur, were much in demand. Even fezzes returned. "A certain free-lance designer was heard to remark, 'Hats are not designed this season, they explode'!"[6] Needless to say, it wasn't the first time. Hairdos of the 1960s didn't go quite that far afield, but "teased" hair was actually a modification of the look of centuries before and became an important adjunct to the fashions, thereby achieving accessorizing status. By mid-decade, hairpieces, like topknots, chignons, falls, and braids, were an acceptable—and, in some cases, necessary—addition to this "lacquered" and frequently overblown look.

Shoes ran the gamut from clunky to glamorous, as did most everything else in this decade of conflicting messages. From flat boots and tied high-tops to "elevator" platform shoes with cork soles, this was the decade of "anything goes." It saw heel heights climb and narrow to unprecedented proportions and, along with the unwieldy platform shoes, start many a young women down the long road to permanent foot problems. These spiky heels also created unexpected maintenance expenses in public places when formerly immaculate carpeting suddenly became riddled with holes from the narrow, almost weapon-like heels that were constantly digging into their surface.

Except for the "flower children," most women weren't about to sacrifice cosmetics, and they remained a permanent member of the female accessorizing family. Cosmetic companies were happy to oblige. A myriad of colors for lipsticks and rouges were offered to complement any outfit, day or night, and elaborate and exotic eye makeup, some harkening back to the "Cleopatra look," added an important finishing touch. Men were also catered to in the toiletries department, and by the 1960s the market for these specialty products —in the form of colognes, shaving lotions, and soaps—grew to massive and profitable proportions, creating an industry onto itself.

Innovation was not lost on marketing moguls during this time of open minds and great change, and the 1960s saw a new trend that would literally revolutionize the industry, eventually trickling down even to infant wear. It was the selling power of designer labels—this time for the population at large. Haute couture had held court in its own select circles for decades, and those names were known and appreciated by fashion mavens worldwide. But designer, celebrity, and company logos rooted more firmly in mass appeal also staked out a claim for the public's dollars, a trend that was destined to grow. These decorative patches and more subtle logos appeared everywhere—on hip pockets and breast pockets, handbags and panties. Even the venerable Hamilton Watch Company sensed a trend that could be successfully addressed in their own business, and in 1969 commissioned Bill Blass to design a watch collection—the industry's first "designer" watches at affordable prices.

In the later years of the decade, a male clothing staple became more than just an undershirt—now it was called a T-shirt and worn by both sexes in lieu of the outer garment that had hidden it from sight. T-shirts served another purpose, becoming "walking billboards" decorated with pictures, slogans, and ornamentation of all kinds. The T-shirt individualized the wearer in a "pop" culture where finding untried avenues of true individuality was becoming more difficult. Another off-beat fashion trend was the short-lived rage for *paper* clothes. This devil-may-care fashion peaked in social events for the elite, like "Paper Balls"—where everyone could wildly follow their imaginations and create disposable "costumes."

Men who shied away from indulging in the laid-back antics of their younger counterparts adopted an Indian-style Nehru jacket with high collar, button front, and no lapels. Although the Nehru jacket fad was roundly ridiculed, it did help to instigate a push toward more relaxed clothing for men in work and social situations. Turtleneck sweaters caught the fancy of men tired of button-down shirts and constricting neckties, even for more formal occasions.

This decade heralded the emergence of an accessories genius whose timeless and innovative designs continue to enchant three decades later. Judith Leiber, known as "the bag lady from Budapest" has consistently added twenty-four or more new handbag designs to her collection *four* times a year, helping her to earn the first Coty Award for accessory design. That one individual is able to keep the creative juices flowing with such dynamic results year after year is a tribute to her training and fertile imagination. It is no surprise that major museums have added her "works of art" to their collections. "One of her first big successes in the 1960's was a black satin envelope with rhinestone handles, which sold for about $40." Three decades later ". . . her jeweled bags start at $800 and go up to $4,000."[7] Priceless Leiber minaudieres have taken on the most fanciful of shapes and designs, from bejeweled animals and mask-like faces to glittering balls of rhinestones and jet with braided silken tassels.

"I have an eye," asserts Judith Leiber, "that discerns things. I don't belabor anything. If I find that a concept doesn't work immediately, it's not worth pursuing. There are too many fantastic ideas out there to waste time on one that's not entirely satisfactory." As it did when she burst on the accessories scene in the 1960s, Mrs. Leiber's inspiration continues to be found in everything around her. Like Poiret and other fashion geniuses, she too observes architecture, paintings and even furniture when contemplating new designs. Workmanship and attention to detail are paramount, and the 1990s find Mrs. Leiber continuing to supervise all aspects of the business, just as she did in the beginning. Harkening back to the great jewelry houses of the 1920s and 1930s, the engineering of the frames and clasps is monumental and painstaking. She designs every frame, makes a wax model, creates a prototype in sterling silver and then transports it to Europe to be cast in brass. Little wonder that each new season is filled with delicious surprises—and that the splendid offerings of Judith Leiber continue to captivate the public decade after decade.

One of the 1960's most revolutionary fashion concepts was the introduction of panty hose. These one-pieced wonders are destined to become, along with jeans, the most indispensable accessory item of the 20th century. Without the ease of pantyhose, women would still be hooking themselves into strap-like contrivances for that daily trek to the office—or dinner on the town. Even some of the "lesser lights" in the decade's fashion picture must be given their due, for many contributed in one way or another to the easing of restrictive clothing.

The fashion "happening" of the 1960s was the overwhelming obsession with *jeans*, that simple pair of trousers in a no-nonsense fabric that had been around for decades became the unisex fashion item of the century. It is, for better or worse, the uniform of our time. While trends come and go, a steady diet of *jeans, jeans, jeans* have become this century's fashion "opiate of the people"—one that has been unfairly assessed as the only real fashion innovation to come out of America. As Kennedy Fraser so delightfully observed in the Seventies, "Unprecedented honor is being given to denim—whose support is already so widespread that a blue haze floats above the pavements of the world . . ."[8]

The Sixties brought us another major fashion influence. As we have seen, reigning heads of state have wielded power when it came to the apparel of their subjects, but never before did the predilections of a First Lady of the United States command so much attention—or exert so much power on fashion worldwide. Jacqueline Kennedy's pillbox hats, Chanel suits, elegant ballgowns, and even casual clothing, enabled women everywhere to share in the magic of haute couture, a mystique that would continue long after the tragedy in Dallas. The fashion sense of Jacqueline Kennedy, launched in the aura of "Camelot," brought to the ordinary woman of ordinary means styles that were copied and reworked for the "ready-to-wear" trade as never before.

From granny dresses, love beads, beehive hairdos, and mini skirts to restrained millinery, understated suits and coats of impeccable tailoring and design, the 1960s were a frenetic roller coaster ride. "It need hardly be said that the sixties opened a lot of floodgates. After that, everything came pouring down: wide skirts, slim skirts, short ones and long; jeans and running shoes one day, teetering heels the next; trousers in every imaginable shape and length . . . Everything and everyone moved back and forth in a single tapestry that constantly unraveled and re-formed. Everything was in style and yet nothing was. Here was freedom or chaos, depending on your point of view."[9] In short, fashion had much to say, and probably said it as successfully as in any previous decade.

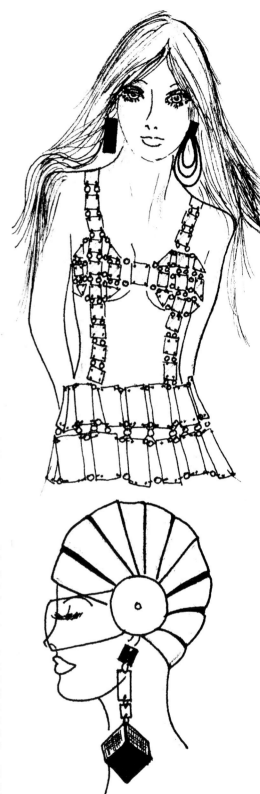

1960-1970
[1] Getting it On: The Clothing of Rock 'n Roll, p. 183
[2] Fashionable Mind, The, p. 242
[3] *Vogue*, September 1, 1963, p. 173
[4] *Vogue*, September 1, 1963, p. 169
[5] *Vogue*, September 1, 1963, p. 165
[6] Historic Costume, p. 275
[7] The New York Times, December 18, 1990
[8] Fashionable Mind, The p. 91
[9] Fashionable Mind, The, p. 241

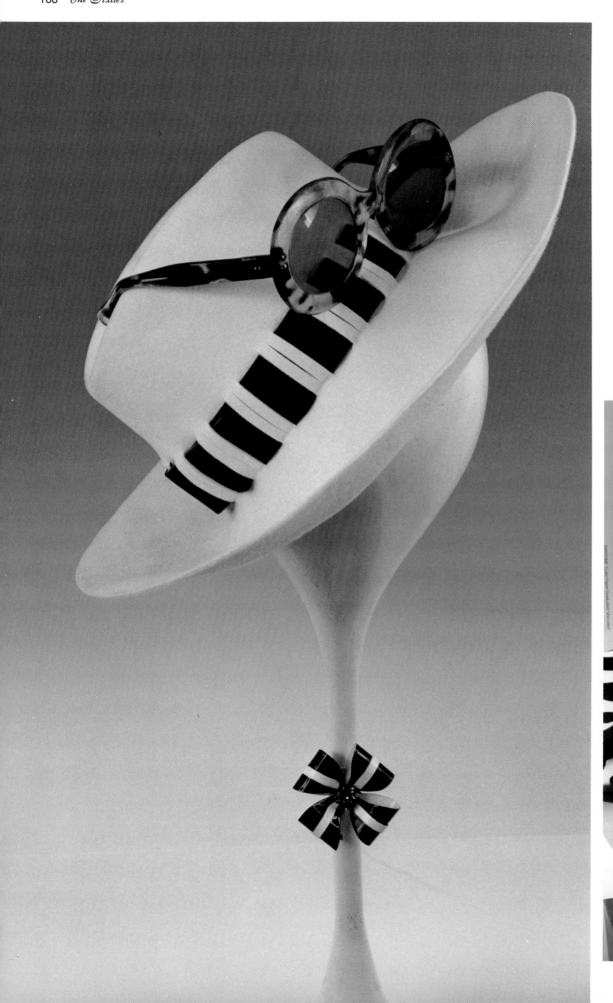

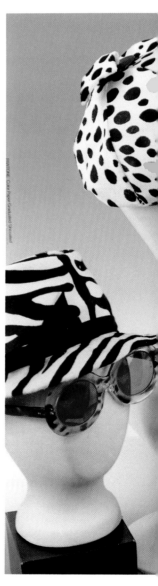

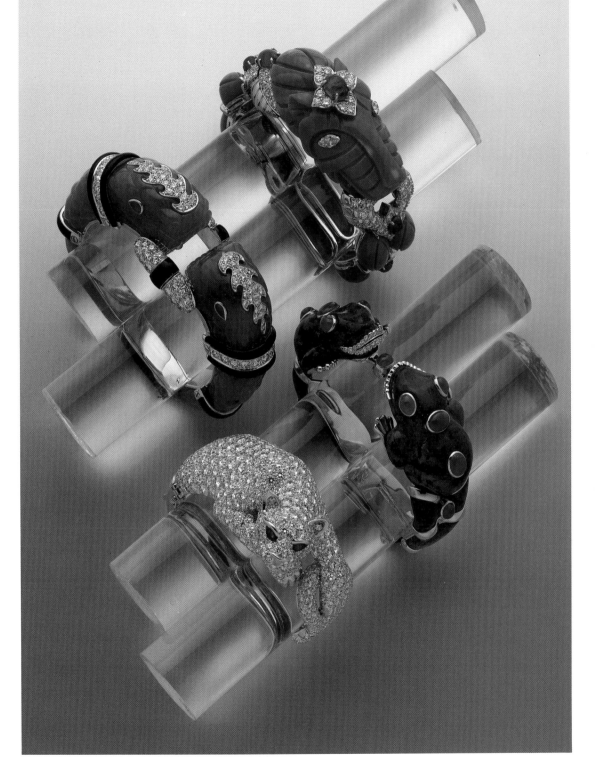

The magic of David Webb.

Yves Saint Laurent hats courtesy of Magi.

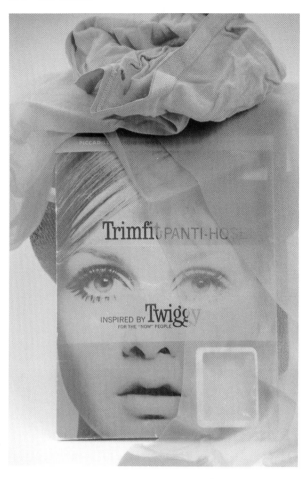

Twiggy Pantyhose for the "now" people.

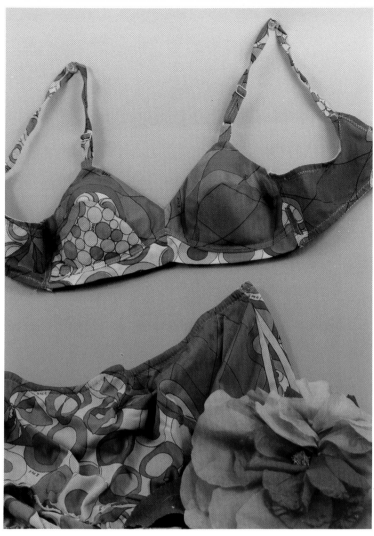

Pucci Amore!

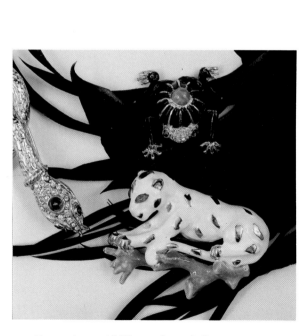

The predators. All KJLane pins and all
ominous! Collection of Rosalind Becker.

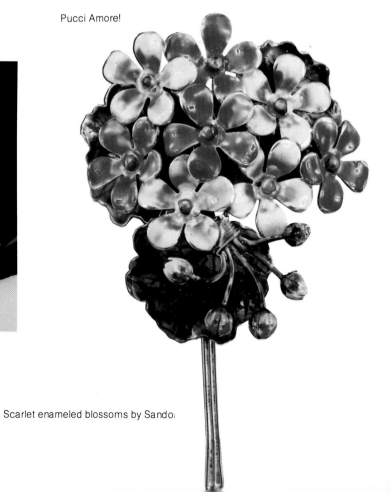

Scarlet enameled blossoms by Sando

Flower Power

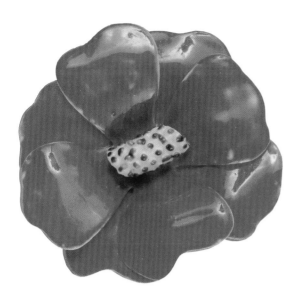

A colorful enameled flower by Robert.

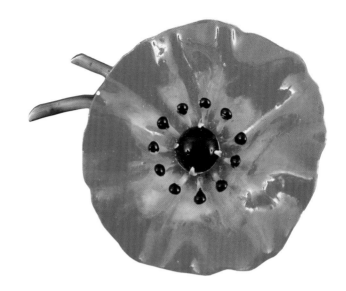

a Robert Original.

A real charmer...this Josephine Baker
pin of Bakelite and base metal by
Sandor.

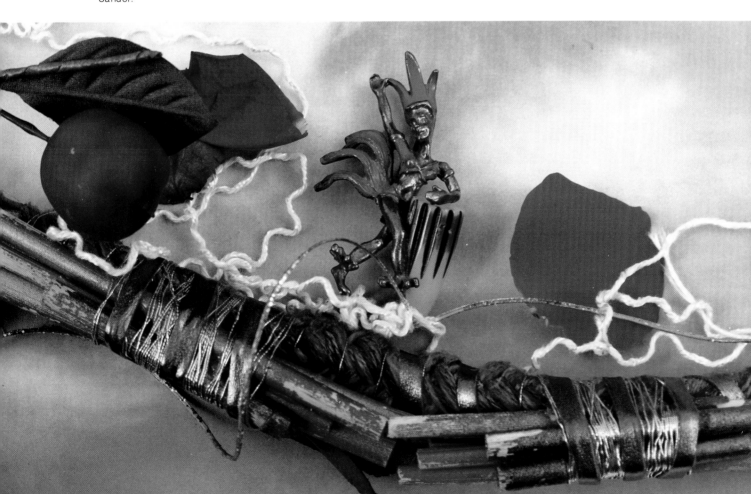

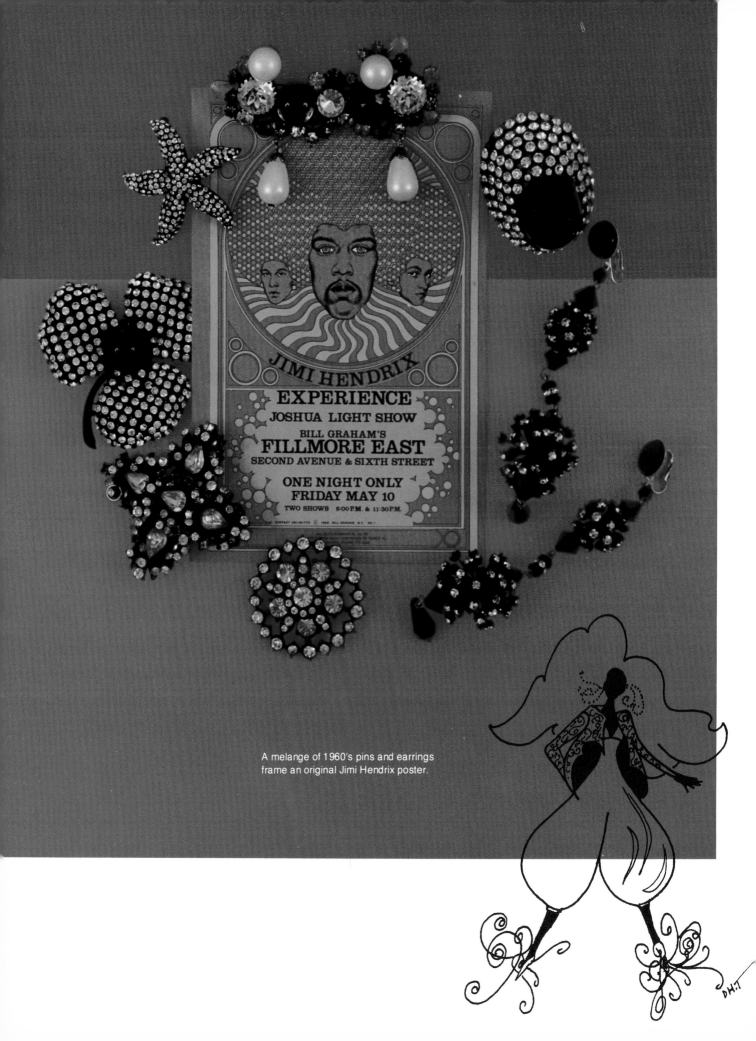

A melange of 1960's pins and earrings
frame an original Jimi Hendrix poster.

In the Shops and on the Avenues

Vogue, January 1961:

"Jewelry in the space race now. This pin, a projection into the highest oval yet, all air and arcs of fake pearls, sapphires, and turquoise, raised about 1-½ inches from the silvery base. By Marvella, $35.

"In the small-and-telling-touches department: a saucer-sized disc of a hat, tipped over one eye . . . a pair of evening slippers with squared-off slender toes and small undershot heels . . . a handbag of lengthy dachshund proportions in a supple leather . . . a tasseled necklace, long enough to knot like a scarf."

Vogue, September 1, 1963:

"Each with the brilliance of an Oriental jewel, sari-silk evening purses in ruby, emerald green, sapphire blue, pearl, and ebony. Handmade in India . . . $12.00."

"A pair of flowers for the hair in a shimmer of ebony-black feathers shaped to evening poinsettias; comb attached. $9.50 each."

"From Italy—hand-knitted mohair sweater with a pebbly look and a big harlequin collar. $22.95"

"White kidskin boots—this year's knockout Courreges signature exquisitely made and fitted. Worn with white leather hat, white leather gloves, the shortest tweed skirts—and the prettiest knees in the world."

"Topping the autumn season; the jacket look, marvelous in . . . down-soft two ply cashmere with braided edging and platter pearl buttons. $40.00."

Vogue, February 1, 1964:

"And, at the very first blush of suntan, we'll reach for some big, bubbly marbleized beads in pink, red, and magenta—stack them high at the neck of a maillot-seamed princess in heavy dead-white pique."

"Wear taupe gloves as pale as white dipped in tea, small narrow-strapped shoulder pouch in green-taupe brown, and naked walking sandals—two broad taupey-beige lizard straps and a lacquery stacked black-leather heel. This is the shoe we'll see walking across the country."

"More than ever, U.S. fashion is on Chanel's wave-length; now it's Chanel right down the line—from the top of the head (rounded, bowed, bangs) to the tips of the fingers (in a short glove—her long, narrow eighteenth-century sleeve has made the one-button glove right as rain again) to the toes (soft and dark, surrounded by a sling of really naked-looking kidskin; stockings of the same pinky beige). All, deliriously pretty and sexy with one of those brawny Chanel tweeds . . . Very correct hang to the jacket, short skirt with a cloche-like slide over hip, lots of action at the hem—couldn't be better."

(British) *Vogue,* December 1967:

"Shades of Sarah Bernhardt and Cleopatra . . . fabulous golden jewelled bracelets twisted into shapes of snakes and leafy trees and legendary beasts. From the new Ken Lane boutique . . ."

"Where the rainbow ends . . . in a scintillating silk striped lame boot, sharp green and gold acid orange red . . . Coffee crepe pump . . . with a gold-orange band of glitter glass beads . . ."

"Razzle dazzle on platform '68 . . . Charles Jourdan's spectacular new evening shoe elevation, platform soles starred with high voltage rings of rhinestone. . . . Black crepe sling-back . . . a fling back to the jazzy tango days of Rogers and Astaire with a Ritz-sized rhinestone buckle, rhinestone rim, and great crepe bow . . . Spinning with glitter, strapped and buttoned with the prettiest pair of diamante flowers . . ."

". . . Three ruffled roses in the hair, all purest white . . . Translucent swinging frond earrings . . . Gossamer glitter white tights . . . slim white crepe shoes . . . Entrancing fragile flowered pierrot . . . Pearly pink voile dress sprinkled with snow and nothing more than a tiny top, a line of little covered buttons and fabulous full pantaloons gathered in at the ankle . . . with the prettiest pale leaf brown and pink periwig in full bloom and matching flowers in ravishing ruffs round throat, arm and ankles. By Jean Muir.

"Luxury by Chanel . . . Reflected like stars from an Eastern night sky, a magical cavern of jewels reflecting Chanel's new inspirations from Siam to Samarkand. Scintillating stones the size of phoenix eggs, almost the real thing—turquoises, sacred river pearls, a ransom of emeralds and pigeon's blood rubies encrusted in gold and turned into star-studded brooches, into flowers and crosses like military orders . . . all handmade in Chanel's workshops . . ."

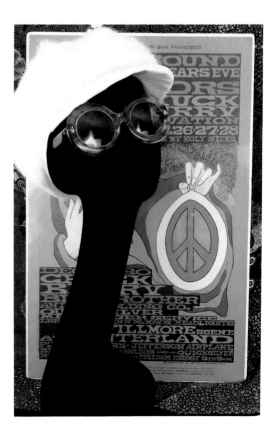

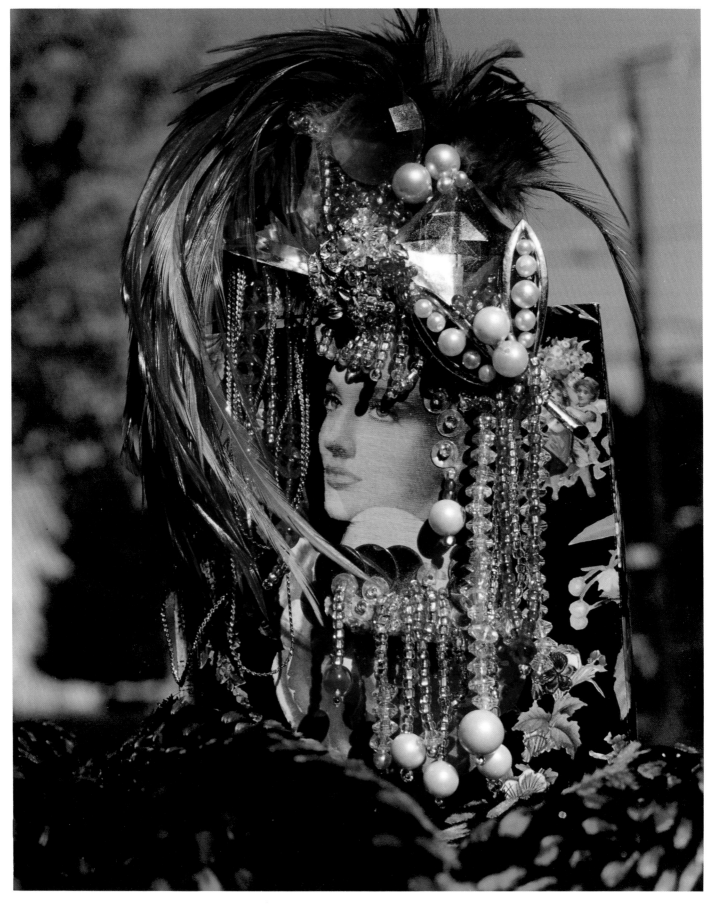

Believe it or not! Like a stately Ziegfeld
girl, a decoupage pin that has absolutely
everything.

The Seventies

"ELEGANCE HAS NOTHING TO DO WITH 'GOOD TASTE,' BECAUSE THE DEFINITION OF GOOD TASTE CAN BE A PRETTY ELASTIC AFFAIR, ABOVE ALL WHEN ONE IS SPEAKING OF FASHION."

Marcel Vertes

Where fashion was concerned, the decade of the 1970s can perhaps best be described as a "hodgepodge" of "something old and something new, something borrowed and all askew." If the fashion bandwagon of the 1970s seems merely a rerun of the 1960s, it is most likely because the "beat generation" was now ten years older and had, understandably, become a tad more conservative.

In describing fashions of the 1970s—and what she aptly called a look of "comic elegance," Kennedy Fraser in an article in *The New Yorker* noted that they were, in some respects "...a complete expression of nostalgia for the sixties.... The fashion tone of the sixties generation prevails in a modified form ... and has shed its original restlessness and frenzy."[1] James Laver expressed much the same opinion when he noted that by the 1970s "...fashion began to look over his shoulder for inspiration, just as after World War II."[2] It was an understandable development, for, with U.S. involvement in Vietnam and the chaos of protests, the 1960s could surely be classified as turbulent times.

In 1971 Yves Saint Laurent, with just such an "over the shoulder" look, added a touch of drama in fashion by basing his collection on the Forties. An article in the November 1983 issue of Harper's Bazaar referred to the decade as "...a particularly dramatic time for fashion in general and for Saint Laurent in particular." The Saint Laurent "look of the Forties" collection "... was naughty and spicy; lots of leg was unbared as dozens of almost brazen-looking mannequins strutted down the runway smoking cigarettes and looking unabashedly sultry."[3]

Far from the houses of haute couture, a personal war was taking place—this time in the lowly gymnasium. This was the war on fat, and it marked the beginning of a health and fitness craze that appears to be a never-ending pursuit. Running, walking, jogging, exercising all require special gear—at least most of the participants prefer to think so. There were loose-fitting jogging outfits and tights for the gym. For outerwear, bomber jackets of leather and suede were seen everywhere, as men—and women—emulated those rugged fellows of several decades back.

Man's companion, that willful young girl of the 1960s, was now a woman in her thirties—or older. Consequently, for a more mature look, some fashion items from the decade before were merely revamped in dressier leathers, luxurious suedes, shiny, wet-look nylon, and bold prints. In accessorizing, *big* was *better*. There were wide studded belts, large handbags, oversized sunglasses—many in the cat's eyes, harlequin shape—and even a continuation of the 1960's body jewelry that literally covered the wearer's chest from neck to waist. There were wide, glittering "dog collar" necklaces and enormous bibs of faux jewels complemented by big, dangling earrings. "Big" shirts, which were later to become a classic, actually made an appearance in the 1970s, but considering that oversized was such a hot ticket, it's surprising that although young people enjoyed parading around in this version of daddy's clothes, women failed to whole-heartedly embrace the look until the following decade.

The coats that had flopped around one's ankles in 1969 were simply shortened an inch or two to mid-calf as the decade began. Regardless of the direction that couture wanted to take them, women, almost en masse, rejected the midi-look. As reported in a *The New York Times Magazine Section* in 1971, "... Now that the furor over hemlines has died down, it's time to have fun with fashion ... to wear a skirt that demurely covers the knees one day, a dress that grazes the ankles the next ... If you like hats wear one that's big brimmed and important. Add strappy shoes ... It's the attitude that counts. And don't worry what men say about not liking the new styles. They always follow the free spirit."[4] Funky accessories, like real rooster feather earrings, kept the legacy of the Sixties alive, but at the opposite end of the accessory spectrum items like folding lorgnettes in tortoise or jet with glittering rhinestone trim also garnered attention.

A note of defiance crept onto the scene—just as it had in other forms a decade or two before. Short shorts called "hot pants"—and worn by teenagers and mothers alike—made their rather shaky appearance in 1971, along with gaucho pants and a plethora of knickers. Fashion ads for 1971 featured evening knickers—a strange "pants dress," sometimes of filmy, printed fabric with bands of smocking that fit tightly on each leg below the knee. Other styles were in traditional plaids for a sportier, daytime look. Wide, bell-bottomed pants appeared everywhere and added a comically nautical look to slacks and jumpsuits. Even the bikini underwent modifications. This time it was the string bikini, which certainly deviated from the "big" look that dominated elsewhere.

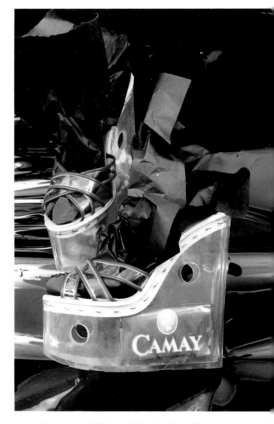

Outrageous! "Pop art" for the feet. The platform shoes to end all platform shoes.

Although music had graduated to punk rock and spawned a trend to wild hairdos, with clothing to match, there was a respite from such frenetic activity in the easy, uncluttered look of many major designers. The British revived the ambiance of the "Romantic period" with camisoles and petticoats replete with lace and flounces. There was renewed interest in cameos and dainty, Victorian jewelry, creating a dichotomy between the "glitz" and the "demure." All in all, the mixed messages in fashion of the 1970s created a new direction. "Individuality did not mean, as in the Sixties, the adoption of a complete look which was itself individual, but arrival at a personally individual style of dressing."[5]

Early in the decade, sweater dresses became enormously popular, and in 1974 soft knits were found in accessories, as well. Especially popular in luxurious mufflers. "... they were around the neck of every mannequin in Paris ... long angora ones, terry ties ... Every outfit had its little knitted glove. Its knitted cap, knitted hat or a soft slouchy felt ..." And for further insight into the fashion scene of Paris 1974, *Vogue, European Ready-to-Wear* goes on, "With pants: tasseled moccasins, Oxford ties ... not a boot in sight ... Belts very narrow ... Bangles luxe, tactile ... ivory, ebony; gold and silver mixed in rows ... Pearls all over the place ... long strands mixed with gold chains ... still lots of rhinestones, still kitsch, but everybody is tired of it."[6]

The T-shirt lengthened into a dress, much in the "granny" tradition. Peasant dresses returned, although not as shapeless or unfeminine as their 1960's counterparts. Opaque tights and patterned pantyhose in bright colors replaced standard nylons, especially when they became part of the layered look, with tights in one shade, above-the-knee stockings of another color on top, clunky shoes or boots with thick heels, and over all, a baggy overblouse billowing around a very short skirt or skimpy shorts.

In many respects, the "girl-woman" of the 1920s seemed to be making a comeback, but on closer look, she didn't emanate the same aura of self-assurance her mother had been so comfortable with 50 years before. The fun of the flapper was lost in this woman of the early Seventies, for the message just never meshed with the clarity and determination shown in the 1920s. Although "... we once adored Courreges's brilliant gaiety; virtually the same ideas now seem clashingly inopportune."[7]

Tired of fashions that failed to inspire, the 1970's woman turned to at-home clothes to assuage her dissatisfaction, just as in decades past. Robes of fleece and quilting were a mainstay of many wardrobes. The working woman popped into one at the end of a busy day, and some were even suitable for at-home entertaining. Long, loose-flowing caftan, palazzo pants with wide bottoms that gave the appearance of a skirt, and even evening pajamas with a sensual 1930's look in sleek prints and bold patterns, were welcomed for their soft, easy appearance and, even better, all were acceptable for evening wear both inside the home and out. "Dressing up" also became a much-needed diversion. Long dresses, and separates like elegant blouses and flowing skirts, were worn not only for formal entertaining and parties but also for informal social occasions and dinner at one's favorite restaurant.

As always, the ever-faithful "classics" never faded from sight—simple Chanel-type suits of luxurious fabrics, carefully tailored coats and, as in the 1960s, furs—both real and fake. The sensuous Pucci undergarments in beautiful prints remained popular. Even makeup got an overhaul of sorts. "The face is treated as a canvas, to be painted with craft and boldness. This trend includes, among extreme exponents, the use of makeup as fantasy and costume and, more moderately, as a visible accessory."[8]

There's always a flip side. This one found some women drawn to a more masculine look, involving fabrics like grey flannel and pinstripes previously reserved for men's clothing shops. For the most part, however, there remained a feminine softness in what could easily have appeared overly masculine if presented with a sterner hand. To complete the outfit, little neckties wound under blouse collars, and berets, some with that old standby, the cockade, complemented the look. A 1971 article stated that "... The hat is gaining because it is an accessory rich in potential comedy, with a wealth of past examples to copy, and because some degree of historical horsing around is by now a necessary element of fashionable dress,"[9] Nevertheless, just one year later *Paris Vogue* reported that, by and large, the covered head was "dead," and hats fell out of favor on a bigger scale than in any other decade. Nonetheless, thanks to Karl Lagerfeld, that element of fun glimpsed earlier in the decade returned in the Fall-Winter of 1978 for, as "W" reported, "... Lagerfeld will show whimsy, tongue-in-cheek elevator attendant hats with chin straps in everything from red patent to black suede ... He is also thinking of piling up junk jewels, which he calls 'theatre jewels' because of their stage proportions. On a day suit, he will pin brooches with paste stones the size of golf balls."[10]

On the more conservative side, the mid-decade saw the emergence of a fashion happening that persevered, in one form or another, throughout the remaining decades. It was the "preppie" look—which later transformed itself into the "yuppie" syndrome when those "preppies" became middle-aged adults. This major trend, which has continued unabated into the 1990s with only minor refinements and variations, was personified in a down-to-earth clothing catalogue from a long-established Maine company named

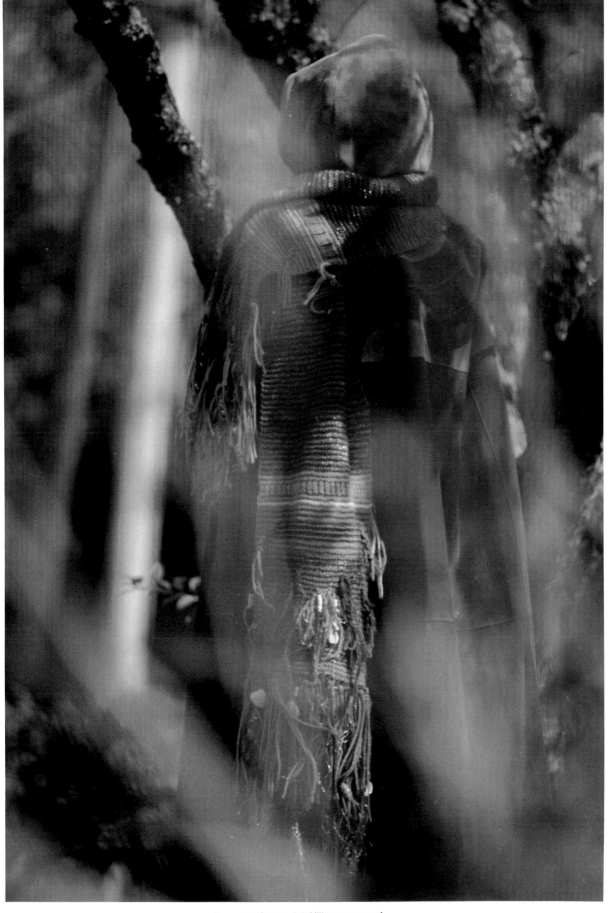

From the Greenwich Village scene of
1970, handmade capes with a
companion hand-knit scarf, replete with
genuine turquoise, shells, and beads.

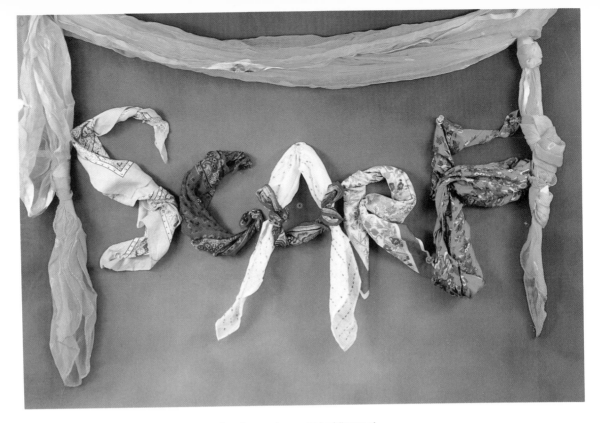

A melange of scarves by Liberty of
London, Echo, Courreges and Ralph
Lauren.

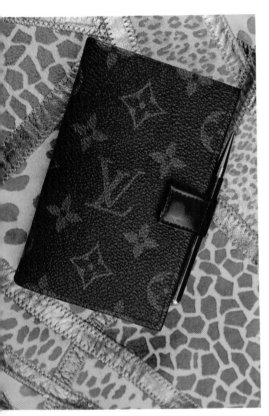

Louis Vuitton address book.

L.L. Bean. From the standard pink and green colors that became the "preppie" flag to the Fair Isle sweaters and rubber "duck" shoes, a new era of fashion comfort had captured the imaginations of both sexes. It melded the simple popularity of the casual cowboy look that intrigued the horsey set in the 1930s with the understated needs of a new breed of "up and coming" suburbanites.

This return to more casual dressing played an adjunct role in the major downturn in accessorizing that began to occur during the 1970s in the fashion jewelry market, building momentum into the mid-1980s. Since early in the century, the popularity of costume jewelry had steadily increased, until by the 1960s it was a burgeoning industry that could barely keep up with the demands of women for "something new and different." However, although big, showy pieces appeared on fashion runways in the late 1970s—and even couturiers like Karl Lagerfeld had the daring and foresight to feature rhinestones with sports clothes, an idea ahead of its time by a decade or so—such sparkling innovations would prove to be one of fashion jewelry's last gasps . . . at least for a while. The "patient" wouldn't be resuscitated until the mid-1980s when a long-overdue appreciation of the imagination and skill displayed by those pioneers of the costume jewelers' art brought about a welcome resurgence of interest.

In the meantime, the death knell was sounding, as world gold prices began their astronomical ascent. Suddenly, there was a frenetic interest in 14-carat gold among the masses who had previously favored the more dramatic, and far less expensive, costume pieces. Their reasons were, for the most part, misadvised. Purchasing simple gold chains and other ordinary items of gold did not constitute an investment in the gold market. Nevertheless, starting then and continuing well into the 1980s, women flocked to department store jewelry counters for supposed bargains in *real* gold and, not to be outdone, males of all ages began hanging chains of gold around the necks of their leisure suits or open collared shirts. Gold chains, separately or in groups, seemed to hang from every neck and wrist.

"There were, of course, that ever-present and vast number of women who refused to be tied to a fashion statement that was, for the most part, not a statement at all. Indeed, the statement was—at least for them—mute! They felt that unless one had enough money to purchase jewelry with heavy links of 14-carat gold or bold and elaborate pieces with gold and gemstones, few outfits would be complemented by what could only be referred to as a smattering of 'ditzy' gold chains, barely discernable to the eye. But . . . enough women chose the path of insignificant gold pieces to send the industry reeling."[11] Many long-standing businesses were forced to close their doors, and others suffered major losses that it took a decade or more to undo.

To add to the disruption, the 1970s were somehow determined to depart kicking and screaming, for one or two fashion pluses seemed to warrant a surfeit of questionable others. By 1978, the layered look had, as might be expected, overdone itself. It was time for bulk, with layer after layer piled one on top of the other. There were buckled leather cummerbunds, leg warmers, and heavy textured pantyhose that tried, unsuccessfully, to appear comfortably correct with strappy sandals.

In welcome contrast, designers like Oscar de la Renta gave fashion glamour a boost in 1978 by featuring some truly breathtaking designs—like down parkas for evening in glorious, stained-glass color combinations. Two years earlier, Saint Laurent did it again with a potpourri of sumptuous designs and accoutrements—like colors ablaze with the look of brilliant gemstones and full skirts that came to mid-calf. There were even embroidered boots and passementerie trims—an ornate, peasant costume feeling. It once again had women breathless, rushing to change their entire wardrobes.[12] Another designer must be given his place of honor, front and center. The gentleman, who deservedly earned the title of the "celebrity" designer, was born in Indiana as Roy Frowick, later known simply as Halston. He personified the elegance and clean lines of his classical, sought-after designs, designs that remained timeless even decades later.

This was the decade that didn't quite "find itself." With the exception of those who slavishly followed haute couture, it is small wonder that most women, who instinctively sensed a fashion conspiracy, revolted and refused to buy much of anything. At least in America, the accepted styles remained generally conservative. Women were understandably baffled—and it showed.

In Paris it was another story. There was a voluminous amount of fabric in just about everything, with a return to capes and shawls and boots with high, high heels. The obsession of French women for these fashions made them appear as "...ankle-wobbling creatures that teetered down the more fashionable streets of Paris like columns of khaki-colored pup tents. This looked suspiciously like the old fashioned, slavish sort of fashion—the delight of cartoonists, the despair of husbands, and the key that unlocked some dark lunatic impulse even in normally sensible women."[13] By 1979, Paris designers were showing coats with football-uniform shoulders and gigantic puffy sleeves, long plaid shawls, and variations on the always faithful Chanel-type suit.

Foresaking all others, if only one item was called upon to signify the fashion "contribution" of this confusing time it would surely be pants suits—and above all, the *polyester* knits of which there were made. A sea of synthetics appeared on ready-to-wear racks, with row upon row of polyester dresses, bell-bottomed slacks, skirts, matching blazers and shirt jackets. Most in bold, multi-hued patterns. Like it or not, polyester was here to stay, but it's unlikely we will again see the fervor or excess of the 1970s.

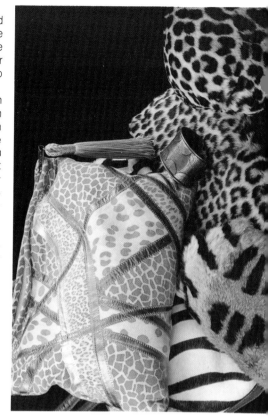

Lisandro Sarasola patchwork jungle suede animal printed leather...over the "real" thing.

Shades of the Twenties...wing tips of the Seventies...and a leopard skin bow tie.

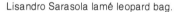
Lisandro Sarasola lamé leopard bag.

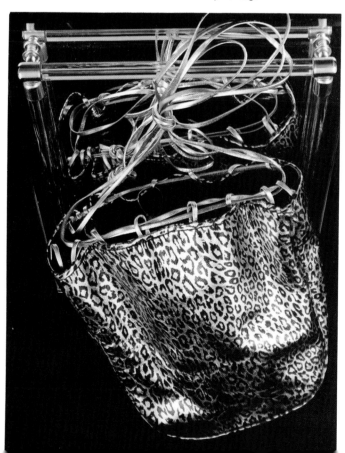

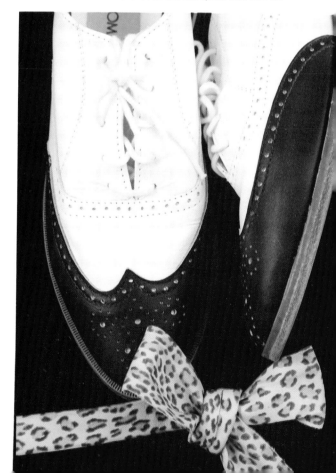

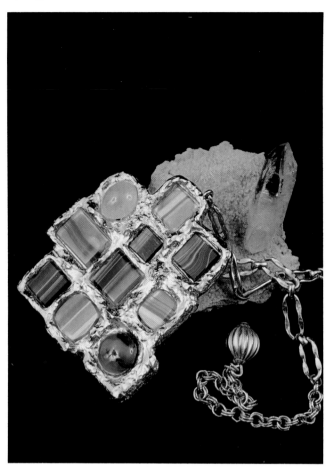

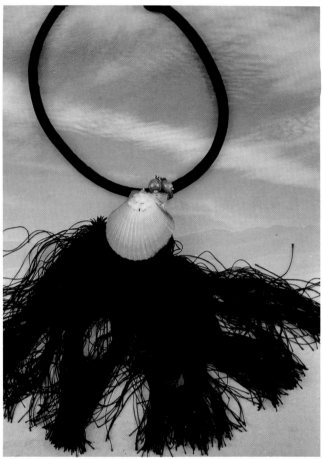

Roughing it with subdued stones and rocks...an unusual KJLane pendant. Collection of Rosalind Becker.

Pariseinne designer necklace of coral and shells with black silk fringe.

The bib to end all bibs. This Selro piece has strands of colorful beads and big multi-hued stones encapsulated by intertwining dragons.

Beaux Jangles . . . Imported from India. A necklace of iridescent glass beads and faux pearls.

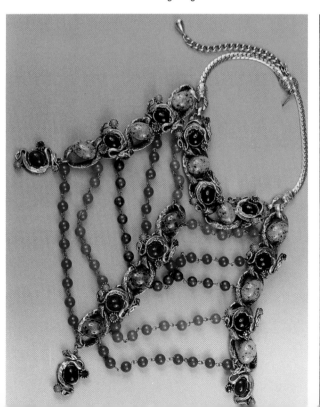

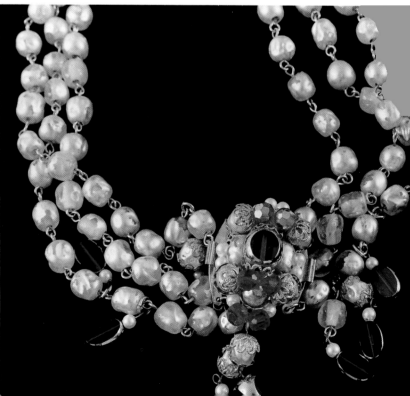

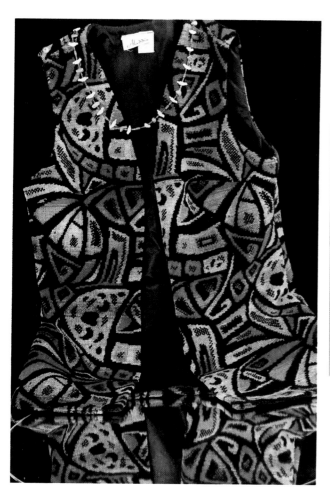

The Seventies' version of the '90s
"grunge" look!

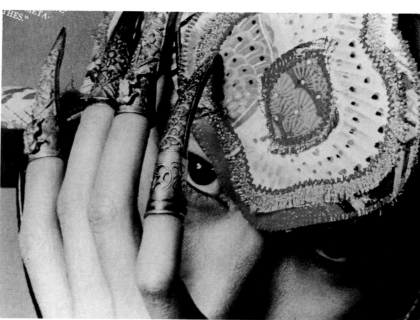

A serpent hood by Kai Sik for Muuntox is
all decked out in Mandarin nail shields.
Harper's Bazaar, 1972.

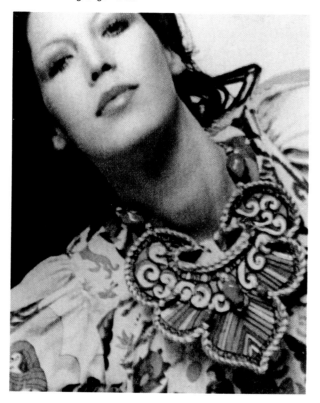

From *Harper's Bazaar*, 1972. An
unbelievable necklace by Lee
Menichetti.

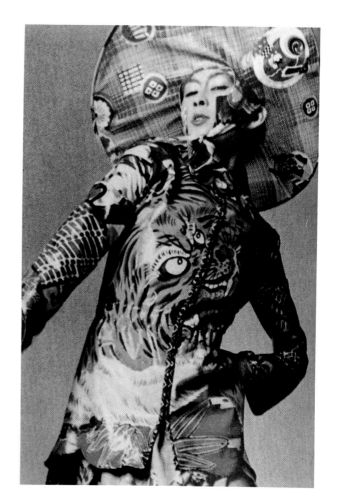

From *Harper's Bazaar*, 1972. Kai Sik for
Muuntox.

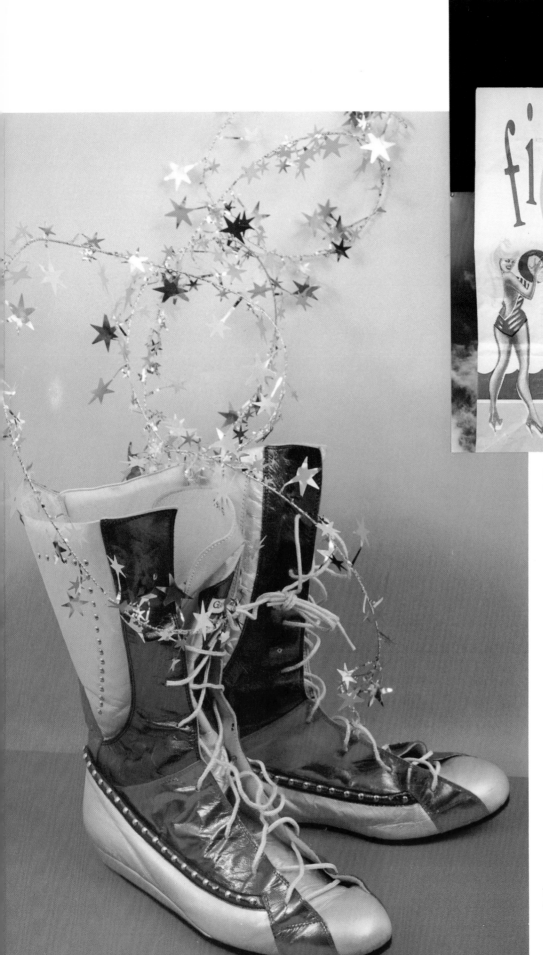

A priceless Fiorucci shopping bag...with detailed "shopping tips" close-ups.

Very Hot Italian! Multo Via Veneto. Courtesy of Magi.

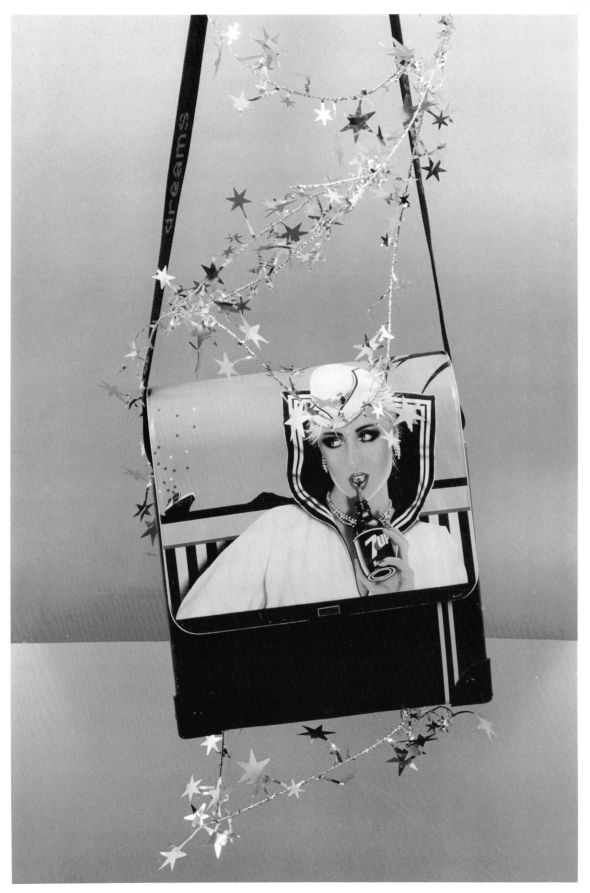

Explicit Fiorucci. Hot summer days and
cool summer nights! Courtesy of Magi.

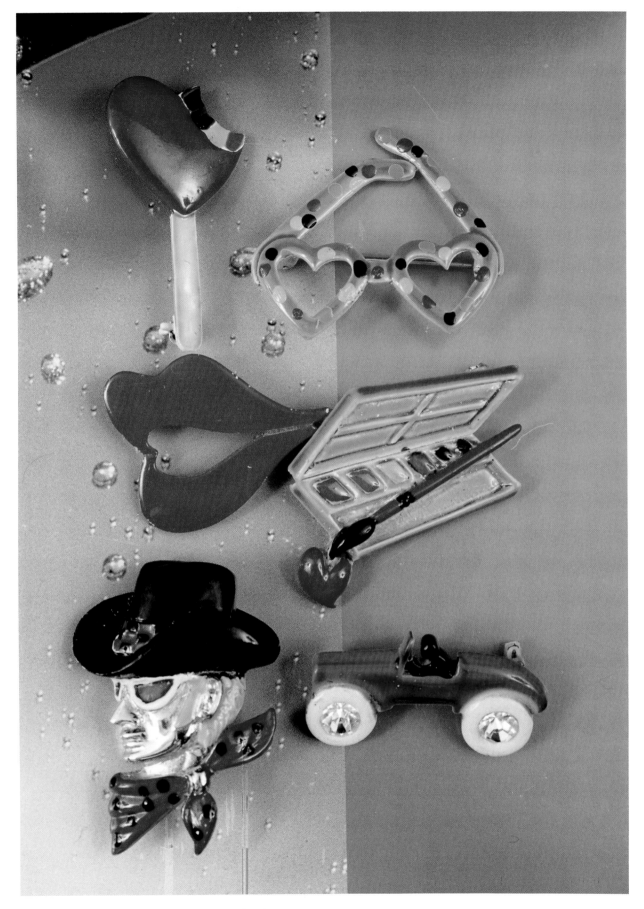

The Sixties aren't dead...they're alive
and well in the Seventies...with hot rods
and kisses!

Harper's Bazaar, January 1972:

"Canvas pants with removable bib which snaps at the waist. Rope suspenders, side lacing. With hand-painted storyboard cartoons."

"The Camelot necklace . . . is a versatile linked adjustable metal chain made with either an antique bronze or pewter finish. A chased design gives it a medieval look, and moveable links allow it to double for a belt . . ."

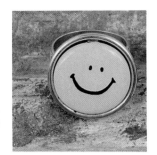

Vogue, August 15, 1972 ("The New Accessories—Night and Day"):

"Soft shiny black satin around the neck, silky black fox muff, and pearly bangles around the wrist—wonderful look with a long bar dress at night."

"the black satin envelope for evening—basic . . . and a natural with ivory satin, K.J.L.'s fake diamond-linked crystal bracelet . . ."

"Fashion essentials: soft ties, mufflers . . . shiny at night. Flat chains, big specs. The bag of the year—the soft, flat envelope."

"The narrow belt, the narrow watch mixed with bangles, pearls, wooden beads, tortoise, crystal. Everything warm and natural . . . texture you want to touch."

Harper's Bazaar, December 1973:

"A single seashell, wrapped in sterling silver, with a link so you can wear it on a chain—or rest it on a table as an oceanic object d'art. $50. By Kenneth J. Lane."

"Envelope bag. Slim. Suede. Sealed with a golden Gucci 'G'. $85. At Gucci."

Harper's Bazaar, December 1974:

"Cinderella Slippers."

"A crisscross of rhinestones . . . a see-through pump of clear vinylite with a narrow band of rhinestones along the edge, criscrossing the toe, and a slim silvery heel."

"A band of silver mesh . . . just a band of silver mesh, a silver kid sling back and heel . . ."

"A gleaming rhinestone buckle . . . The barest—a simple strapped sandal of all-clear vinyl, except for a buckle of rhinestones, a sliver of silver kid heel . . ."

"Cinderella rhinestones . . a classic satin evening pump completely paved with rhinestones . . . sensational. And to give your legs a sexy, silvery gleam—Christian Dior pantyhose."

Vogue, August 15, 1974 ("European Ready to Wear"):

"Speaking of mufflers, they were around the neck of every mannequin in Paris . . . long angora ones, tiny ties . . . every outfit had its little knitted glove. Its knitted cap, knitted hat or a soft, slouchy felt . . . With pants: tasseled moccasins, Oxford ties . . . not a boot in sight . . . Belts very narrow . . . Bangles luxe, tactile . . . ivory, ebony; gold and silver mixed in rows . . . Pearls all over the place . . . long strands mixed with gold chains . . . Still lots of rhinestones, still kitsch, but everybody is tired of it."

Harper's Bazaar, December 1974 ("Guide and Gifts"):

"Six-in-one ring for almost every day of the week. Hinged dome opens to change the cabochon shaped stones of ivory, tortoise, lapis lazuli, turquoise matrix, apple jade and blood coral colors. Set (ring and six stones), $10.

Vogue, August 15, 1974:

". . . the whole 'thirties-'forties-'fifties thing has taken a long time to die but when the trendy, super-looking girls like Marisa Berenson begin to be seen in easy, straightforward, classically simple clothes, you don't have to be hit over the head to get the message: the masquerade is over. Just as we've seen it happen in America, fashion here has come to life . . . real life."

1970-1980
[1] Fashionable Mind, The p. 166-167
[2] Fashion & Costume, p. 268
[3] Harper's Bazaar, November 1983, p. 157
[4] The New York Times, Fashions of the Times, February 28, 1971
[5] Fashion & Costume, p. 276
[6] Vogue, European Ready-to-Wear, August 15, 1974
[7] Fashionable Mind, The p. 9
[8] Fashionable Mind, The p. 20
[9] Fashionable Mind, The p. 57
[10] "W" March 31-April 7, 1978 p. 30
[11] Costume Jewelers The Golden Age of Design, p. 49
[12] Marian McEvoy Brandsma, Harper's Bazaar, November 1983
[13] Fashionable Mind, The p. 121

Resplendent on a Louis XIV chair,
Robert Lee Morris art wear transports us
to other times, other places...and into the
future.

The Eighties

"NOTHING SUCCEEDS LIKE EXCESS."
Oscar Wilde

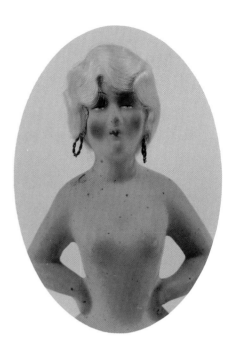

From just about any vantage point, the 1980s must be viewed as the decade of excess, and with this excess came a surge of indulgence in high-quality, high-ticket items, ranging from luxury penthouses and automobiles to what we wore and the accessories to complement them.

Names were everywhere and on everything. Yves Saint Laurent even had a cigarette brand with his famous YSL logo on a high-gloss designer package. These designer identifications and labels assumed more importance for more people than ever before. Just as that hip patch on a favorite pair of jeans or the pocket patch on a comfortable shirt became status symbols, so did the names associated with more extravagant purchases. The odds had shifted, however, for more people could indulge in items like Rolex watches, Gucci shoes, Chanel handbags, Hermes scarves, and status symbol items *ad infinitum*. There were, of course, other "goodies" like diamond "tennis" bracelets or even a bauble from the Duchess of Windsor's collection at the Sotheby auction.

The early years of the decade ushered in another round of interest in the Southwestern look, with its muted shades of turquoise, tans, and corals. The "horsey," countrified look was back—if it had ever really left—and to satisfy that plain, old cowboy instinct, there were elaborately tooled Western boots and belts, along with variations on the big cowboy hats, giving us the sophisticated cowgirl and cowboy from head to toe. These buckaroos may not have "made it" on a ranch in the old West, but they sure looked great on Fifth Avenue or Main Street, U.S.A.. Indian jewelry in bold designs, like those found in chased belts of glittering silver and squash blossom necklaces, was also high on the list of "must haves."

Ralph Lauren, with his gentrified "Polo" logo, elevated sportswear and casual clothing to "400" status. His boutiques were aimed not only at the society set but that vast majority of consumers who simply wanted an element of sophistication mixed with their day-to-day endeavors. Whether it's polo or tennis—or a stroll down Rodeo Drive—Lauren continues to provide something for everyone. One may not be "to the manor born," but he manages to imbue his offerings with an ambiance that has much to say in defense of "understated elegance" for every day . . . of every year. Lauren was in tune to the needs of the 1980s, and with an uncanny sense of timing created a casual yet lush world that the privileged and not-so-privileged could enjoy when they pushed open those shiny doors of Ralph Lauren's *Polo*. From a different angle, Calvin Klein brought the "lowly" blue jean to designer status, intermingling the formerly simple jean fabric with liveable, easy designs in a host of sportswear and accessories items . . . but, above all, generating a worldwide frenzy for a pair of "Calvins."

From straightforward and simple to quilted and designer inspired, down coats and parkas wrapped their occupants as few coats had before. This look complemented the skiing craze that went schussing out of control as "singles" searched for weekend and vacation playgrounds, and families strove to extend their "quality" time. This updated look required "special" accoutrements for that "special" impression. From just the right skis, to just the right jacket, gloves, hat, and sunglasses, everything was important. The sun didn't just reflect off the hard-packed snow—it also reflected the chic image of the skiing enthusiast as he or she whizzed down the slopes. With a "Tyrolean" Swiss Alps look, the short, boiled wool jacket was another fashion that seemed "just right" for the times, especially since it fit so well with the longer skirts and boots. It was a fashion that would continue, with variations, throughout the decade and into the next.

The first half of the 1980s also saw soft leathers in skirts, coats, belts, bags, and gloves. There were ponchos as big as blankets, high boots, wide-waled corduroys, and bulky knits in sweaters and coats. Skirts reflected a myriad of lengths, ranging from above the knee to ankle-length pants-skirts with wide bottoms. There were argyle knee socks, brightly colored pantyhose, pearls, little ties at the neck, and soft shoes that were light on style but heavy on comfort, except for the high, slip-on mules for evening.

Although there were exceptions, especially in couturier lines, truly exciting accessories seemed to take a "back seat" in the general fashion picture early in the decade. The look was tailored, conservative, and somewhat boring . . . with a tentative, almost insecure air about it. By mid-decade, however *big* was back—along with all the bold, fun, and assertive baubles that represented. As the Eighties progressed, accessories were once again "front and center." There was lots of jewelry, with arms covered with bangles, some with a medieval look; large, flat-brimmed hats; gold-chained designer handbags; and big disc and hoop earrings. The strength of names like Gucci, Cardin, and Chanel continued unabated, in both fashion and accessorizing. With a theme of Persian opulence, evening

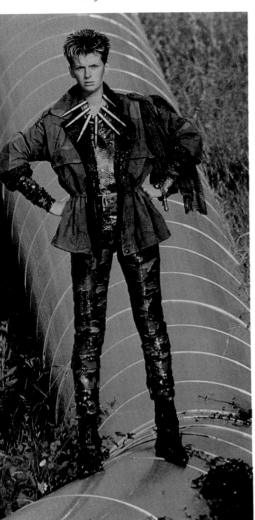

Early Jean Paul Gaultier...chain mail, feathers, sequins, mesh...and boots!

brought us satins, silk taffeta, heavy brocades, and jeweled belts. From Milan came the ever-popular Italian knits. Paris fashions included leather suits by Yves Saint Laurent, ankle-length skirts, jockey caps, and countless variations on those little short jackets. Above all, the large, mass audience had become more intrigued by the message of designer fashions. "In the Eighties, the mystique of couture evaporated. Women knew more about cut and fabric than at any time since World War II, and every woman was well equipped to design her own look."[1]

The artistic philosophy necessary to achieve that *look* was well represented in Paloma Picasso's eclectic sense of color and creativity—displaying, in another realm, the bold genius of a Picasso masterpiece. Mirrored in her designs for fashion accessories, as well as decorative accents for the home, are the imaginative images that come to mind when she observes, "Accessories should reflect classicism as well as a sense of timelessness."[2] Much of what has endured in fashion of this century, and Picasso's contributions to this art, mirror just that—a return to the past, a firm rooting in the here and now, and an imaginative look to the future.

There was another important adjunct to the feel of the 1980s—one that seemed to grow and grow. The decade saw an astounding increase in the popularity of antique and collectibles shows, including those featuring vintage clothing, jewelry and other accessories. Magazines on antiques, as well as periodicals to keep the professional in tune to the market, and also to whet the appetite of beginners, enjoyed tremendous popularity. Although stores were crammed with an endless array of new merchandise, the public also yearned for a taste of nostalgia. There was not only an interest in fine antiques, but a deepening appreciation for items that "smacked" of quality, beauty, and superior workmanship but were only 20 or 30 years old—like jewelry, perfume bottles, and dressing table items. "Collecting" became a national mania, and was heavily represented in what people wore and the accoutrements they chose to have around them. It all had a direct impact on fashion and accessorizing, with many upscale department stores and boutiques promoting special sections devoted to baubles from 20, 30 or 40 years ago. Although "big" jewelry was everywhere, as in previous decades, the Victorian and Art Nouveau influence remained popular, especially for collectors and those who felt a special bond toward those less frenetic, more gracious times.

Hand in hand with antique shows and upscale antiques and collectibles magazines and periodicals came a boom in the business of auction houses, both large and small. In fact, "In one fantastic fortnight in early May (1989) in New York alone, more than $670 million worth of artworks and objects changed hands..."[3] Collecting and investing in the antique market was in its heyday, most likely reaching a greater level of interest and, mort importantly, a broader audience than ever before.

As women's place in the work force grew, so did a revitalization of "dressing for success." Although the look of the Seventies had been subdued and somewhat unisex, a more relaxed, feminine attitude pervaded the Eighties. Happily, there was a "surfeit of goodies," not only in the variety of styles but in the brighter, more feminine colors. The result was an ambiance of renewed individuality in lieu of the copycat "uniform" look that many females on various rungs of the career ladder had considered necessary in their "dress for success." This reversal called for bolder jewelry and accessories, creating a more self-assured look than women had displayed in the office climate of the Seventies, somewhat like the message her sisters in those hard-driving, career-track movies of the 1940s had flashed on the *silver screen*.

Silver bells and cockle shells. Art wear by Robert Lee Morris.

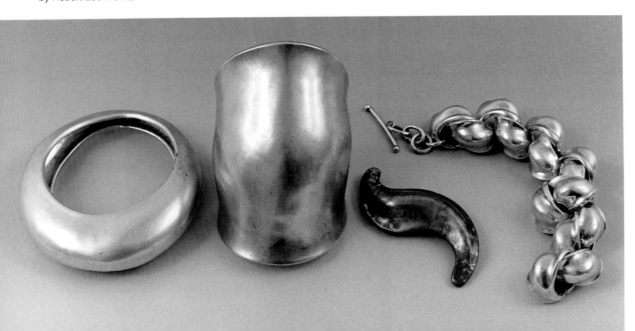

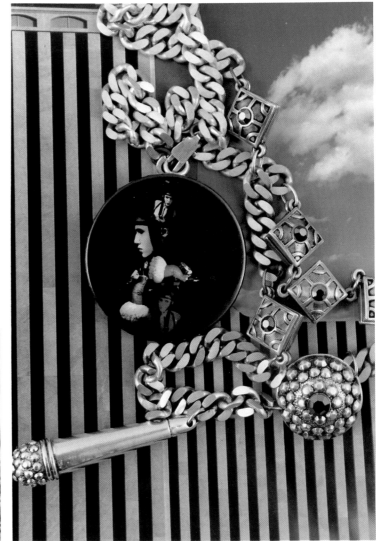

Necklace and pin-back button by Jean Paul Gualtier—the "cutting edge" of the '80s.

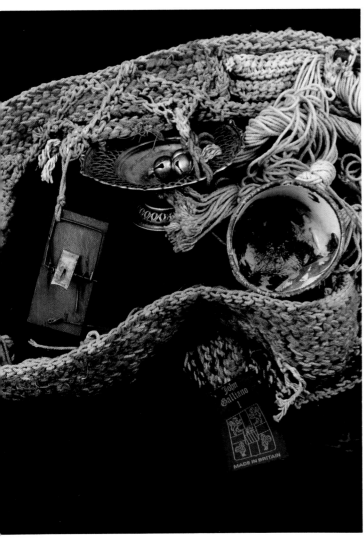

"Build a better mousetrap"? England's John Galliano already did, with this "mousetrap" belt . . . not to be worn by the squeamish!

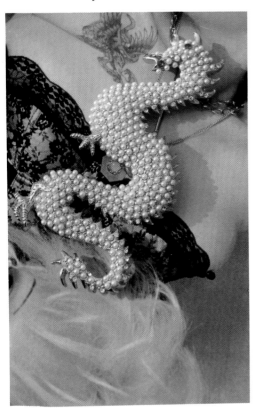

Could this be "Puff the Magic Dragon"? Richelieu brooch, model by Keith Cerio. Courtesy of Herman Gold, President, Richelieu.

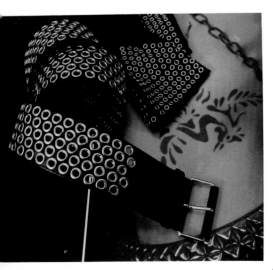

Azzedine Alaia belt and gloves, both of studded leather.

In discussing executive dressing in an August 1986 article for the *New York Times Magazine* "Fashion of the Times" section, it was noted that "These are several steps up from the suit, skirt and bow tie uniform of yesteryear. They range from softened versions of this formula to quite racy suggestions that involve body suits, tights, soft suede boots and wrapped and tied skirts." [4] And the article continued, "...a new young customer elite appears to be forming, firm in outlook, open to fresh fashion thinking and most importantly, eager to dress up." [5]

This new life of office-by-day brought about many additions and revisions to formerly straightforward accessories. Handbags were now outfitted with organizers that included business items like calculators, pens, and rulers, along with handy calendar books to record an hour-by-hour rundown of one's busy day, as well as keeping addresses and phone numbers of clients and friends at one's fingertips. Many handbags also contained items that would have seemed unnecessary, and even unthinkable, short decades before—like pocket flashlights, whistles, and even cans of mace—or a firearm! The formerly boring briefcase gained new life and accessory status—somewhere between an elegant, oversized handbag and a business-like catch-all for paperwork—when it was "dressed up" for the female trade in soft leathers and designer-inspired styling.

But in the world of bags, one old favorite became an Eighties' standout. This time the lowly gym bag, usually reserved for high school and college athletics, assumed a whole new persona. With a sleek new image, it was now a duffle bag of sorts, in many styles, colors, and shapes. The fitness craze that had begun in the 1970s had widened into "big business," and now both men and women proudly carried work-out togs like a badge of honor . . . a testimonial to their determination to achieve the perfect body. As they struggled with body building equipment and aerobic exercises, that ugly zippered "thing" that was formerly pushed to the back of a dank gym locker now became an important accessory. Although many fought a losing battle, each strove to put these new fashions on a body that successfully emulated the muscular young man or slim-hipped young woman who paraded down couture runways or filled the pages of slick magazines.

This obsession with body image caused casual clothing to become even more important, with jeans leading the way as they continued their march into denim heaven. Denim fabric continued to fight for respectability in the dressier category, and appeared in a barrage of chic suits and dresses, some in shades rarely seen in yesteryear's simpler designs, and many decorated with studs and faux jewels. There were also sleek jumpsuits and a return to stirrup pants with under-the-foot straps to keep everything tightly in place.

As it had for decades, the influence of the media cannot be overlooked when one is discussing fashion. In the 1980s, however, television played a major role in fashion and dethroned the "place of honor" formerly held by movies, at least so far as dictating fashion via a "screen." Nighttime "soaps" like *Dallas*, *Dynasty* and *Falcon Crest* brought glamour to American—and foreign—living rooms. Kenneth Jay Lane and Joseff "jewels" complemented Bob Mackie and Nolan Miller gowns, and offshoot bibelots like "celebrity" fragrances created a boom for more than just the sponsor's product. What viewers watched in their homes was reflected in what they bought—and wore—next Saturday night. Soft, metallic-look fabrics, including brocades, with a matching look in high-style, burnished jewelry and glittering stones created a whole new genre in the history of motivation for "dressing up."

From the "drawing rooms" of *Dynasty* to the sidewalks of everyday existence, the closing years of the decade saw ankle brushing, oversized trench coats for both men and women. Some sported military-style epaulets, and were in shimmery fabrics of muted pewters and bronze. Fur linings were "in" again, with big fur, or faux fur, collars. Hat styles ranged from flat, broad brims to soft upturned numbers. Fun was everywhere and head coverings joined in the frivolity. Some of those upturned brims were available with colorful plastic buttons or brooch-like ornaments, but if the hat was unadorned, it offered a great opportunity to display whatever "pin-on" collectibles had captured one's fancy.

Above all else, the 1980s should be credited with expanding on—and glamorizing—the look of easy dressing, but this time ease of dress didn't mean just "plain and simple." For "easy" had some dashing surprises—in color, imaginative styles, and dynamic accessories. In short, the confusion was gone. The 1980s became comfortable with what the folks in the Seventies probably had in mind but couldn't quite get themselves "together" enough to wholeheartedly endorse. Soft flowing lines caressed the body, with fabrics to match. Waistlines were cinched with big belts, and crystals and faux jewels glittered like a spectacular light show on ears, wrists, and necks, and added verve and glamour to sweaters, coats, belts, hats, and shoes.

Everything we surrounded ourselves with became an accessory of sorts. Even the umbrella was no longer a simple, uninteresting and solely utilitarian item, regaining some of the importance given it in decades long past, for the 1980s saw a revival of the umbrella as a complementary accessory. Fabrics were of lush designs and brilliant prints, and handles were eye-catching works of art in fanciful shapes of unusual materials like frosted lucite. No longer to be folded and hidden in a desk drawer or shoved in the office closet, these hearty rain protectors also became a personal reflection of the "carrier."

In much the same way, luggage graduated from utilitarian to designer-inspired, with all manner of coverings, from Oriental tapestries to butter-soft leathers. Travel for both business and pleasure increased tremendously in the hectic Eighties, as both sexes rushed from home to airport to destination and back. It was understandable that whether "checked in" or "carried on" most placed great importance on this luggage of the 1980s for, as with other appendages, these pieces became an adjunct to one's individual fashion "imprint."

Few if any accessories, however, can claim to be more personal or revealing than eyeglasses—and their "offspring" the "always important, never be without" sunglasses. Eyes are reputed to be the "windows to the soul" of the individual. It's a long journey from the type of eyeglasses first written about in Confucius' time to those made *au courant* by movie stars and other celebrities of the Thirties and Forties. But for two innovative artists, Barbara McReynolds and Gai Gherardi, it was a short hop. These two Californians, who founded the *l.a. Eyeworks* in 1979, became a vital link in the chain that separated eye glasses from the "prothesis" mentality, thereby catapulting them into the world of fashion. Their marketing strategy may seem strange by the tenets of most standard marketing guides, for they took the supposedly "bad" and turned in into *desirable*. Touring European markets, this "far-sighted" duo asked designers and manufacturers to show them the frames that *didn't* sell. Defying the rules of successful entrepreneurship, they wanted what everybody else *wasn't* buying! The result became a generic optical statement, so to speak, for they took these "orphan" frames, dyed and sandblasted them, and even mirrored the lenses.

But in some instances they, surprisingly, did *nothing* at all. Those plain gold or silver frames of the "older folks" became a hot fashion statement when worn by a beautiful twenty-two year old model. Voila! Suddenly, the face became the focal point . . . the whole face, not covered with the hair of the Sixties. A concept was born, and that concept led to an advertising campaign that continues to receive accolades: *A face is like a work of art. It deserves a great frame. l.a. Eyeworks* has been instrumental in giving the public "great frames" for their faces. They have also become the guardians of many of those sometimes beautiful, sometimes outrageous sunglasses from the past that were unique and individual works of art. Over the years, these partners have amassed an eclectic collection of vintage eyeglasses that have toured the world and been displayed in design shows and museums, most recently in 1992 when the Shiseido Corporation featured their collection at the Ginza Art Space Gallery. It's a "double bonanza," for McReynolds and Gherardi have not only given the fashion world their own "out of sight" designs, but they've preserved those wonderful glasses from the past for all to see and exclaim over.

The car as an accessory? Well, in some instances you might call it that, for they too became symbols of what and who we were . . . and are. Like the luggage we shuffled through airports, and the watch we glanced nervously at as we trudged through those vast caverns and seemingly endless corridors, a Mercedes, BMW, or sleek, high-powered sports car also reflected the "high-powered" man or woman who drove one. Harkening back to media images that tantalized us with an open convertible, and a beautiful young thing with long locks catching the wind, a car can appear to wrap itself around the occupant in much the same way as an opulent fur or satin evening coat. In fact, this young lady could be remembered as "the girl in the red convertible" just as easily as "the woman in the blue satin evening coat."

And so, as that dashing middle-aged gentleman of the 1980s tools down the freeway in a jazzy sports car named for some sleek jungle animal, and we watch him quickly disappear over a distant hill . . . just remember—he'll come into view again at the top of the next rise and continue his fast-paced journey into the unpredictable 1990s!

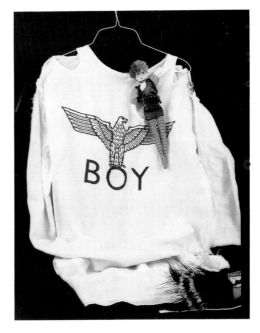

Punk Rock from *Boy* of London...with a handmade punk doll.

1980-1990
[1] Costume & Fashion, p. 72
[2] *Style*, Cable News Network, January 25, 1992
[3] Conoisseur, August 1989, p. 30
[4] New York Times Magazine, Donovan, Carrie, August 1986
[5] New York Times Magazine, Donovan, Carrie, August 1986

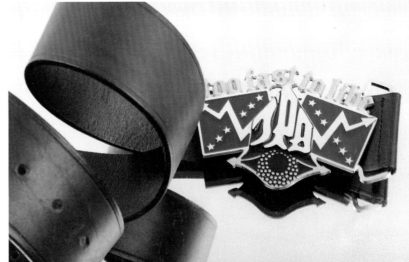

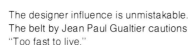

The designer influence is unmistakable. The belt by Jean Paul Gaultier cautions "Too fast to live."

Giorgio Armani

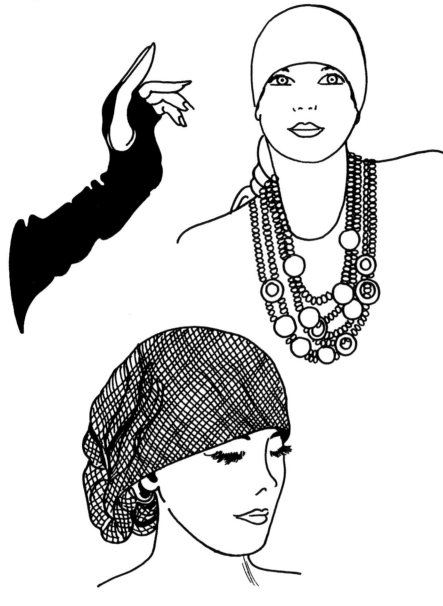

Bulgari

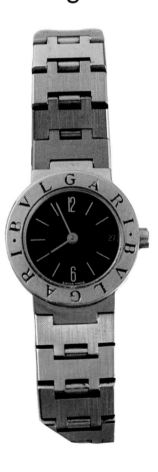

Belleissima!
Italian Fashions

A priceless timepiece by Bulgari.

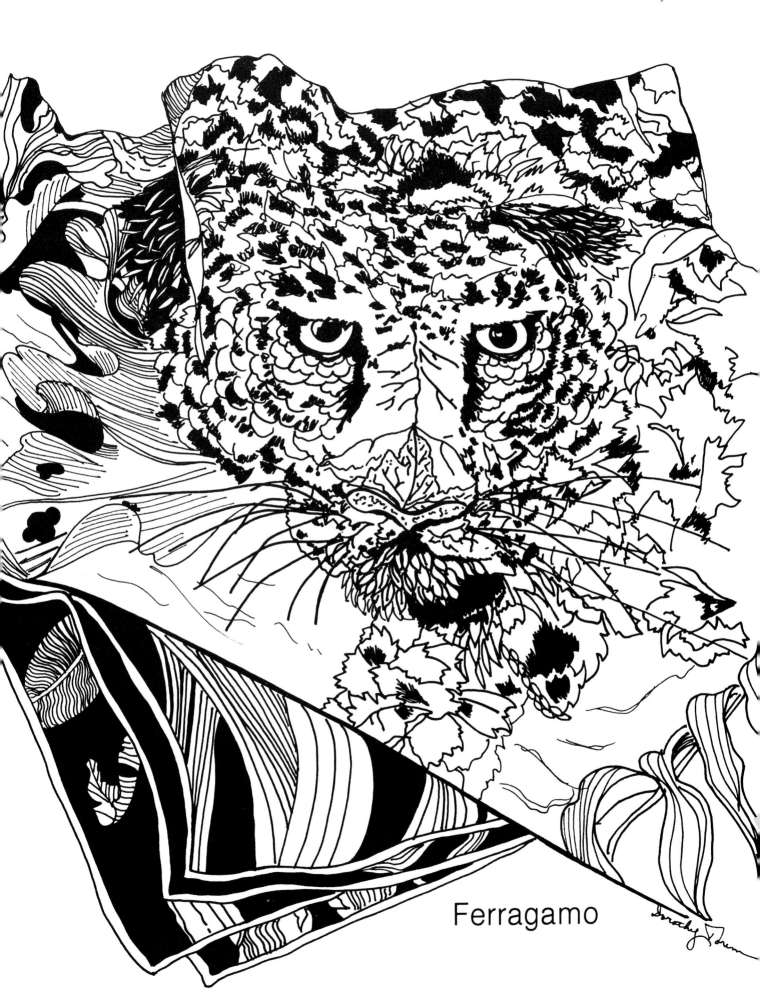

Ferragamo

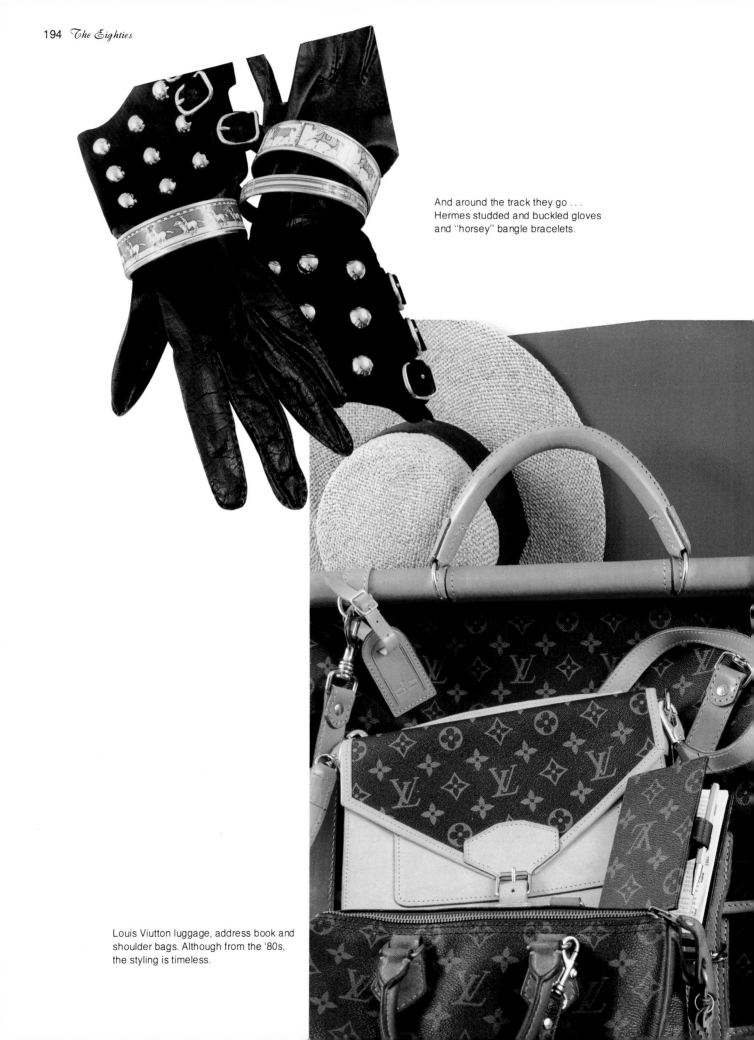

And around the track they go . . .
Hermes studded and buckled gloves
and ''horsey'' bangle bracelets.

Louis Viutton luggage, address book and
shoulder bags. Although from the '80s,
the styling is timeless.

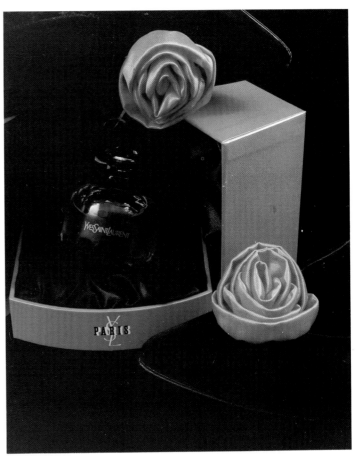

From Paris—YSL perfume adds an exotic touch to panne velvet Yves Saint Laurant shoes, flamboyantly topped with a brilliant red satin rose.

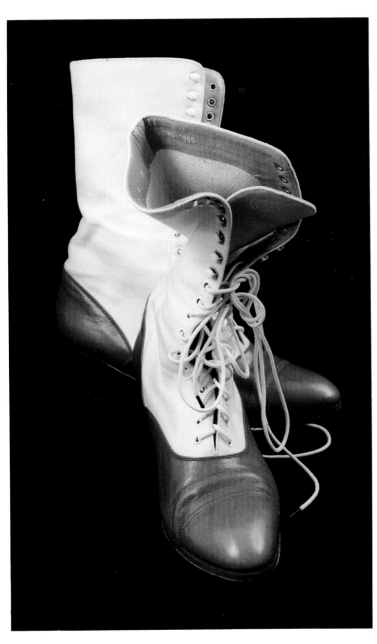

This style of boot keeps reappearing...Classics by Ralph Lauren.

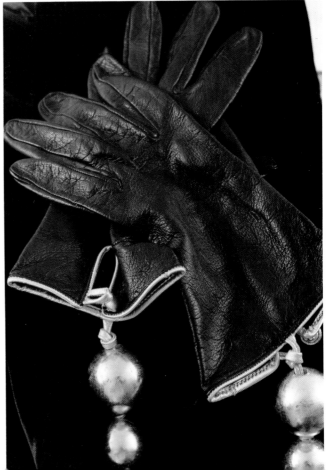

Up close and wonderful! Gloves by Paloma Picasso with gold leaf trim and wooden ball drops.

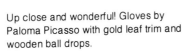

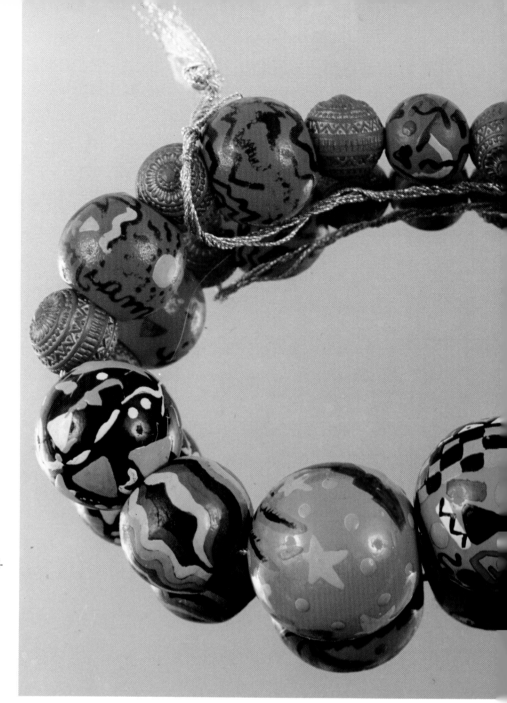

Frenetic. Graffiti style beads in hand-painted "street" jewelry.

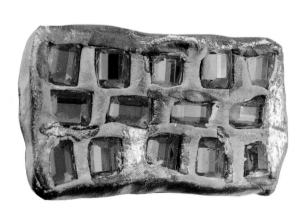

By Billy Boy, a brooch that's a fine example of sculptee, decoupage, New Wave jewelry.

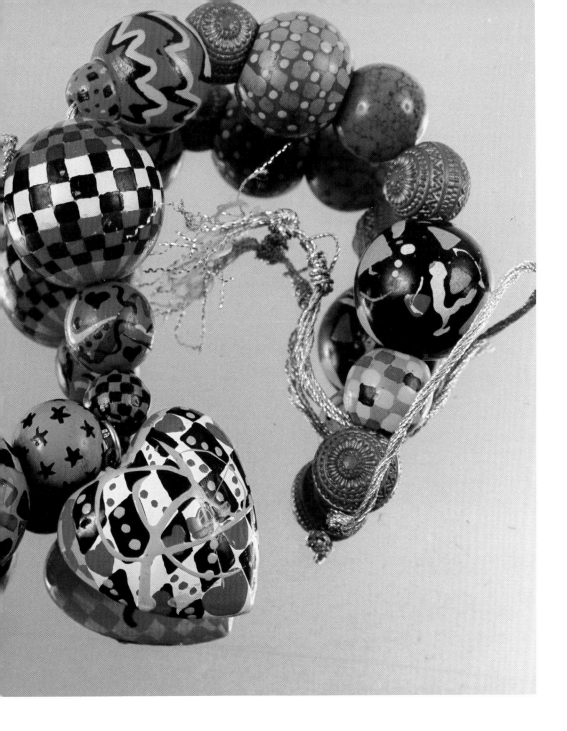

A 1983 neon Artwear brooch by
Japanese artist Sachiko Uozumi.

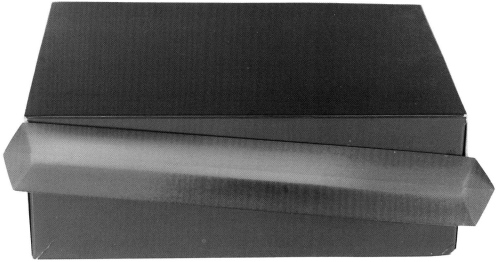

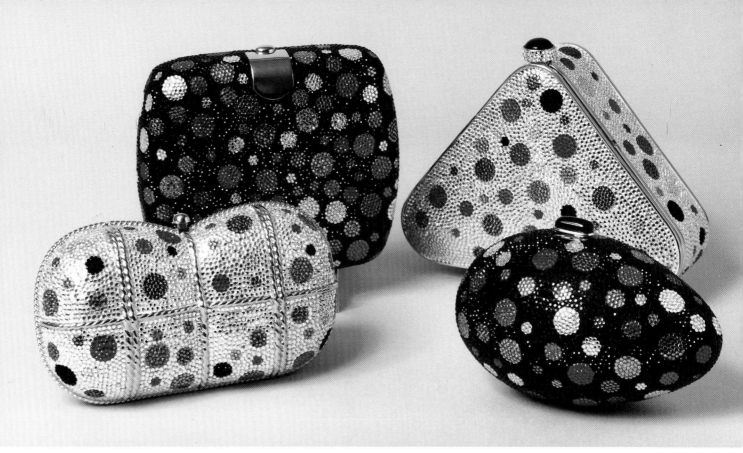

Following the trend of renewed interest in all things Oriental, Judith Leiber presented this glorious Japanese Obi handbag in 1983. Photo courtesy of Judith Leiber, Inc.

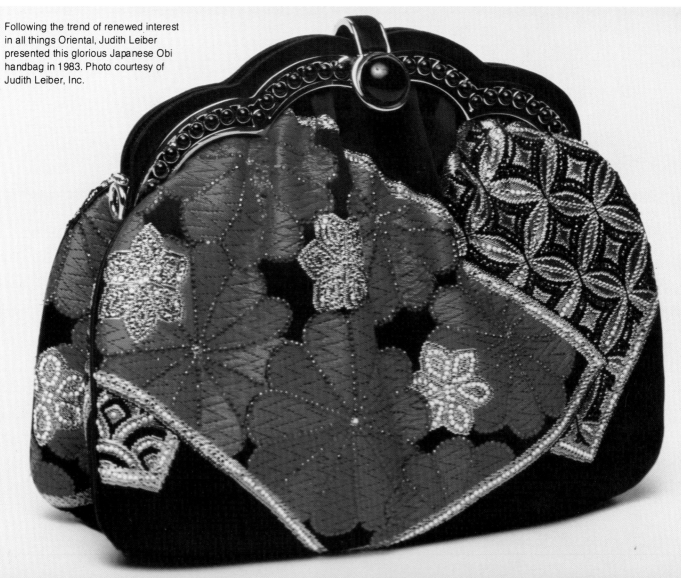

A feast for the eyes, these multi-dot Judith Leiber bags glitter like confectioners' baubles. All but the white triangular one, which is from Leiber's 1991 collection were presented in the 1980s. From 1982, the black egg, the black multi-dot in the left rear appeared in 1984; the white one with braided trim in front is from 1989. Photo courtesy of Judith Leiber, Inc.

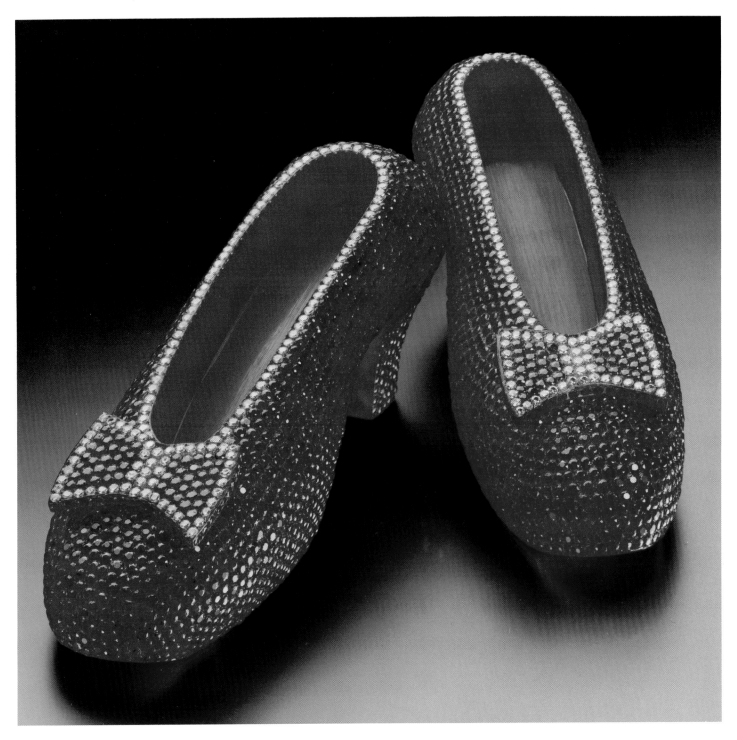

The ultimate "dream accessory," these life-size ruby slippers were designed by Ronald Winston, CEO and President of Harry Winston Inc., to commemorate the 50th anniversary of the classic film *The Wizard of Oz*. It took two months for Winston craftsman Javier Barerra to painstakingly set the 4,600 rubies (totaling 1,350 carats) and 50 carats of diamond trimming into the Lucite base of the shoes. Perhaps if Dorothy clicks her heels three more times . . . well, maybe . . . just maybe . . .! Photo courtesy Harry Winston, Inc.

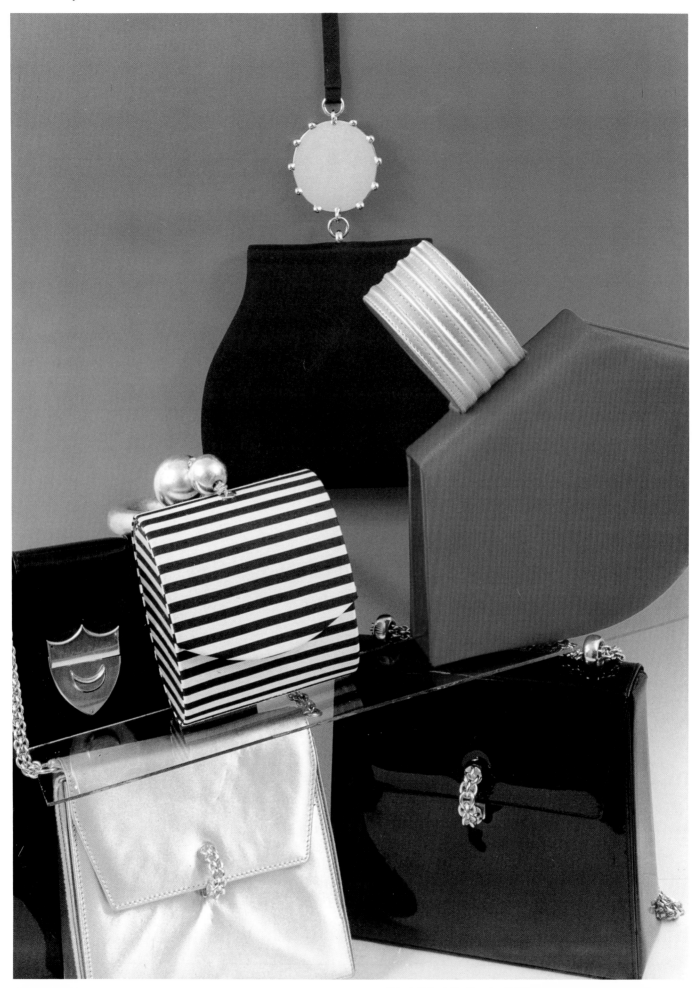

In the Shops and on the Avenue

Harper's Bazaar, November 1981:

"18K gold pillbox in stunning mask shapes—great for storing lip glosses, too . . . $1,500."

"For the class-conscious man . . . let him store his toiletries in Cartier's antique leather-bound case with three lapis-topped bottles. $6,700."

"18K yellow gold antique purse with special compartments for powder, lipstick, lip gloss, perfume . . . anything at all! Cartier. $15,000."

"All the rich, romantic associations we make with gold are poured into the best nighttime clothes right now. Gold is precious . . . it's glamorous, it's sexy, it's hot."

"A fur-trimmed gold jacket . . . or a surprisingly golden duffel coat add something breathtakingly beautiful to basic black"!

"There's something magical about the 18th century . . . he (Adolfo) says. And you can see that bygone grandeur in his signature bows, opulently beaded bodices, the ruffles and lace, the royal colors . . . "

"Precious stone colors . . . in bugle beads and sequins. By Halston, camisole-topped by hip-skimming jacket . . . velvet pants."

"What makes the difference in nighttime dressing are the little things . . . the wonderful new shoes that combine texture with glitter; the jewelry that's nothing less than sheer extravagance"!

Harper's Bazaar, November 1983:

"Far from plain geometry: black ribbed rubber bags, by Pierre Cardin Handbags. About $50."

"Stars are really shining now. The rhinestone star pin by Chanel, about $220."

"This year's perfect pale fur: natural Russian lynx in a notched collar, full length coat . . . about $150,000."

Harper's Bazaar, September 1987:

"Cropped short, outrageously dyed-fur turns razzle-dazzle in these cool-weather jackets and coats." (Turpoise, olive and bright yellow)

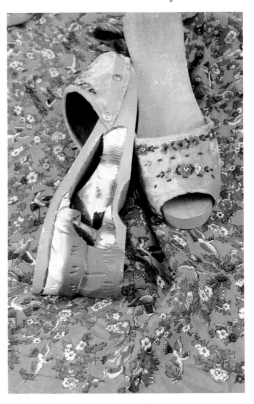

Clogs...with a South American flair.

The exciting neon-like look of acrylic and plastic Artwear pieces, signed and numbered, complement a vivacious 1960's Marilyn Monroe.

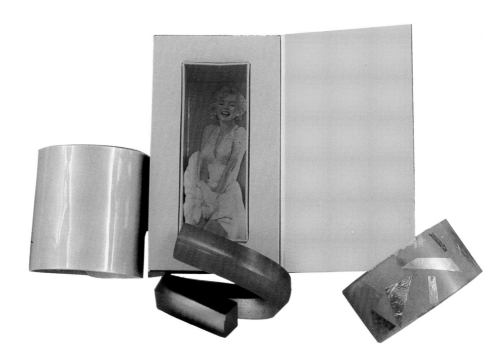

The refined beauty of Paloma Picasso handbags. Courtesy of Lois Lewis; Carole Satmary; Alyson Torem-French.

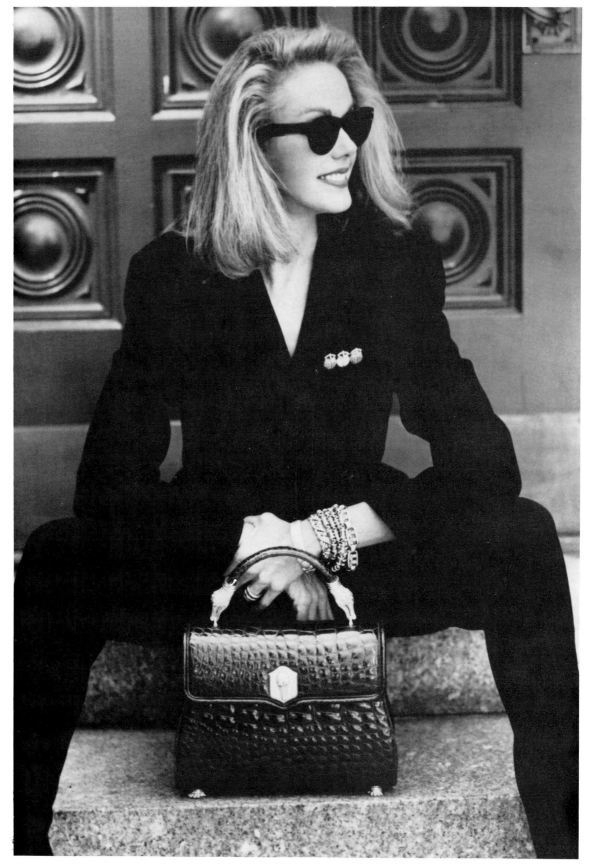

Ce Ce Kieselstein-Cord at rest.
Accessories by Barry Kieselstein-Cord.
Photograph courtesy of Barry
Kieselstein-Cord.

The Nineties

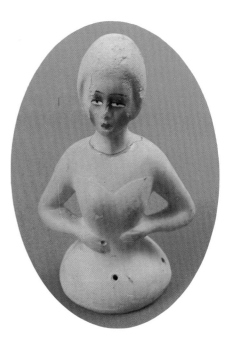

"CLOTHES MAKE THE MAN."
                    Anon
or said another way . . .
"NAKED PEOPLE HAVE LITTLE OR NO INFLUENCE ON SOCIETY."
                    Mark Twain

As we begin our journey through the last ten years of the 20th century, the fashion legacy of the 1990s must remain an "unfinished symphony." Unlike the decades that went before, they cannot yet be synopsized. Much remains ahead of us, and only a few short years are now history.

Nevertheless, the first few years inspired a vast array of dazzling fashions, from snappy and sexy to sophisticated and demure to playful and splashy. *Anything* and *everything* reflected the importance of the individual needs of women and men in all walks of life and all age groups. Probably never before in this century has there been more opportunity to "cover so many bases" for so many people with such diversified tastes.

Collecting and wearing vintage clothing and accessories came into its own during the latter years of the century. Our love affair with the glories and, yes, even those endearing idiosyncrasies of the past, intrigued us, and inspired designers anew. This look of old and new gave the early years of the 1990s a distinctive ambiance. Walk down the streets of any major city and see in a short span of blocks mini-skirted suits with long jackets, big shirts and ankle-length skirts, kelly bags and giant carryalls, decorative hats with upturned brims, or no hat at all, jeans and athletic shoes, sky-high four inch heels, or flat ballerina shoes, short swingy trapeze coats, or long, floppy ones brushing the tops of designer "work" boots, gigantic floral brooches, and understated gold and gemstone pins, arms full of bangles, designer watches, giant hair bows, flashy neckties and preppy knits.

Much of fashion is, after all, a theatrical presentation in both content and style. In the early Nineties, haute couture met that challenge, and in the process provided a tantalizing glimpse of what's just over the horizon, as well as what's "hot" today. Thus far, we've been privy to the birth of a triumphal fashion exodus as the remaining years of the Nineties march swiftly onward—and the promise of an equally triumphal entrance into the uncharted waters of the 21st century. Witness the following:

The early years of the decade continued the strong fashions of the 1980s, replete with jeweled, metallic looks, airy, sometimes see-through fabrics, short skirts and long jackets and big, decorative hats. Couture designs featured footwear that ran the gamut. There were openwork laced-to-the-knees boots, much like those of Roman gladiators, and more feminine versions with giant platform soles and leather thongs laced around the leg. Glamorous mules, harkening back to the 1930s, and wide-strapped and T-strapped pumps and sandals also dominated shoe styles.

In the Fall of 1991, Karl Lagerfeld covered us in reversible furs and an updated version of the "cocoon look" that had wrapped our mothers and grandmothers so long ago. Once again, Paris dazzled with avant garde fashions reminiscent of the space-age look of Cardin. For Spring 1992, Jean-Paul Gaultier, considered the "cutting edge" in "far out" design, brought us the "miracle" jacket with a concealed metal belt that held the jacket open to the waist with no buttons. For Lanvin, Claude Montana ". . . made a strong case for pure, clean, uncluttered clothes that express many people's conception of modern fashion."[1]

Traveling another path, Ungaro featured slim-waisted peplum jackets with puffy, leg-o'-mutton sleeves that enfolded the audience into the romance of Victorian times, and Romeo Gigli's offerings transported us even farther back, with fashions exuding a Renaissance flavor. Bob Mackie, with a sharp eye to the century's end, featured nostalgic styles of the 20th century as worn by its legendary women, with many capturing the big, full-skirted look of the 1950s.

In a modern-day version of the slashed garments of centuries ago, Valentino courageously did the same to hemlines, but with an updated variation, for these folded under, surrounding the hips with large loops of fabric. In sharp contrast, ". . . serious hats and marcel hairdos make the models look as if they have stepped out of an old movie."[2] In his line for Chanel, Lagerfeld also exhibited his playful view of fashion, including ". . . sheer skirts with the hems painstakingly shredded to flutter like straws in the wind."[3]

Indeed, straw found a fashion niche in 1992 that differed greatly from the homespun look of the past. Gianfranco Ferre used decorative edgings of straw or raffia but with a new twist—a quick dip in gold paint. High gloves had straw cuffs, and there were farmer-style hats with shiny lacquer-finished brims. Even the tops of evening gowns were decorated with raffia and wooden beads. By converting one standard fashion item into another unlikely one, Ferre showed real versatility—and showmanship—when he

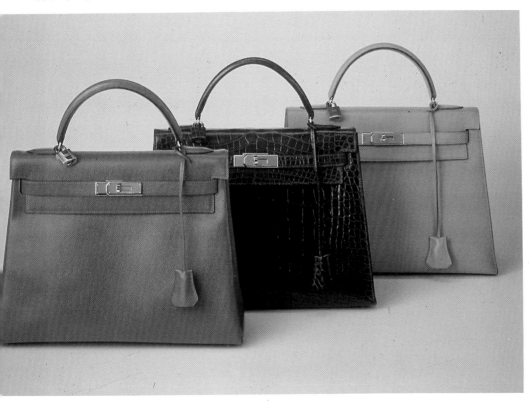

Hermes created these classic designs—Constance, Bugatti, and (Grace) Kelly. The history of the Hermes "Kelly" bag is a long and illustrious one, inspired as it was by a much larger original called a "sac haut a courroie" or "high-handle," which was used as a carrying case for saddles. Third generation family member Emile-Maurice Hermes used the bag to take his saddles on the road to sell to distant kings, tsars and other patrons. Hermes craftsmen later scaled down the proportions to suit a woman's needs, little knowing that it would later become the namesake of a princess. Grace Kelly loved its size and shape and owned many. When she was photographed in the Fifties for *Life* magazine holding little Princess Caroline with one hand and covering her newly pregnant tummy with her purse, the bag was renamed "Kelly" and has been known as such ever since.

Even today, it takes a craftsperson eighteen hours to build an Hermes "Kelly" bag. Cut and stitched entirely by hand, as are all Hermes leather products, each is made from start to finish by the same craftsman, who dates and initials it so that if refurbishing is ever needed, the bag can be sent back to the same careful hands that created it. Photographs courtesy of Hermes.

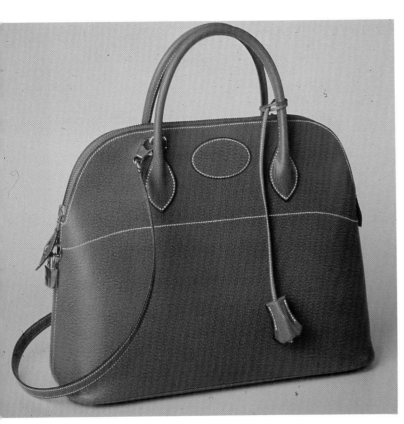

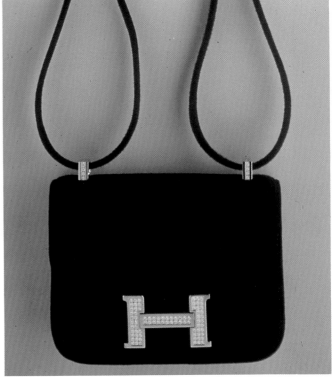

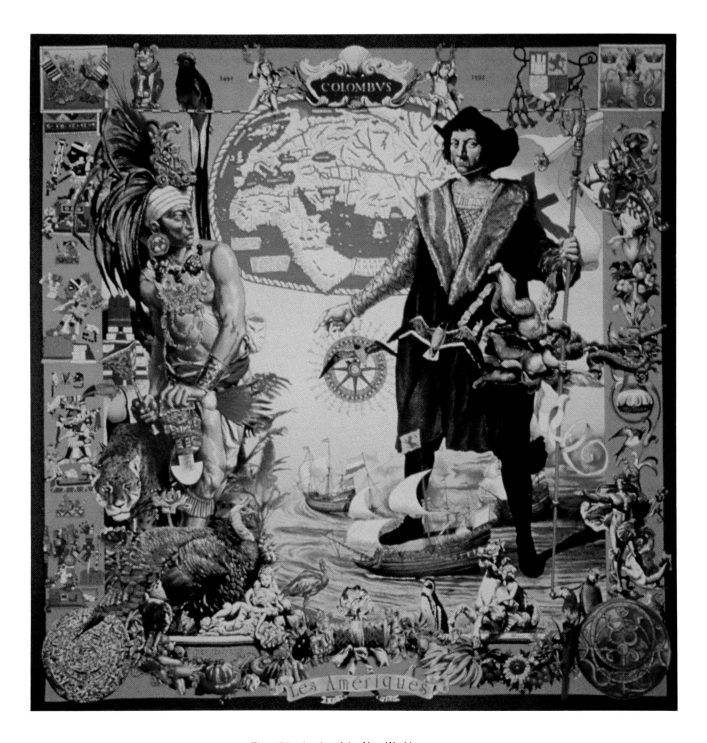

The wild splendor of the New World
meets the classic civilization of the Old
World in "Les Ameriques," Hermes' lush
1992 tribute to the 500th Anniversary of
Columbus' voyage. Photograph courtesy
of Hermes.

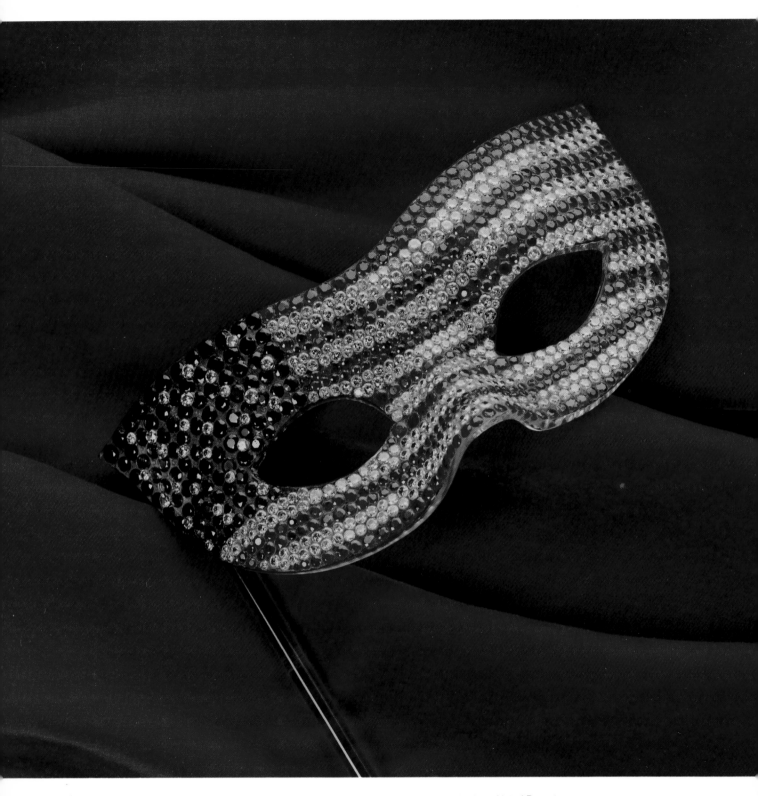

This jeweled mask by Harry Winston, Inc. made its debut at the Dallas Museum of Art's Grand Bal Masque des Beaux Arts in 1991 and was appropriately christened "Peace '91." A rendition of the American flag, this one, set on a Lucite base, billowed with a collection of 383 rubies, 463 diamonds, and 100 sapphires, with a total carat weight of 119. In the midst of Desert Storm, Ronald Winston, CEO and President of Harry Winston, Inc. captured the upbeat mood and unity of the American people when he said, "I feel that the mask is a symbol of the renaissance of American patriotism." And long may she wave! Photograph courtesy of Harry Winston, Inc.

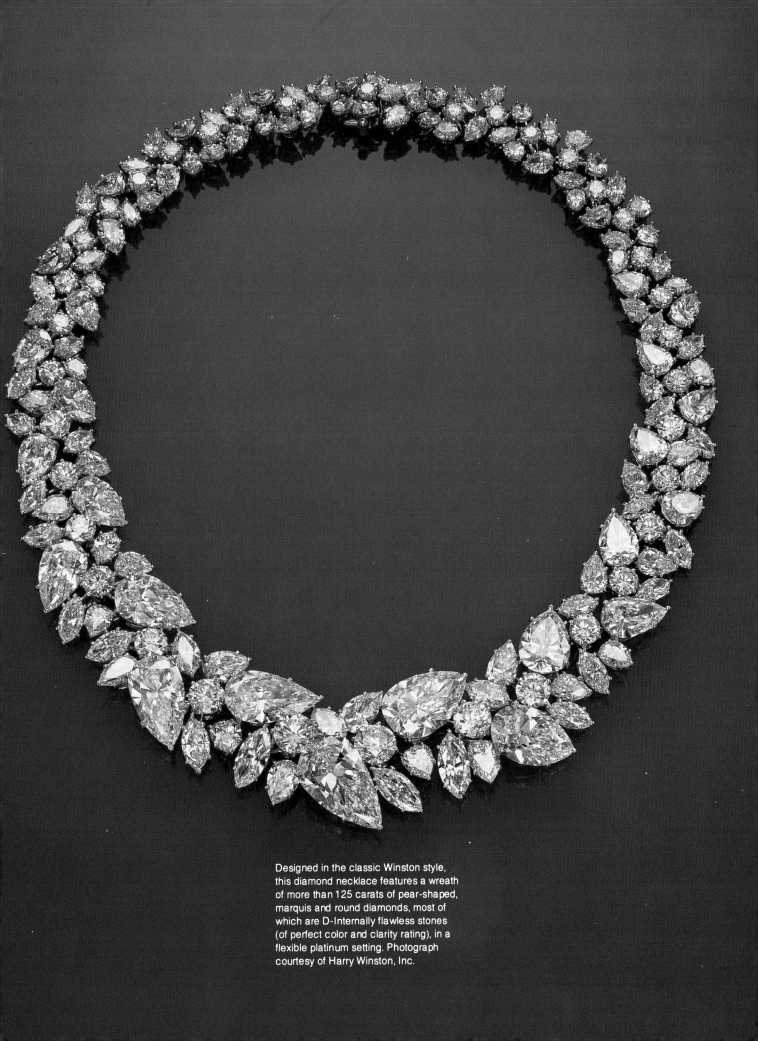

Designed in the classic Winston style, this diamond necklace features a wreath of more than 125 carats of pear-shaped, marquis and round diamonds, most of which are D-Internally flawless stones (of perfect color and clarity rating), in a flexible platinum setting. Photograph courtesy of Harry Winston, Inc.

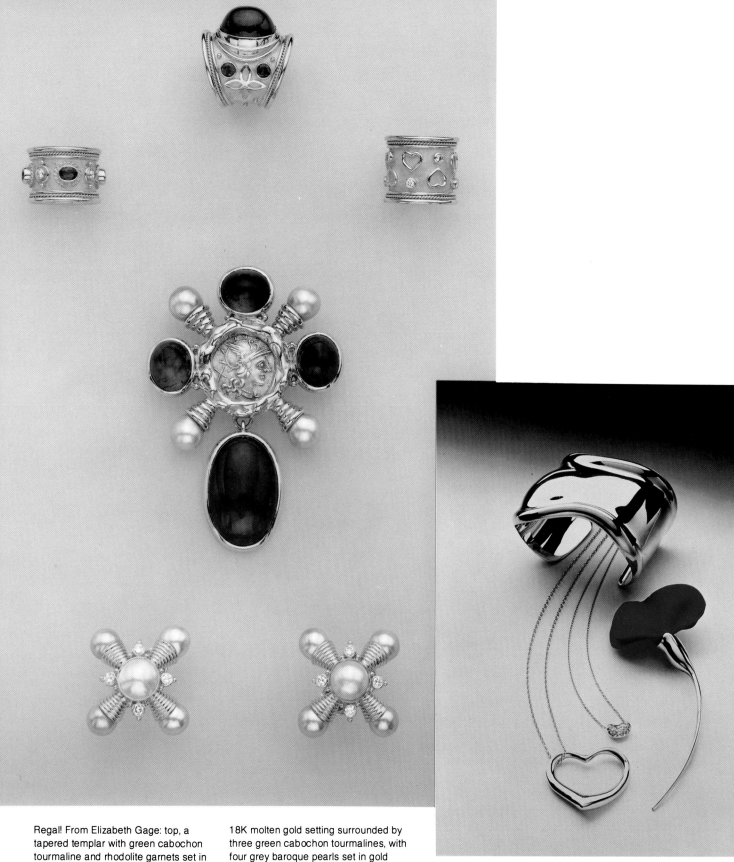

Regal! From Elizabeth Gage: top, a tapered templar with green cabochon tourmaline and rhodolite garnets set in 18K gold; top left, narrow templar band with diamonds set between rubies and sapphires; top right, templar band with diamonds alternating with heart shapes, in 18K gold; centre, Aurelius Pin with a silver coin (Aurelius Rufus 40BC) in an 18K molten gold setting surrounded by three green cabochon tourmalines, with four grey baroque pearls set in gold cones between, and a deep red tourmaline pendant. bottom, Pearl Kiss earrings, made with a Mabe pearl in the centre, diamonds, and grey baroque pearls set in 18K gold cones. Photograph courtesy of Elizabeth Gage.

Timeless into the 1990s and beyond. These pieces introduced by Elsa Paretti in the Seventies are much in demand at Tiffany today. Photograph courtesy of Tiffany & Co.

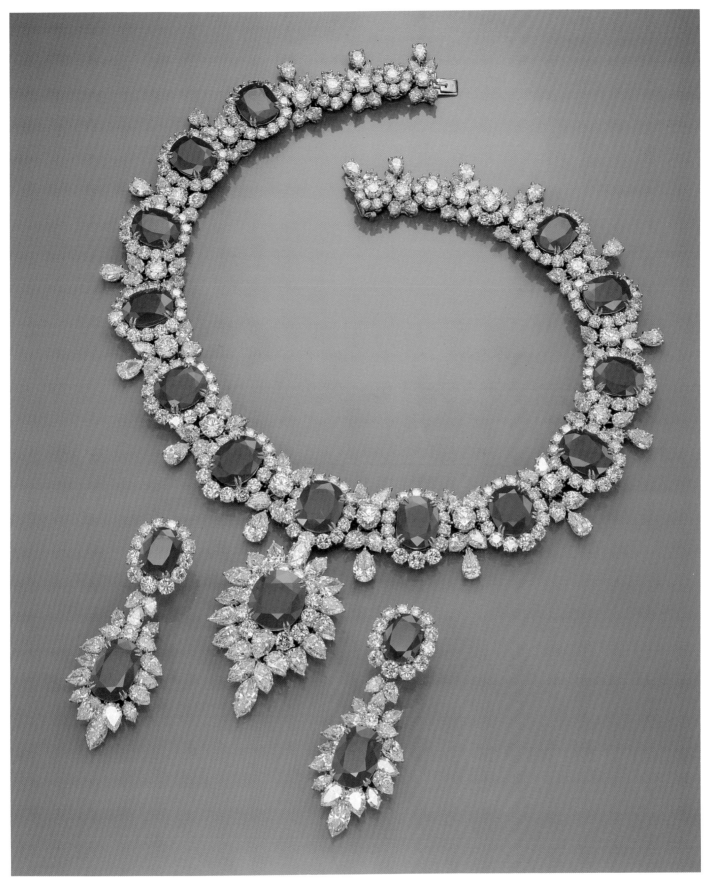

This magnificent suite of necklace and earrings boasts 175 carats of Burmese rubies set among more than 145 carats of diamonds, in platinum and 18 karat yellow gold. Photograph courtesy of Harry Winston, Inc.

offered up a sleeveless jacket that had been made from a big straw hat. Reversing direction, he also transported us to an under-the-sea paradise, with prints that reflected water and sky, many aglitter with beading and sequins, long filmy scarves covered with sparkling paillettes, and baubles like silvered nautilus necklaces, wide matching bracelets on *each* arm or simply armfuls of bangles. Discoveries from the "briny deep" were the inspiration for the jewelry featured on the models of Gianni Versace.

The theme of sea and sky was evident when Oscar de la Renta teased the audience with vibrant colors striking enough to lure them onto the next cruise ship bound for the Caribbean. These fashions were accented by bold jewelry with a Colombian-look, shiny Madras-inspired plaids, feathers, ruffles, turbans with big bows, giant hoop earrings—and even snappy "cowgirl" hats.

Dior concentrated on ". . . long slender evening dresses, some pleated to look like Greek columns . . . bustle effects in the form of bows, poufs and pleats turn up . . . on a few of the dressier clothes. How will the wearer sit down to dinner?"[4] Bustles aside, ". . . for the most part, the designer sticks to a realistic game plan. If there are a few excesses, remember that this is top-of-the-line fashion: They come with the territory."[5] Other Dior designs for 1992 were accentuated with oversized belts, some with attached purses that looked like updated versions of those trolley conductors wore at their waists decades ago. There were opulent earrings, shorty gloves, and dynamic masses of artificial flowers at shoulders and bosoms, as well as a return to the "daisy" craze of the 1960s. In fact, many fashions shown in the early 1990s reflected updated, but more controlled versions of the fun and imagination of the 1960s. This encompassed everything from lace, macrame, and mesh to provocative cut-outs and bold fabrics—like the abstract prints and 3-D embroideries shown by Scassi, who also accessorized his garments with flowers that were "bigger than life."

Big handbags were even bigger in 1992. Chanel bags featured quilted terrycloth for washability, and LaCroix ". . . covered shopping bags in bright gingham and Ungaro splashed bold rainbow stripes across straw beach baskets."[6] As did others, Lacroix also showed some longer lengths for Spring 1992, but they were either wrapped or strategically slit to show an enticing expanse of leg. Again, unusual fabrics, like those with the glimmer of stained glass windows, highlighted the collection, as did the eye-catching jewelry.

Adolfo continued to enchant with wonderful understated designs of "controlled elegance," all with impeccable tailoring and fabrics. For evening, there were gossamer skirts slit into wide "ribbon" strips that fluttered seductively. And he too displayed a version of the long overskirt or pannier.

At the other end of the spectrum was the "sparse" concept. Armani sections, with the ambiance of a glorified Army PX, opened in a series of upscale stores. At Bloomingdale's, an electronic billboard flashed *Store. Men's. Women's. Clothing. Jeans. Basics. Period.* The words, spit out like an old telegram message, give an idea of what fashion is coming to: utilitarian, economical, splendidly null."[7]

There's utilitarian sparse, and then there's just plain sparse. That was the swimwear story, more or less, with many designs bearing the strong, not unintentional, look of lingerie. Above all, with suntanning no longer considered a healthy pastime, swimwear followed the trend set in the Eighties, and was elevated to "clothing" status. Harmful rays or not, we were obviously never going to return to the bulky covered-up styles seen earlier in the century, for bathing suits had developed a style and importance that enfolded them even more firmly into fashion importance. It was equally obvious that the bikini, in one form or another, was here to stay. Styles ranged from the standard skimpy look to new, higher-waisted versions to designs featuring strategically placed "thongs," leaving even less to the imagination.

There was, nonetheless, an atmosphere of nostalgia at the beginning of the decade that magically brought about the look and feel of the 1940s. This heralded the revival of such diverse fashion elements as gingham, full flowing skirts, ruffles, those strappy platform shoes, sleek tank-style bathing suits amid the plethora of skimpy little numbers, halter tops, and neat, saucy shorts reminiscent of the look the gorgeous legs of Betty Grable helped to make popular in the 1940s. As a March 1992 *Mirabella* article mused, "Maybe we're ready to reverse the direction in which fashion influence flows. For the past three decades, mothers have been taking fashion cues from their daughters. In reviving forties fashion, many women are going back to styles that looked great on their mothers fifty years ago."[8]

Fall 1992 gave us another side to couturier designs—a somber, bizarre one that cannot be overlooked although, hopefully, will not be taken too seriously. "The avante garde designers have turned away from the glitz and glamour of the 1980s. They also seem to have rejected whimsy, bright colors and obvious sexuality. Gone are the flaunt-the-body tight miniskirts . . . and vibrant yellow and turquoise peacock colors of recent years." Instead they ". . . served up a somber stew: black or earthtoned skirts that droop to the ankles, unevenly cut layers of protective clothing that cover the body, and

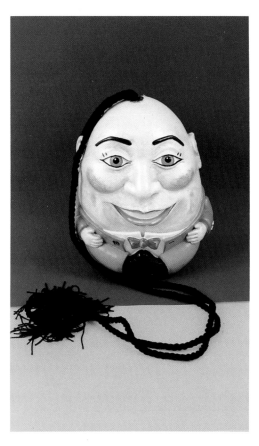

Humpty Dumpty sat on a wall; Humpty Dumpty went to the ball! An evening bag by Kazo that's sure to "rev up" a dull evening.

unfinished slice-and-dice hems and seams."[9] "All of this—the frayed hems, exposed seams, and overall tattered look has created a mood (that) is so serious, it's depressing... these clothes are the ultimate anti-fashion statement."[10] Who could dispute it when they view gloomy black dresses like mourning outfits with huge bunches of fabric where the sleeves have been put in backwards? "'They have to hope there are a lot of suicidal millionaires out there,' said a European fashion critic."[11]

But not to worry. Most of the couturier collections gave us much to exclaim over—and keep our mood gay. For instance, in his 1992 Fall/Winter line for Chanel, Lagerfeld featured "...handbags the size of overnight bags, Chanel's trademark bows now placed at the back of the head instead of the top, models chained up like Prometheus to his rock, and everything bearing the interlocking CC initials."[12] Christian LaCroix chose pantyhose as an accessorizing challenge, embroidering a bouquet of flowers just above the knee, thereby making it mandatory to wear short skirts if these decorative fancies were to be seen. Couturier skirt lengths for these Fall/Winter showings were *up and down*, giving plenty of leeway to individual preference.

With a standing ovation reserved exclusively for one of Paris' most venerated masters of couture, the 1992 fall/winter collection of Yves Saint Laurent featured wide brimmed hats that swept off the face in "Gigi-like" fashion, ascot-style ties, and moderately platformed shoes. Creating a sensation—and giving this usually simple piece of lingerie a daring ambiance—exquisitely beaded and fringed bras left midriffs bare and were, not surprisingly, the focus of attention beneath elegant evening jackets. Building on a decades-long tradition, Paris once again did not disappoint. "Creativity begets creativity. This is where the fashion action starts."[13]

And on couture runways, not only dresses but also *tresses* became a part of that action. For instance, from "...Karl Lagerfeld's painted hair to Valentino's shoulder length page boys, the hairstyles created for the Mori show (Hanae Mori) by Alexander of Paris were notable. He swept the models' hair into top knots and then lacquered it into arresting shapes." [14] Should we fear that Marie Antoinette's monstrosities lurk just around the corner? Doubtful. But it does serve to illustrate that, with modified variations, even hair goes "'round and 'round'" on *more* than the top of the head!

Of course, not all Parisienne couture is wholly French-inspired. Although an integral part of Paris couture since the 1980s, the boundless energy and stark beauty of Japanese minimalists like Issey Miyake, Johji Yamamoto, and Reikawa of Kubo for Comme des Garcons are imbedded in their roots thousands of miles to the East. Indeed, minimalist or not, their influence on couture cannot be *minimized*, even into the 1990s.

Not all fashion happenings occur on the fashion runways either. On the streets of Paris, young people were at the core of a "hot" new jewelry trend. A fad for clusters of lapel pins began in the early Nineties and grew in popularity as the decade progressed, eventually covering not only lapels but entire jackets and even hats. At first merely small pins of stamped metal like those handed out by airlines, they rapidly escalated to couture status. In July 1991, "... Christian Lacroix made a designer version to give to buyers and journalists at his haute couture show. Soon Boucheron and Cartier, the top-drawer jewelers, had their own version ... Chanel sells letters spelling out its name ... the most desirable pins fetch up to 12,000 francs, about $200."[16]

Expanding on the nostalgia movement that had begun in earnest in the 1980s, the Nineties' woman continued to search for bold costume jewelry pieces from the mid-century. All of this served to strengthen the market for interesting costume pieces, whether new *or* old, for, heeding the ground swell, many of the giants in the industry took a second look at their fashion jewelry lines.

Trifari, for instance, recognized the appeal of their early designs and, in the late 1980s, began reissuing some of them. To better address these needs, the Napier Company, a mainstay in costume jewelry for decades, decided to take a different approach in 1991. "'There's always a certain respect one brings to anything that's survived 20 years,' said Neil Calet...of Calet, Hirsch.... Yet research the company conducted determined that'... there had been a significant change in what women think about costume jewelry.' Previously ... the purpose of costume jewelry, or fashion jewelry, 'was to imitate the real thing.' But no longer is such jewelry part of what Mr. Calet called 'a *tasteful lady* category,' adding that women now regard wearing costume jewelry as 'a fun, enjoyable, imaginative exercise.'"[15]

The public's fascination with incorporating animals and insects into their fashions didn't wane in the Nineties, and for 1992 the bees were back. This time they were swarming over everything from wallpaper and fabrics to costume and fine jewelry. Continuing the legacy of its founder, the Duke di Verdura, E.L Landrigen, Inc./Verdura playfully labelled these diligent workers as "...'decorative, omnipresent and hard-working'"[17] when they elevated these "buzzing beauties" to new heights by studding them with diamonds, rubies and sapphires—a treasure for any hive.

Taking a walk on the wild side, Fall of 1992 was a spotty one indeed. Animal prints paraded from one end of the fashion spectrum to the other, encompassing dresses,

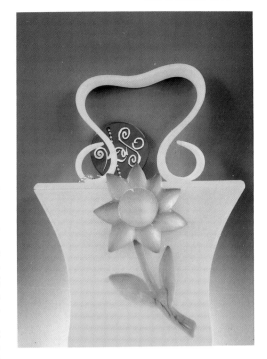

Plastics of the Nineties.

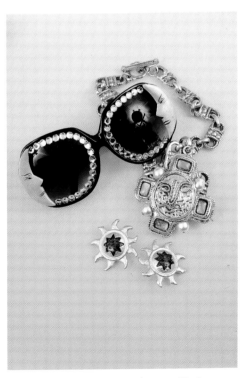

The sun, the moon, and some glittering rhinestone "stars." Half-moon sunglasses, with the look of Hollywood's golden years, Robert Rose earrings, and a topaz/pearl pendant.

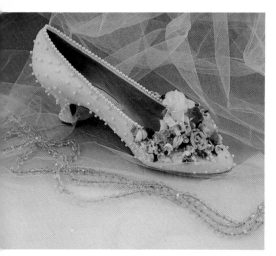

For a special party . . . or the bride to be. Here are fairyland "shoes to order." Courtesy of Barbara Music Designs, New York.

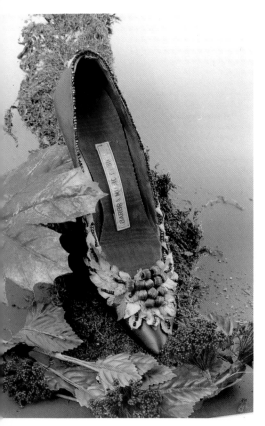

Autumn in New York . . . in a glorious pair of green satin pumps. Courtesy of Barbara Music Designs, New York.

sportswear, coats, and all manner of accessories—like calfskin bags stenciled with leopard markings or, in striped zebra on white calf, ". . . Bruno Magli ankle-high calfskin boots with witchy pointed toes and sexy black stacked wooden heels . . ."[18] creating a stampede for clothing with the excitement of a safari to the Serengeti Plains. In the wild animal sweepstakes, zebra ran a close second, but leopard "leaped ahead" in this spotted and striped menagerie.

Of course, it's not only what's "buzzing around" or lurking behind a bush on the African plains that captures our "fashion fancy." The sights and sounds we absorb daily are major players in determining where our dollars go—and why. For just as movies of the Thirties and Forties, and television programs like *American Bandstand* in the Fifties and Sixties, played an explosive role in influencing fashions of the time, the power of MTV was enormous in the 1990s. What was portrayed on those television screens in millions of homes created a stampede for a myriad of fads, many of which achieved more than mere "here today, gone tomorrow" status—like hats covered with little pins or decorated with one big brooch, wide belts, shredded jeans, studded leather, cowboy boots, and even "rap" pendants by "status" names like Chanel. They all became an indelible part of "street scenes" from the "Big Apple" to St. Tropez. Thus, along with the ever-present influence of the media, fashions of the 1990s whether startlingly new, or taking us back—with modifications—to Forties or Sixties retro, a touch of the Fifties or an eclectic mix of every decade before, created a happy union of garments and accessories.

"My accessories are not meant to be fashion . . . they are designed to augment fashion. Things made of precious metal are meant to last forever and a day.'"[19] Thus Barry Kieselstein-Cord, an American original, states his view of the role of accessories, and especially those representative of his craft, until recently limited to the very finest in jewelry and belts. His jewelry is of 18, 22, or 24 karat gold, and each piece is signed, dated, and copyrighted. It is a pride of workmanship and design that is well-deserving of the accolades he's received both from his peers (he is a two-time winner of the coveted Coty Fashion Award) and his entourage of loyal customers and admirers. Kieselstein-Cord numbers hundred of "celebrities"—who come back again and again to sample his new offerings—among his clients. His jewelry creations made their first "public appearance" at Georg Jensen, New York in 1973. Since then Kieselstein-Cord has reigned over in-store boutiques at Bergdorf Goodman in New York, Neiman Marcus in Beverly Hills, and Mitsukoshi in Tokyo, and he plans additional major introductions in Hawaii and Milan, as well as other European locations.

In 1976 Kieselstein-Cord introduced his classic belt buckle, the Winchester, and followed it year after year with others in either 18 karat gold or sterling silver, all hand-cast and, as with his jewelry, signed, dated and copyrighted. Seeing the Nineties as a time to have fun with accessories, Kieselstein-Cord recently expanded his repertoire to include handbags and gloves, with further accessory additions on the "drawing board." Once again, nothing less than the very highest of standards will suffice. Handbags, for instance, are given their stiffening only with leather and they are all lined in green pig suede.

Interestingly, Kieselstein-Cord prefers to call his offerings "concepts" rather than collections. "'Using the word collection limits you. A concept you can constantly enhance."[20] That these concepts are bona fide works of art is not debatable, for some ten years ago Kieselstein-Cord's exasperation with "knock-offs" of his designs led to a U.S. Circuit Court awarding him a precedent-setting copyright ruling. It stated that his designs were not merely functional—they were art. This protection of an artist's rights won international acclaim as the single most important legal decision for artists in 50 years. One has only to look at a Kieselstein-Cord original to understand the wisdom of that Circuit Court decision.

Such works of art are also the province of the always exciting jewelry designer, Robert Lee Morris. His creations, with their rich patinas and sometimes mystical concepts are not unlike an artist's brush strokes to canvas. For instance, early in the decade he wound his audience in chain jewelry—this time, yards and yards of chains that became body art, a veritable sculpture to be worn. Morris referred to it as having a ". . . massive heavy metal, super-glamour, super rock star kind of image."[21] Other of his designs had an organic, prehistoric construction with lines resembling the vertebrae from animals, snakes and birds. Morris is comfortably at home in the present, but he is able to travel to ancient times and places that bring his jewelry miraculously to life. In a twinkling we can be transported from the age of dinosaurs to the glory of the Byzantine, with its massive settings and sparkling stones.

In contrast to the Byzantine influence, and with a playful eye to less genteel and more fashionably "funky" times, "Lagerfeld took the idea of chunky necklaces literally and ran with it. For his spaghetti-western collection for Fendi, he cooked up huge, brightly colored plastic pasta pieces and strung them with African-inspired gold beads."[22] Thus, there is art in the breathtakingly beautiful and the playfully amusingly.

Few accessory designers of this or any century have allowed their imaginations fuller rein than Isabel Canovas. In 1982, Canovas, who was to become one of the most influential figures in the world of fashion accessories, chose Paris as the site for the opening of her first boutique. Formerly an accessory designer for Dior and Louis Vuitton, Paris-born Canovas brought a wealth of expertise and a daring artistry to her new venture. Then as now, Canovas had long recognized the exciting role accessories can play in the wardrobe choices of fashion-conscious women—not as an "afterthought" but instead a focal point—thereby elevating haute couture accessories, as well as accessories in general, to a "place of honor" in the world of fashion. "Easy-going to elegant . . . serene to seductive . . . flirtatious to flamboyant . . . these contradictions can be achieved visually through one's choice of accessories." With those words, Canovas conveys her view of the versatility of a *well-chosen accessory.*

With boutiques bearing her name dotting the thoroughfares of major cities like New York and Madrid, Canovas' craft, presented in two collections yearly, is indicative of her unflagging perfectionism. That insistence on unqualified excellence has taken her to places like the Far East for semi-precious stones, Thailand for silks, and Africa for exotic woods, resulting in an eclectic mix of materials, such as Bakelite with bronze or silk with kidskin, all combined to dazzle the eye with startlingly beautiful results. Imbued in the splendor and opulence of her Spanish heritage, vibrant colors also add a lush beauty to these flawless masterpieces.

As the 1990s began, men were certainly not relegated to a back seat on the "fashion bandwagon." "There are many wardrobe basics, including accessories, that can put you right on fashion's edge. . . . The look for contemporary men of the Nineties has its roots in Euro-style, but it also is heavily influenced by the hip-hop culture and the casualness of American sportswear."[23] Again, individuality was king, with enough flexibility in wardrobe choices to give any man who chose to do so an opportunity to tastefully tailor-make his own wardrobe. Sports items were supreme, from quilted baseball jackets to what Roy Campbell of Knight-Ridder Newspapers called the #1 accessory—the baseball cap. It gives the wearer plenty of leeway to advertise, on his head no less, that *his* team is the best bar none, or just enjoy the cap for what it is—a simple headcovering. As Campbell instructs, "You can sport the logo of your favorite college or professional sports team or just wear a basic black cap."[24]

Traveling from the male head to his waist, one is apt to see wide leather belts with big, big buckles, either going through the standard belt loops or cinched at the waist of soft, unstructured slacks; wrists may sport fun timepieces, like fossil watches with granite-looking faces; and at least one of the footwear fashion statements for the rugged male of the 1990s appears to be laced-up black boots.

And—no surprise here—the cowboy-Western influence again surged forward in the early 1990s. Always popular, the worldwide interest in this American-inspired phenomenon rides on waves of popularity decade after decade, and the Nineties are spawning another *Big Kahuna.* Whether off-the-rack or designer inspired, the trend toward cowboy hats, boots, jewelry, scarves, and belts echoed the same resounding theme for both sexes. The public loved the mystique of the cowboy in 1900—and they were just as enthusiastic about the heroes and villains of the Old West during this century-ending decade.

Even the seemingly simple necktie was graced with the couturier touch, like the luxurious silk print cravats by Chanel for the discerning, upwardly mobile male. Less conservative, but certainly not to be overlooked, were the scarves and ties of Nicole Miller, in splashy, wild prints. When a tie is necessary—and even when it's not—with these Miller creations, gentlemen are able to choose from a vast array of designs to please even the most particular. This amusing yet surprisingly sophisticated neckwear does everything that much of couture has been urging for decades: to simply enjoy fashion for what it can be—a lighthearted romp that needn't be taken too seriously. Men of the 1990s seem eager to comply—and women are equally enthusiastic when they sport one of Miller's eye-catching scarves.

Miller's talents have produced more than accessories, for season after season she's also given women stunning choices in imaginative fashions. Her Spring 1992 collection "scored a triumph,"[25] with models decked out in feminine, hour-glass and "fit and flare" shapes—and not a baggy look in sight. Although her witty signature prints have generally been relegated to the accessory lines only, this Spring fashion collection also featured a smattering of amusing prints and beautiful florals—all with the magical Nicole Miller touch.

Strenthening the power—and wit—to be found in accessories, one of the most whimsical trends early in the decade was to feature accessories on all manner of items. Inspired by eye-catching and amusing shirts by the Italian designer Moschino, scarves, vests, hats, and even hatboxes made of fabrics splashed with illustrations of shoes, hats, gloves, and jewelry soon appeared—and then, reversing itself, jewelry brought us elements of these same accessories, with brooches and charms in the shape of hats, gloves, and shoes! Suddenly, accessories were no longer just items of ornamentation but instead were used to *decorate* each other in their own image! Fittingly, this category,

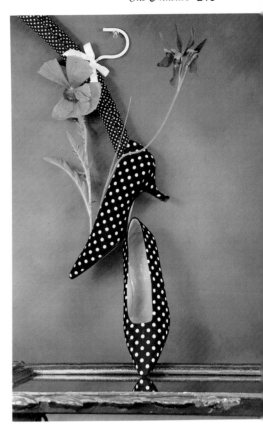

Dot happy . . . Phillipe Model shoes.

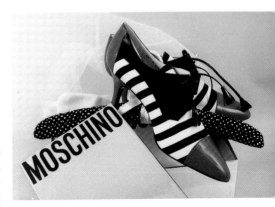

Moschino does Rodeo Drive! Were there ever a more glorious pair of shoes than these?

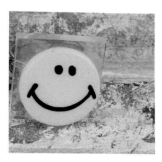

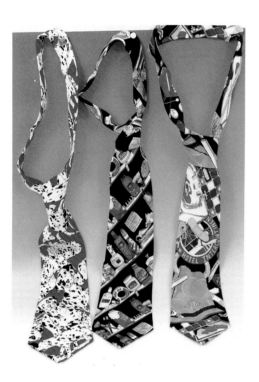

Nicole Miller ties . . . a choice for every man! Courtesy of Nicole Miller.

always ripe for those with fertile imaginations, had extended itself to yet another plateau.

Moschino must also be credited with starting the trend toward displaying designer names on fashions in a daring and tongue-in-cheek way. Elsa Klensch referred to him as ". . . the designer whose sense of humor never fails."[26] His Spring 1992 line didn't disappoint, featuring, for instance, a stunning jacket that had emblazoned on the back, THIS IS NOT A MOSCHINO JACKET. And, on an even lighter note, he is also responsible for the return of those 1960's "smiley faces." Humor aside, Moschino's designs are impeccably presented and neatly tied together with beauty of line and detail, most often in his signature colors of red, black, and white.

A woman who has taken risks that the faint of heart, and even many of bolder ilk, would have considered far too dangerous is Vivienne Westwood. Like the legendary Pied Piper, she leads the way down a path filled with beauty, merriment, and frequently outrageous fun . . . and her legion of faithful followers gladly accompany her on a journey that has opened many new and exciting fashion pathways. In a most positive way, she may be regarded as eccentric, but it is that courage to take a step or two . . . or even more . . . beyond the safe and secure that has brought Westwood's art to the apex of security in individual expression. "Experts on style the world over consider Westwood to be the most influential and original figure working in the fashion business today,"[27] and "John Fairchild, the editor of *Women's Wear Daily* and *W* . . . has called her one of the six greatest designers of the latter half of the 20th century."[28] High praise indeed for a tiny Englishwoman who flaunts six-inch platform heels and often wears her red-pink hair in pincurls.

Since rock 'n roll's heyday, the trends attributable to Westwood are enormous. With one foot planted in the culture of the Sixties and the other well prepared to conquer the challenge of the future, it is no surprise that she presents an intriguing dichotomy . . . taking her designs from the "far-out, man" look of punk to an albeit sometimes unrestrained inventiveness awash with visions of the future. It seems fitting that the company she formed with Malcolm McLaren in the 1970s was named "World's End," so visionary were the designs. But in this case "end" is *followed* by "beginning" . . . for that is what Vivienne Westwood continues to bring to the world of fashion—new concepts that are unhampered by convention and restrictive barriers.

As Westwood has so remarkably shown, the theme of couture fashion and upscale accessory designs of this decade and many before it must be regarded as a paean to individuality. Karl Lagerfeld expressed it most succinctly. In 1992, when asked his advice about fashion, this recipient of the Council of Fashion Design of America "Accessory Designer of the Year" Award, answered, "Dress the way you want, mix the way you want."[29] The major designers lead, and the trickle-down effect leaves behind ripples of fashion trends as diversified as one could possibly imagine.

Just as those merry revelers waited expectantly as the clock ticked its last seconds between December 31, 1899 and January 1, 1900, so too will 20th century party-goers welcome the 21st. Those charming ladies of 1899 attended their New Year's Eve galas with capes of opulent fur, full, bustled skirts of rustling fabrics, with only the tips of their black shoes peeking beneath, plumes in their hair, an intricately beaded bag in one hand and perhaps a glittering mask fan clasped in the other, and a dainty cameo or sparkling gemstones fastened at their milky-white throats. Their companions wore shiny top hats, black waistcoats above which rose rigid white collars, and black ties to match the sheen of their black shoes. From virtually every vest pocket hung a chain that was attached to that precious gold pocket watch. Most likely the only other adornment these gentlemen sported was a diamond stick pin.

By way of contrast, we can but speculate on the tableau that revelers on New Year's Eve 1999 will present. The decade has already shown us bits and pieces of every ten-year span since the century began. There are panniers and "lampshade" hats bedecked with flowers that are modernized versions of turn-of-the-century styles. Drop-waist dresses and ropes of beads transport us back to the Twenties, and daring re-creations of the sexy silk chameuse "lingerie look" harken back to the sultry glamour of Jean Harlow in a 1930's movie. There are echoes of every other decade, including the kerchiefs Louis Del'Olio wrapped around his models' heads in his collection for Anne Klein; as well as sleek turbans from the Forties; beaded sweaters, nipped-in waists, and even "Barbie Doll" inspired fashions by Ana Sui, from the Fifties; and fabrics of faux leopard and animal prints that scream "Seventies." And, never to be ignored, on any stroll through the local mall will be hangers-on from the Sixties shoulder to shoulder with younger folks giving it a whirl for the first time, as if they invented ripped jeans and mismatched outfits.

Traveling much farther back in time—and giving solid credence to the excitement that fashionable twists and turns can ignite as we journey to other times and places—Christian Francis Roth's Fall 1992 collection emulated the best features of that mainstay of sartorial splendor—the Edwardian dandy. But this time the fashions were aimed at female clients. With models making their entrance through a gentleman's armoire, there

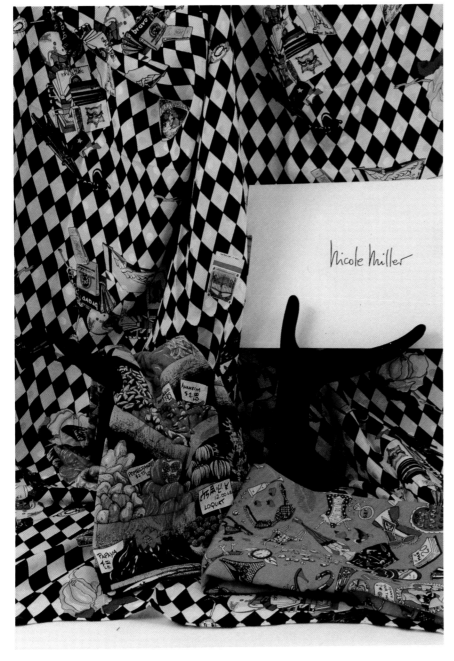

Giant Nicole Miller scarves...dynamite!
Courtesy of Nicole Miller.

were charming high crowned hats bedecked with giant feathers, long skirts with softly gathered, very modified, semi-bustle effects, and even saucy canes to accompany their outfits. Roth's view of the gender mixtures in fashion spoke not only to the Nineties but to decades and even centuries before, as well as those to follow, when he made the provocative observation, "It's all about masculine and feminine fighting for real estate on the body."[30]

So whether it be glittery ball gowns and tuxedos or cozy jogging suits and athletic shoes, the past ten decades have clearly shown that at the drop of a hat—whether bowler or fancy chapeau—everything changes. What goes up, comes down. What comes down, goes back up—and what folks choose to wear on that magical night when they usher in the 21st century is anybody's guess.

In the meantime, however, we must expectantly wait for those final chords of this century's "fashion symphony." Will it end with a vibrant drumbeat and clashing symbols or the soothing notes of a flute?—the haunting melody of a violin or the tinkling piano of the jazz-age?—an animated trombone, or the understated rhythms of a foot-tapping banjo? In light of what's gone before, we'll probably be lucky enough to hear—and see—them all.

. . . And may the band play on . . . and on!

1990—
[1] Bernadine Morris, New York Times, January 29, 1992
[2] Bernadine Morris, "In Paris, Diverse Dreams," New York Times, January 28, 1992
[3] "By Design," New York Times, January 28, 1992
[4] New York Times, January 28, 1992
[5] New York Times, January 28, 1992
[6] Vogue, January 1992, p. 52
[7] New York Times, February 18, 1992, Patterns, Woody Hockswender
[8] Mirabella, March 1992
[9] Nina Darnton, Newsweek, April 6, 1992, p. 50
[10] Nina Darnton, Newsweek, April 6, 1992, p. 51
[11] Nina Darnton, Newsweek, April 6, 1992, p. 51
[12] Bernadine Morris, The New York Times, March 31, 1992
[13] Bernadine Morris, The New York Times, March 31, 1992
[14] Bernadine Morris, *The New York Times*, July 30, 1992
[15] The New York Times, September 11, 1991
[16] Woody Hochswender, The New York Times, March 27, 1992
[17] *USA Today, Arlene Vigoda, May 13, 1992*
[18] *The New York Times*, "By Design," Carrie Donovan, June 23, 1992.
[19] Jill Newman, *WWD*, January 1990, p. 8
[20] Jill Newman, *WWD*, January 1990, p. 9
[21] *Style*, Cable News Network, January 25, 1992
[22] *Vogue*, January 1992, p. 52
[23] Roy H. Campbell, Knight-Ridder Newspapers, *The Hartford Courant*, January 21, 1992
[24] Roy H. Campbell, Knight-Ridder Newspapers, *The Hartford Courant*, January 21, 1992
[25] "Style, with Elsa Klensch," Cable News Network, May, 1992
[26] "Style, with Elsa Klensch," Cable News Network, June 1992
[27] Sally Brampton, *Elle*, February 1992, p. 144
[28] Sally Brampton, *Elle*, February, 1992, p. 144
[29] "Style, with Elsa Klensch," Cable News Network, February 1992
[30] "Style, with Elsa Klensch," Cable News Network, July 11, 1992

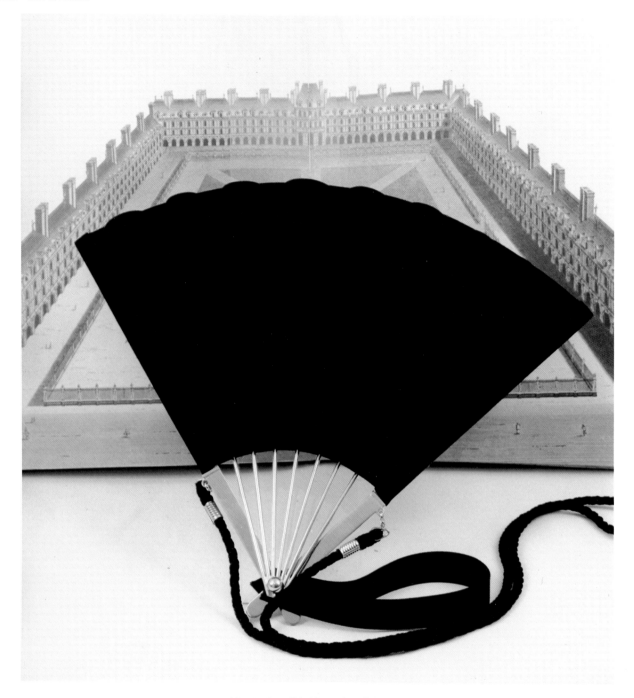

Like the fan of Karl Lagerfeld. This time
a stunning handbag reminiscent of the
French court.

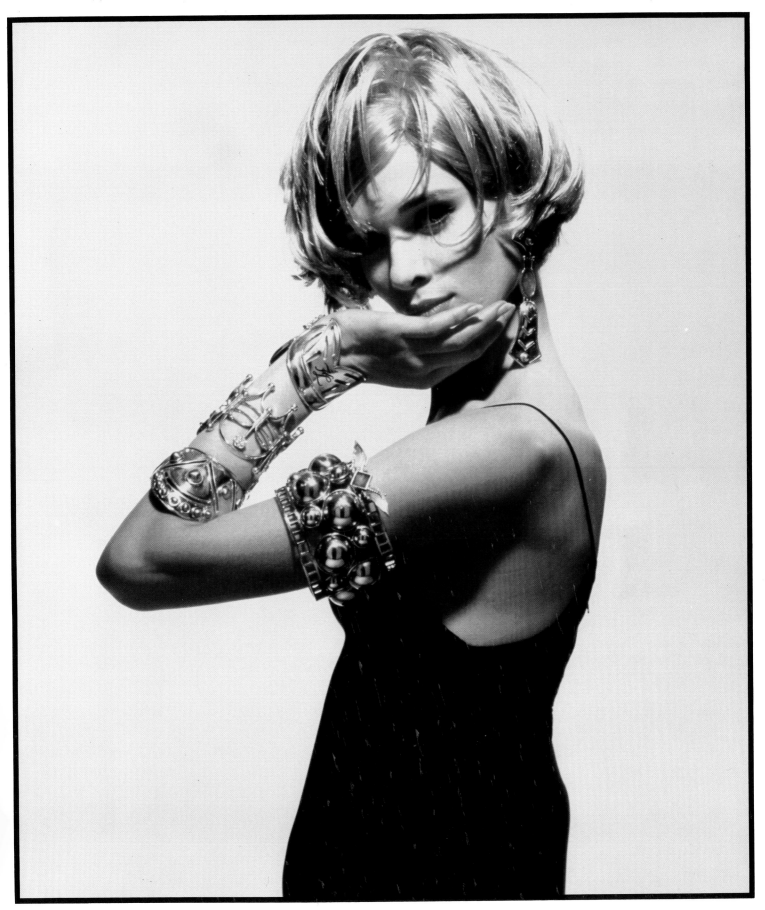

A glorious preview! Both photographs
courtesy of Karl Lagerfeld in July 1992,
from his upcoming 1993 collection.

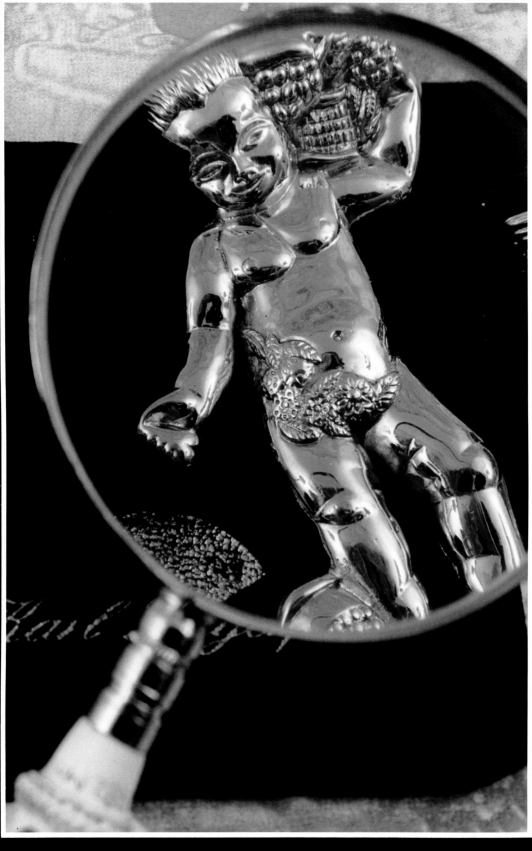

Thru the looking glass . . . Karl
Lagerfeld's "Bacchus" brooch.

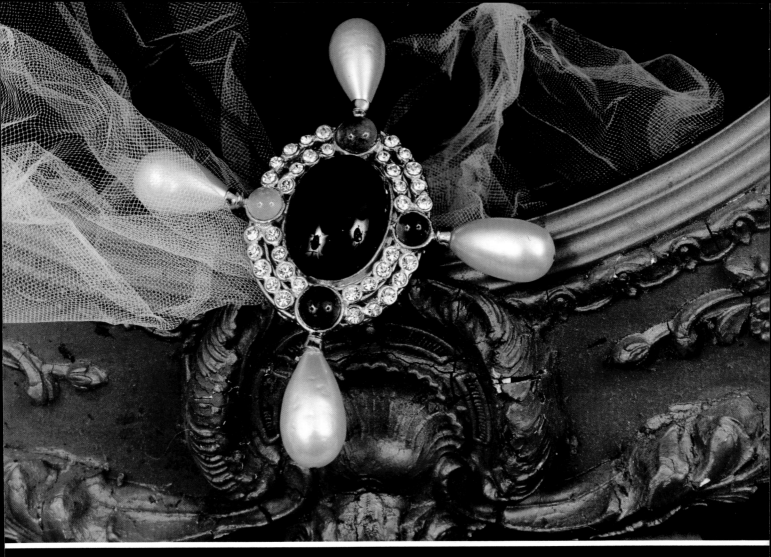

Elegant, as always...a 1992 Chanel
brooch of cabochons and pearls.

Heavy metal heaven! Handmade by
Susan Clausen.

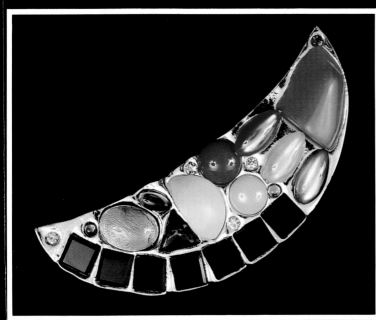

A rugged "stonescape" on a surrealistic
crescent moon. By Chanel.

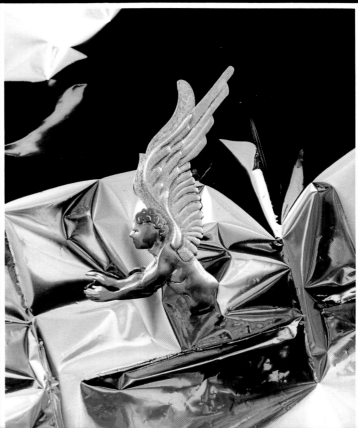

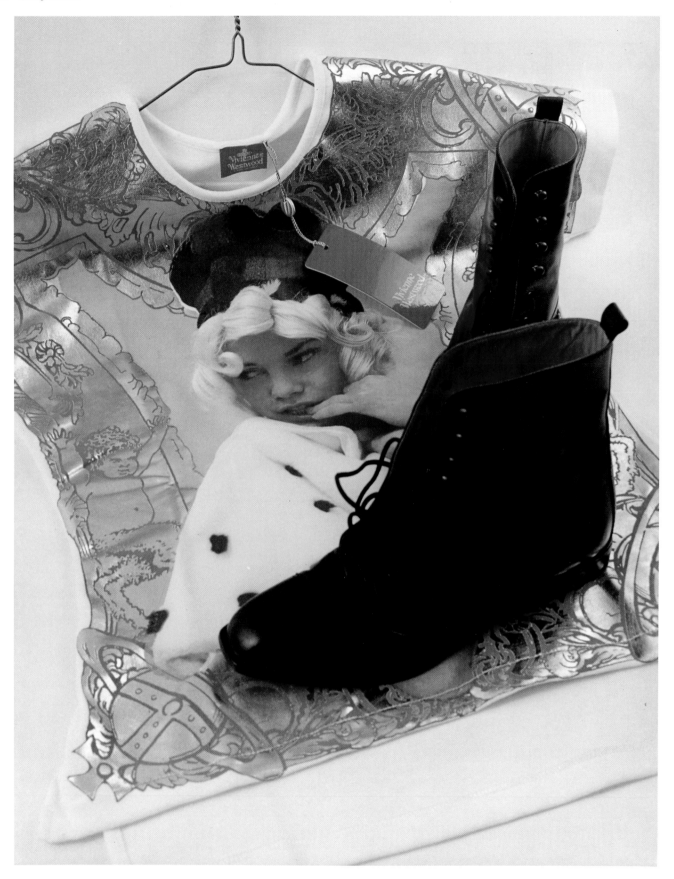

London and Paris: Pensive young lady is
the focal point of Vivienne Westwood
"golden" tee shirt. The boots are French.

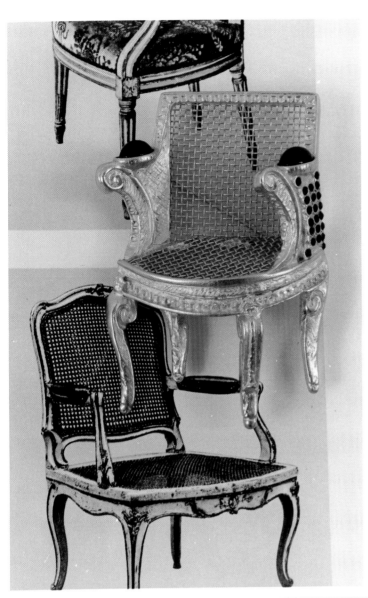

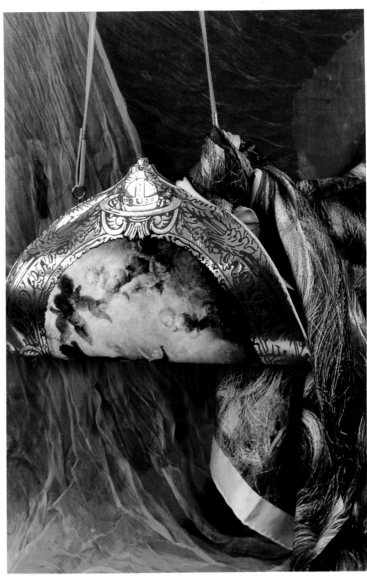

A "heavenly" Vivienne Westwood bag
and delightfully daring blonde hair scarf.

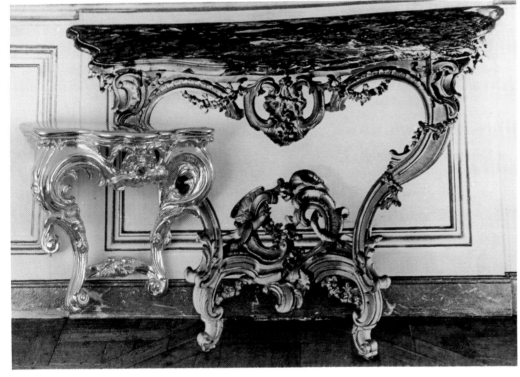

From Karl Lagerfeld...miniature gilded
chair and console brooches against
their French drawing room counterparts.

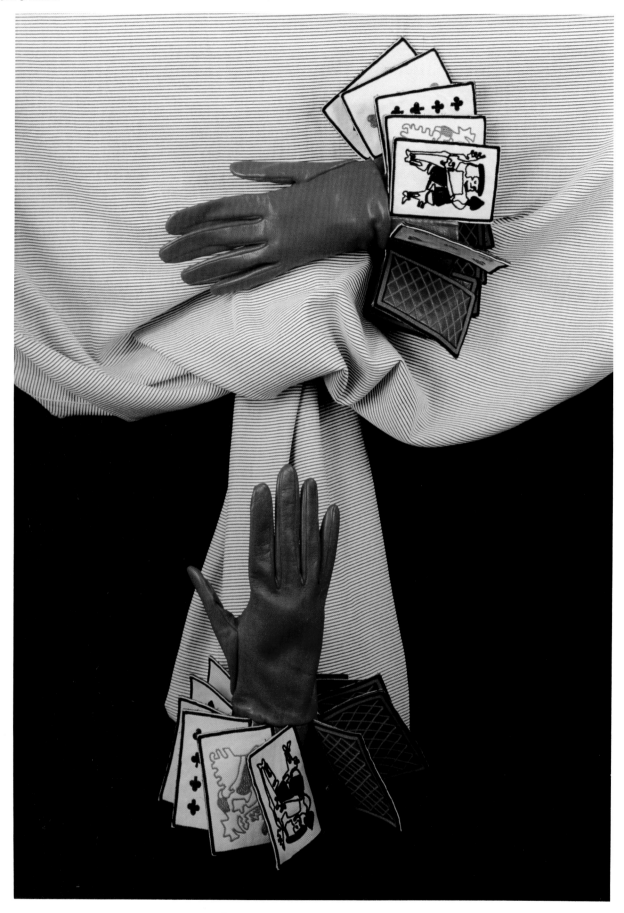

Gant Whist gloves. Courtesy of Isabel
Canovas.

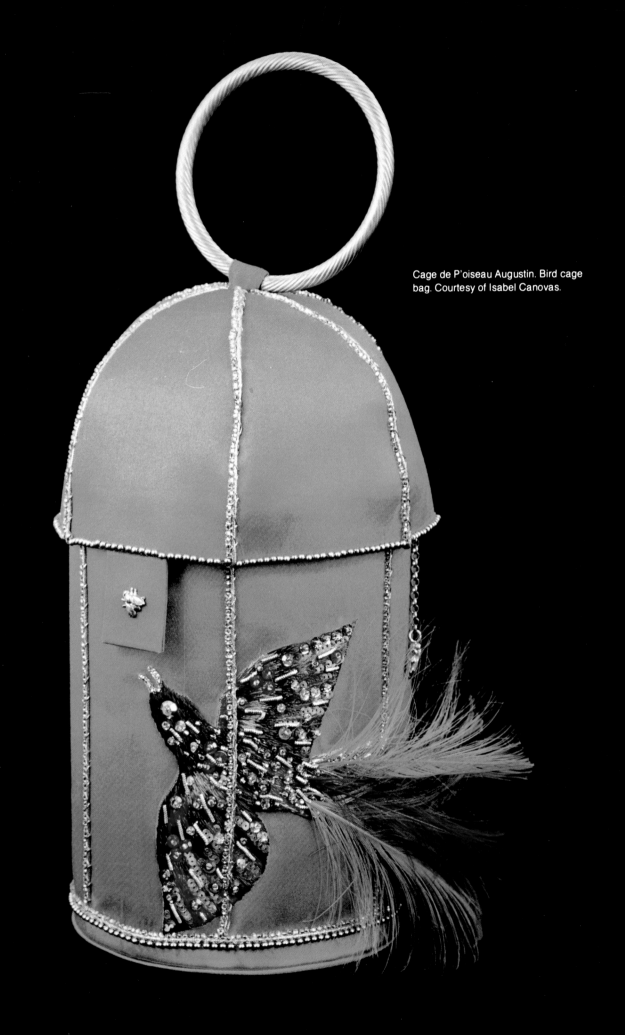

Cage de P'oiseau Augustin. Bird cage bag. Courtesy of Isabel Canovas.

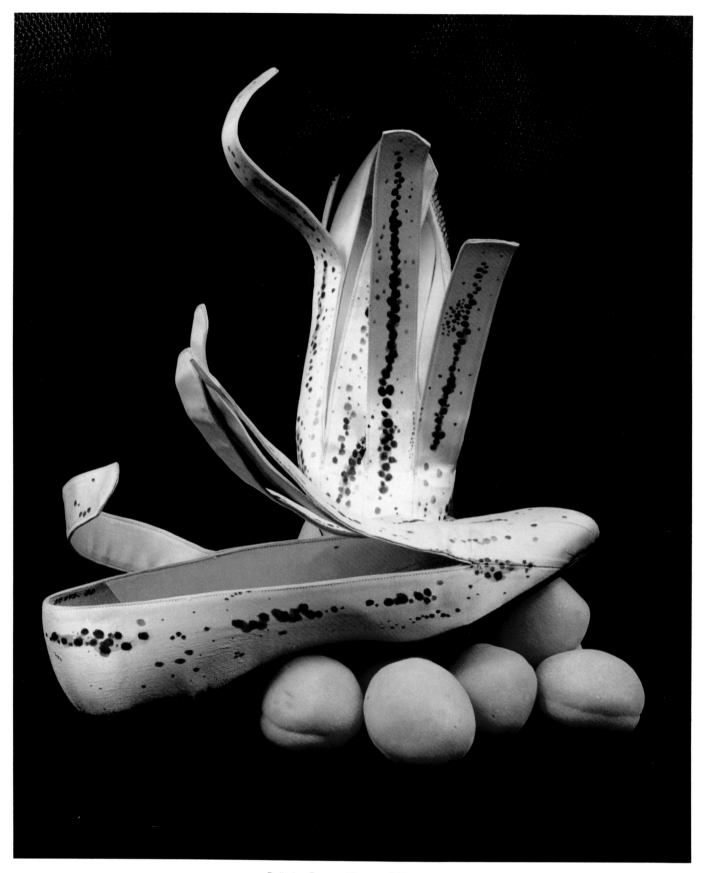

Ballerine Banane Viana . . . Without a
"slip" in sight, these banana peel shoes
were made for walkin'! Courtesy of
Isabel Canovas.

Le Magicien Gino...This bunny in a magician's hat, courtesy of Isabel Canovas, is a clever handbag—his ears are the handles.

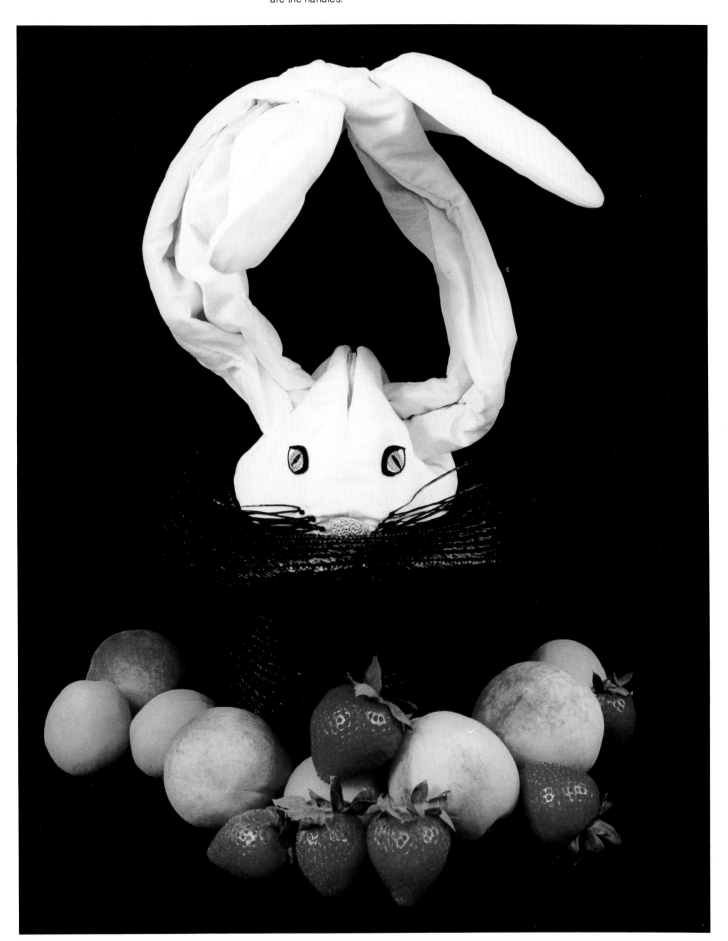

Le Chapiteau brodé. Circus tent bag.
Courtesy of Isabel Canovas.

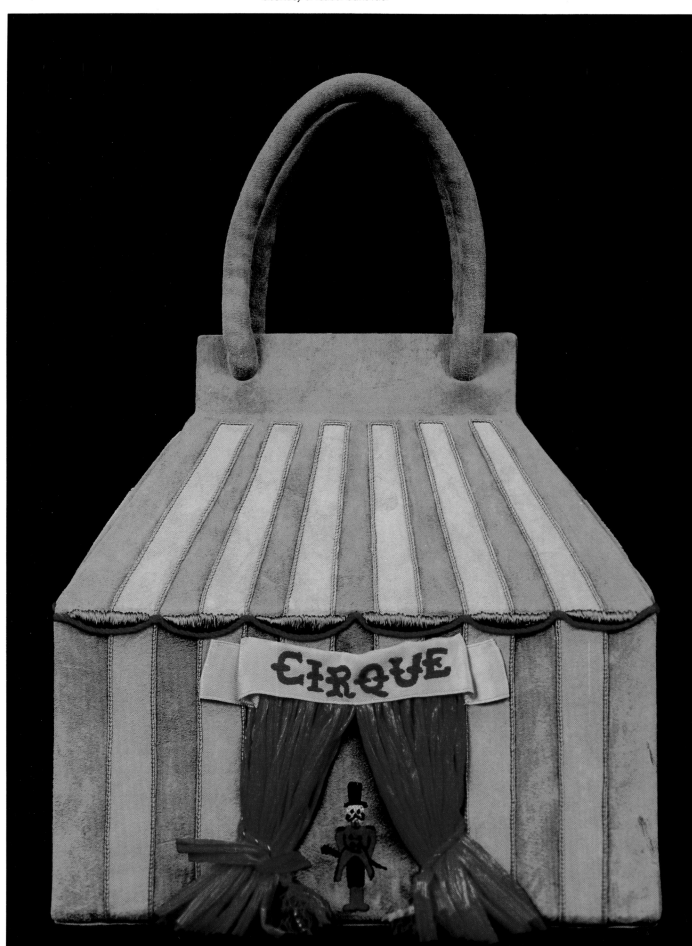

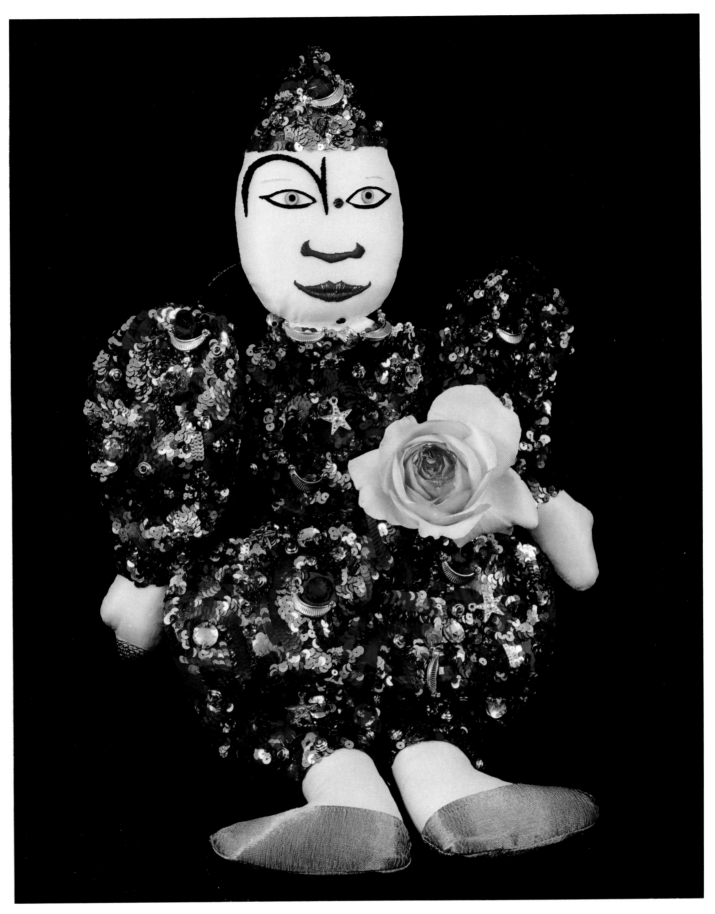

La clown blanc...the most elegant clown
ever, this sequinned bag with one
tasteful rose! Courtesy of Isabel
Canovas.

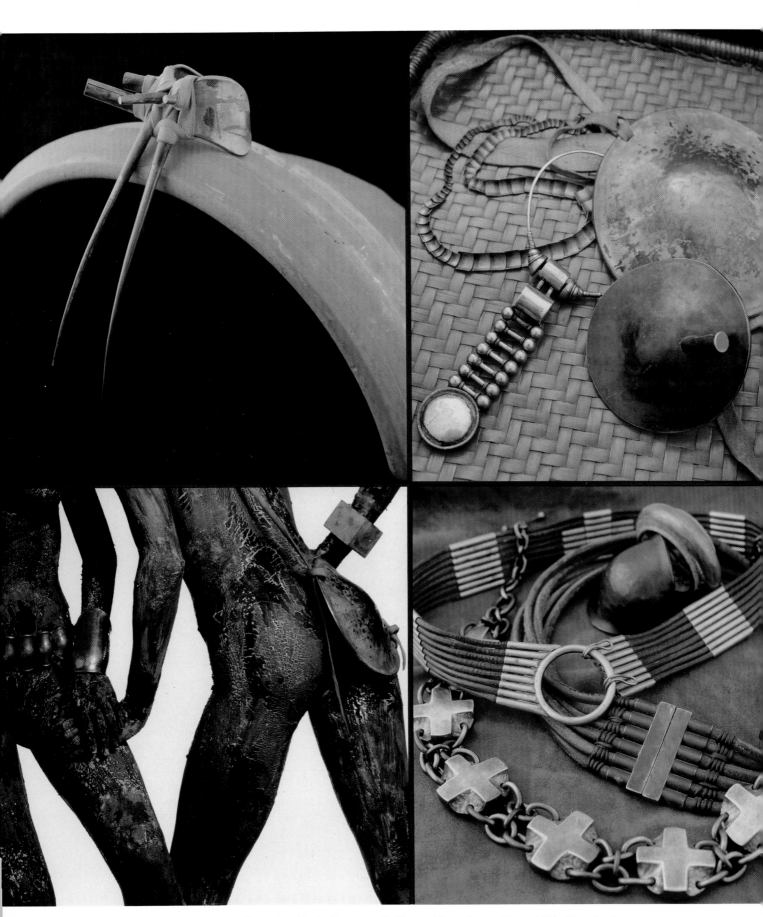

Photographs courtesy of Robert Lee Morris. Photos credits: Teresa Masagal except lower left by Klaus Laubmayer.

Contemplations on the Past and Present . . . and Glimpses into the 21st Century

My jewelry is a distant cousin of ancient armor (those smooth sensual body conscious constructions that employ ingenious mechanics to allow for fluid movement). My inspiration has never been clothing or fashion trends, but rather, the human need for personal intimacy with tokens of spiritual potential that amulets and talismans provide.

I constantly seek to fine tune, focus, purify, and strengthen my style; to make it more clear, more recognizable and more understandable by people of any and all cultures.

Mass fashion jewelry in my mind is purely decorative, employing a cacophony of glittery values to achieve a dazzling effect. This is as much a part of human culture as the bright plumage of birds and will remain with us as it should. But, it has always been against this world that I design my work; placing value on classicism and heirloom status over the thrill of temporary trends. My forms and shapes lead my concepts. My concepts are generally anthropological and my attitude is less is more.

My forecast for accessories in the future is that micro technology will invade everywhere, and the computer will be in our chains and in our shoes, bags, and belts. The telephone bracelet will come in hundreds of varieties. The scarf will provide vitamins and nutrition through skin contact and shoes will have super conductive soles for high speed travel. Eye glasses will convert to T.V. screens with a flip of a switch. It's going to get more exciting than ever.

Robert Lee Morris (For *The Art of Fashion Accessories*)
June 1992

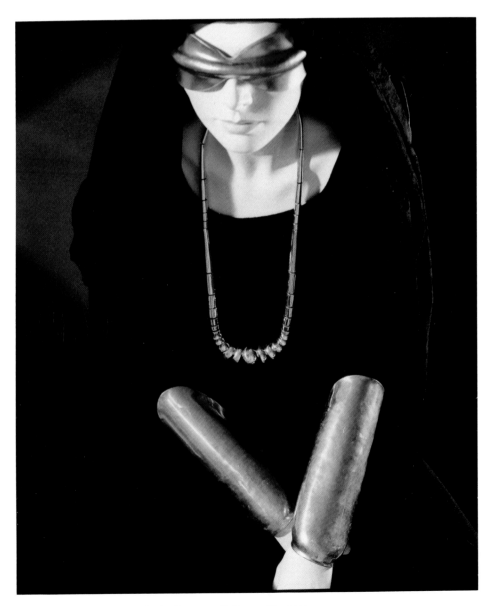

Copyright by Robert Lee Morris. Photo credit: Teresa Masagal.

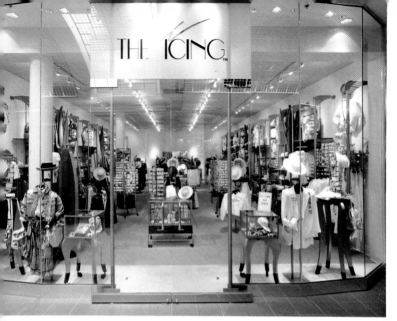

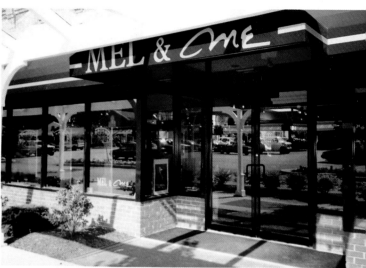

Photograph by Steve Howes, courtesy of
The Icing.

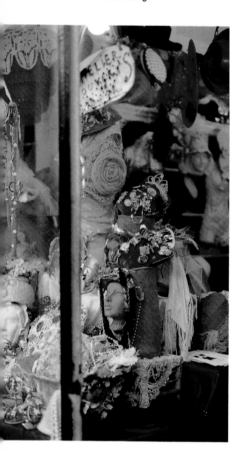

Gay Paree . . . 1991.

Contemplation on the Past, Present, and Future

In the past..."accessories were for decoration, ornamentation, and adornment and had mystical, spiritual, and religious connotations." In the future..."accessories will have therapeutic and ecological implications, i.e., hosiery with a moisturizer in it or insect repellent. Based on the marketing concept of 'cocooning'—activities focused around the home—people will want to accessorize their environment, as well as their wardrobes. There will be specialty stores that will have a totally integrated accessory collection—accessories for the *home,* as well as accessories for one's *wardrobe.* (Elida Olsen, spokesperson, *The Icing,* June 1992.)

"Designers for the 21st century will need to utilize more natural fabricating techniques. Plastics and other non-degradable substances shall have become illegal, due to their polluting tendencies. Hopefully, the next generation of artisans will explore fashion and accessories that respect nature and reinforce goodwill, while still keeping a sense of humor." (Rosalind Becker of *Roz and Sherm*)

"...One of the best things we have done is being able to put together great collections of jewelry that have the look of being family possessions—beautiful old pieces, with each having a personality of its own, like the quality of an old jacket—elegant, classic, yet fun and accessible fashion-wise. That's our niche in the world of jewelry and accessories—we are not creators per se; we have created 'a look, a corner.'" (Fred Leighton, Fred Leighton, N.Y., from a telephone interview, Paris, June 1992)

In the past,..."When people dressed they considered every detail. Gloves for example were always the mark of a gentleman or gentlewoman. Nowadays, people's dress is simplified and more graphic...for anybody who can afford the cost and time involved, to consider accessories and to make it work...is always worthwhile." (Vivienne Westwood, April 1992)

"We make bold jewelry, jewelry that makes a statement, jewelry that's meant to work. It becomes a part of your look, your style. There's nothing worse than a collection of jewelry that sits in a vault. Our overall goal is wearability—to make jewelry to wear, to travel with...As a women at our Boutique remarked, 'It's got character, guts, and femininity all at the same time.'" (Stanley Silberstein, President, David Webb, 1992.)

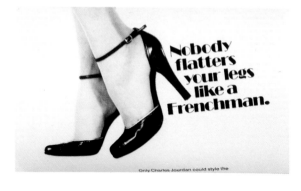

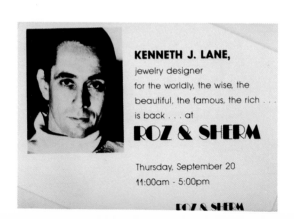

KENNETH J. LANE,
jewelry designer
for the worldly, the wise, the
beautiful, the famous, the rich . . .
is back . . . at

ROZ & SHERM

Thursday, September 20
11:00am - 5:00pm

ROZ & SHERM

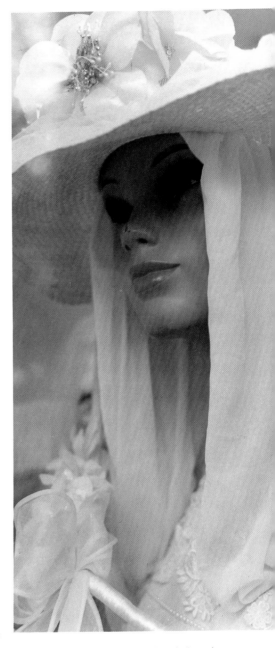

Among, of course, many others, there are three outstanding examples of the emphasis by retail shops on the importance of accessories.   Whether in a mall or on a more intimate basis, *The Icing*, *Mel and Me*, and *Roz and Sherm* stand as gleaming monuments of retailing entrepreneurship in the field of accessories.

The Icing

The Icing is a group of nationwide stores that brings all manner of great accessories to the public. Situated in shopping centers throughout the United States, this is quite simply "an accessories store." But simple it's not! For from jewelry to belts to hair ornaments, one cannot help but be bedazzled by the "spendiferous" array awaiting browsers of all tastes when they enter those inviting portals. As Elida Olsen, spokesperson for *The Icing* explained, "Accessories are an integral part of a woman's wardrobe. They *complete* a look. An outfit without accessories is like a blank canvas, waiting for the artist to apply his creative touches . . . The results become an extension of one's persona and mood. They reveal a woman's personal style—*Bold and Strong* vs. *Delicate and Demure*—or lack of it, which equates to *Boring*. Accessories should be *Fun and Amusing* . . . a distraction that reminds one of happy . . . simple, childlike days . . ."

Mel and Me

"Accessories can be the difference between a dress and a fashion statement." It is this philosophy that has placed *Mel and Me*, a Cranston, Rhode Island boutique founded in June of 1991, squarely in the world of upscale fashion. With the value of accessorizing at the heart of their merchandising philosophy, partners Mel Baker and Brenda Bedrick have intuitively cultivated that ever-present cadre of women who insist on incorporating accessories into the "feeling" of the garment, thereby creating a *total* effect.

That such attention to an individualized "head to toe" look is a highly sought commodity becomes apparent when one views the success achieved by this stellar operation in such a very short time: witness the fact that *Mel and Me* is frequently featured in *Harpers Bazaar*'s "panel" section, and that in the corridor between New York City and Boston they are the only operation of its kind to boast trunk showings by fashion giants like Karl Lagerfeld, Georgio Armani, and Donna Karan.

Going even further into the realm of the "unexpected," *Mel and Me* also offers their clients the opportunity to enjoy a unique, "once in a lifetime" experience. Each year the renowned French fashion photographer Michel Colombo is commissioned to spend a day at their Cranston store photographing these women just as he photographs fashion models worldwide. This is yet another example of how the interaction of imaginative marketing, innovative presentations, and an innate understanding of what most women *truly* want but generally have little assistance in achieving, can create success stories—both for the store *and* for the lucky customer who recognizes the value of all three!

Roz and Sherm

With hands-on management of three shops that vibrate with the excitement of dynamic presentations, the husband and wife team of Rosalind and Sherman Becker of *Roz and Sherm* in Birmingham, Michigan, are nationally and internationally renowned for their innovative promotions and advertising. Above all, they exemplify the apex to which fashion and accessorizing in a boutique atmosphere can soar.

From their beginnings in the mid-1970s, when they concentrated solely on the very best and most exciting in shoes, their shops now feature great fashions by established designers and promising innovators alike. But amidst all of it is their undying passion for elevating accessories to a prominent place in couture. With their infectious enthusiasm and dynamic presentations, Rosalind and Sherman Becker have built a following of loyal, "fashion-savvy" customers who revel in the family atmosphere of cordiality and personalized service that awaits them when they enter the doors of *Roz and Sherm*—a welcome oasis far from today's oftentimes hectic and frustrating shopping experience. It's that philosophy of being willing to go the extra mile—in a great pair of shoes, of course—that keeps *Roz and Sherm* and their lucky customers "on top of the world."

As Rosalind Becker, and forward-thinking designers and retailers recognized early on, accessories are the "frosting on the cake." But a cake without the yummy delight on top and oozing between the layers is just that . . . a cake!

The options are many, for you can decorate that cake any way you like—with chocolate fudge or fluffy marshmallow, colored shots or candied violets—or you can discreetly tuck that ornamentation between the layers—like a mysterious epicurean delight just waiting to be discovered! That's what well-conceived accents are all about—satisfying the need for individual expression in all of us. Remember, we can each carry the same plain white cake to the charity bazaar, but how we deal with what's on top is the all-important element that separate *us* from every other white cake baker in the world!

A study in beauty from the window of a Paris salon.

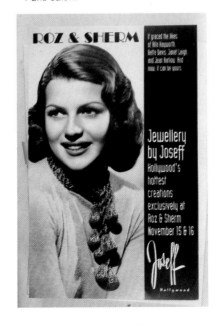

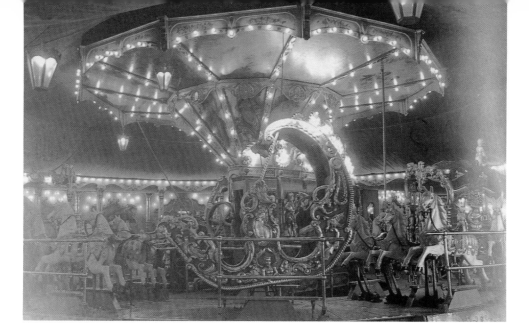

Epilogue

"We are by nature all as one, all alike, if you see us naked; let us wear theirs and they our clothes, and what is the difference?"

Robert Burton

As we begin our journey through this last decade of the 20th century, with January 1, 2000 rapidly approaching, one thing is apparent: that is, the truth of the old saying that, "What goes around, comes around."

Whirling through centuries and decades past is much like a fashion merry-go-round that slowly gains speed as the music cranks out joyously, and riders revolve before our eyes. The gaily decorated animals they perch upon either duplicate real creatures or are fantasy-land creations. Some of the riders laugh and sing, cavorting like children, while others sit demurely and the remainder appear uncomfortable, even anxious. A few come close to catching that brass ring, others miss by a mile! As a group they present a kaleidoscopic panorama of the past, as the gaily-colored platform revolves and carries them from sight. But never fear, mere seconds later this magical calliope brings its occupants around again, and we can catch another glimpse, perhaps seeing some tiny detail that escaped us before. In fact, is it our imaginations, or do these people look somewhat different each time they come into view? Didn't that lady with the big flowered hat have a rooster on her head the last time? And didn't the fellow with the knickers and shiny hair transform himself several revolutions back into a strange looking young man with a broad-brimmed hat and a funny, long chain that fell to the knees of his pegged, knicker-like pants? They do indeed seem to change themselves ever so slightly—back and forth, back and forth—with each revolution. Here they come again . . .

Atop the black stallion sits a crusty gentleman with cowboy hat and leather boots, a polka-dotted kerchief tied nonchalantly around the neck of his flannel shirt. On the giraffe to his left perches an elegant, long-necked lady with feathered headband, billowing chiffon skirt, and jeweled cigarette holder poised languidly between her fingers. The sleek panther behind her presents a study in black and white, for on his back rides a gentleman in formal attire, his top hat falling jauntily over one eye as he struggles to keep it in place while his long, white scarf catches the rushing air and ripples behind him. To his right, trying mightily to maintain her dignity, is a tight-lipped matron whose bustle makes sitting on a long-legged antelope well nigh impossible, as she clutches the gigantic flowered hat perched precariously atop her head.

Behind her, one hand gripped tightly around a unicorn's horn, is a young male with a brightly polished guitar slung over his shoulder. His hair stands wildly on end like zig-zagging electrical charges, and the glitter of his lone earring matches the brightly sequined top above his skin-tight trousers. To his left is a girl with twinkling eyes and a broad smile. As she gaily tosses her waist-length hair, it tickles the back of the dappled pony she rides upon. Her denim jacket is covered with hand-embroidered flowers, emblems, and words like "love" and "peace," and her long skirt flies freely over the tops of her simple, round-toed boots. Peering over her shoulder is a tanned young lady sitting side-saddle on a graceful white swan, lithe legs draped seductively over its feathered side. She wears a tiny, yellow polka dot bikini and ankle strap platform sandals on her gaily tapping feet. Big yellow earrings swing saucily as her head sways from side to side in tune to the music. The gentleman riding the striped tiger to her right is wide-eyed and enthralled, although obviously disbelieving of this nearly naked vision beside him. The stiff-brimmed straw hat sitting far back on the crown of his head gives him a rakish air, but the high white collar is so stiff with starch it creases his neck as he turns to admire her. His handlebar mustache hides a smile of delight, and he snaps his suspenders while the music ebbs and flows.

The sophisticated lady to his rear looks somewhat bemused as she struggles to sit properly erect on the back of a snarling leopard. One is hard pressed to tell where the leopard ends and the lady begins, for her leopard "look-alike" coat and matching hat meld harmoniously with his spotted body. Like him, she is polished and sleek, but obviously a matron from the suburbs who was lured onto this ride and would much prefer a trip on the escalator of a big city department store! She rather envies the innocent young girl on her left—a mirror to her past—who sits, hands demurely in her lap, on one half of high-sided wooden seats with outer panels decorated in the likeness of a giant snail enfolding the occupants securely in its shell. Her blonde hair turns under in a soft pageboy, and a peter pan collar peeks above the top of a cozy shetland sweater. The pleated plaid skirt beneath it is carefully pressed, and her thick white anklets turn down neatly above the immaculate brown and white saddle shoes. A nervous smile flickers across her lips as she tries to appear oblivious to the strange fellow on the seat opposite her. His hair has a brilliantine finish, and the tight band of his voluminous knickers meets the patterned knee-high socks tucked under them. He waves one arm—strangely weighted down with a wide silver bracelet—in a friendly gesture to the young couple behind him. Both are astride a bucking bronco, the girl's arms wrapped tightly around her companion's waist. Each wears tattered denim jeans, a designer name resting securely on a leather strip above the back pocket. Their once-white shoes are identical. Well-worn and bulky they were obviously meant for running or jogging, and yet another name is emblazoned across the side. She wishes she had worn her leather mini-skirt; he wishes his black motorcycle jacket wasn't so hot—but both seem to be enjoying the ride!

Suddenly all heads turn. Look! Instead of a brass ring, the stationary pole that flies by with every revolution now contains a host of numbers. First the gentleman on the stallion grabs for one—it's a 2. He smiles broadly! The matron on the antelope tries to keep from sliding off as she quickly reaches out. A zero falls, as if by magic, into her outstretched hand. She beams in disbelief! The sequinned male is confidence personified. Leaning forward, he holds onto the pole protruding from the back of the unicorn with his left hand and grabs another zero with his right. "Way to go!", he yells. The straw-hatted fellow behind him is swept up in the excitement. The right arm of his white, elastic-gartered sleeve takes a mad swipe at the flying ring within inches of his grasp. Another zero. "We're on our way," he shouts! The calliope revolves once again, and each lucky rider holds his prize aloft for the crowd to see.

2 0 0 0 flashes in front of them in bold, bright numbers.

But wait! That demure bobby-soxer seizes the moment. She jumps from her seat and, grabbing the poles of the animals between her, sways to the edge of the platform. The spectators grow silent and all eyes are riveted on the figure charging toward them—but alas, no numbers remain. Not to worry . . . as if by magic, the brass ring materializes, glittering like precious gold. Flushed with expectation, she grabs wildly, but in a twinkling the loop of brass slips from her grip. The crowd groans. With only a split second remaining, she makes a last valiant lunge and the ring slides miraculously over her hand! The spectators cheer, while her companions breathe a collective sigh of relief . . . for now the image of each will indelibly whirl ever onward—and carry them merrily into the 21st century!

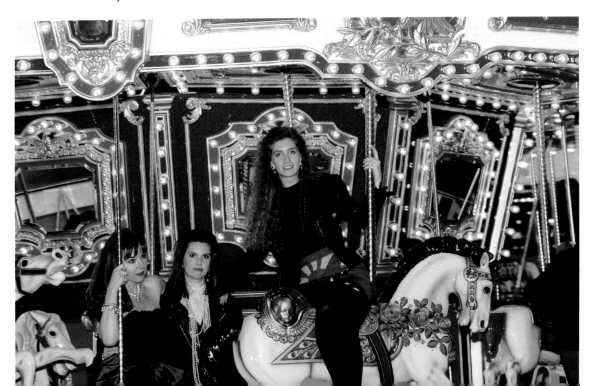

Bibliography

Ball, Joanne Dubbs, "Costume Jewelers, The Golden Age of Design," Schiffer Publishing Ltd., West Chester, Pa., 1990

_____, Jewelry of the Stars, Creations from Joseff of Hollywood," Schiffer Publishing Ltd., West Chester, Pa., 1991

Ball, Robert W. D. and Vebell, Ed, "Cowboy Collectibles and Western Memorabilia," Schiffer Publishing Ltd., West Chester, Pa., 1991

Baseman, Andrew, "Scarf, The," Stewart Tabori & Chang, New York, 1989

Battersberry, Michael and Ariane, "Fashion The Mirror of History," Greenwich House (Crown Publishers, Inc.,) New York, 1977

Blum, Stella, "Designs by Erte, Fashion Drawings and Illustrations from Harper's Bazar," Dover Publications, Inc., New York 1976

Cable News Network, "Style, with Elsa Klensch"

Cassin-Scott, Jack, "Costume and Fashion," Blandford Press, Ltd., London, England, 1971

Churchill, Allen, "Remember When," Golden Press, Inc., New York, 1967

Conoisseur, The Hearst Corporation, New York, August 1989

Culmer, John and Rayner, Nicholas, "The Jewels of the Duchess of Windsor," Vendome Press, New York, in association with Sotheby's, 1987

Davenport, Millia, "The Book of Costume, Volume I," Crown Publishers, N.Y. 1948

Delineator, The Butterick Publishing Company, New York

Deslandres, Yvonne, "Poiret," Rizzoli, New York, 1987

Dorner, Jane, "Fashion (The Changing Shape of Fashion Through the Years)," Octopus Books Ltd., London, England, 1974

Elle, Elle Publishing, Hachette Magazines, Inc., New York, February 1992

Esquire, New York, September 1947

Fraser, Kennedy, "The Fashionable Mind: Reflections on Fashion 1970—1981," Alfred A. Knopf, New York, 1981

Harper's Bazaar, New York

Hartford Courant, The, Hartford, Connecticut

Jones, Mablen, "Getting it On: The Clothing of Rock 'n Roll," Abbeville Press, New York, 1987

Ladies' Home Journal, The, The Curtis Publishing Co., Philadelphia, Pennsylvania

LaCroix, Paul, "Arts of the Middle Ages, The," Bickers & Son, London, England, 1870

Laver, James, "Costume and Fashion," Thames & Hudson, Inc., New York, 1985.

Lubke, Prof. Dr. W. and Lutzow, Prof. Dr. L.C., "Denkmaler der Kunst," Klassikes, Ausgabe, Stuttgart, Germany, 1893.

Lester, Katherine and Kerr, Rose, "Historic Costume," Chas. A. Bennett Co., Peoria, Illinois, 1925

McCalls, The McCalls Co., New York (1930-1935)

Mirabella, New York, March 1992

Motion Picture Magazine, Fawcett Publications, Inc., Greenwich, Connecticut, February 1948

Mulvagh, Jane, "Vogue History of 20th Century Fashion," Viking Press, London, England, 1988

New York Times, New York Times Magazine, New York

Robinson, Julian, *The Golden Age of Style,* Harcourt Brace Jovanovich, 1976

Ross, Josephine, *Beaton in Vogue,* Clarkson N. Potter, Inc., New York 1986

Schroeder, Joseph J., Jr., Editor, "Sears Roebuck and Co., Fall 1900," DBI Books, Inc., Northfield, Illinois, 1970

"This Fabulous Century, 1930-1940," Time-Life Books, Inc., New York, 1988

USA Today, Arlington, Virginia (May 13, 1992)

Vogue, New York

Vertes, Marcel, and Byam Holme, *Art and Fashion,* Studio Publications Inc., New York and London, and Plantin Press and Albert Davis, 1944.

Webb, Wilfred Mark, *The Heritage of Dress,* E. Grant Richards, London, England, 1907

Yarwood, Doreen, *The Encyclopedia of World Costume,* Scribner Book Co., New York, 1978

Index

Adolfo, 201, 210
Alaia, Azzedine, 190
Alexander of Paris, 211
Altman, B. & Co., 109, 115
American Bandstand, 160, 212
Antoinette, Marie, 18, 211
Armani, Georgio, 192, 210, 233
Astaire, Fred, 93

Baker, Josephine, 171
Baker, Mel, 233
Balenciaga, 109, 135
Barbier, George, 50
Barclay, McClelland, 91, 106
Barerra, Javier, 199
Bean, L. L., 178
Beaton, Cecil, 87, 90
Becker, Rosalind, 232, 233
Becker, Sherman, 233
Bedrick, Brenda, 233
Bell DeLuxe, 149
Berenson, Marisa, 185
Bergdorf Goodman, 109, 135, 138
Bernhardt, Sarah, 173
Billy Boy, 196
Black Starr & Frost, 137
Blass, Bill, 166
Bloomingdale's, 210
Bogart, Humphrey, 115
Bonaparte, Napolean, 19
Bonnie and Clyde, 94
Bonwit Teller, 135
Boucher, Marcel and Sandra, 114, 152
Boucheron, 211
Bourjois, 116
Boy of London, 191
Brummell, Beau, 19, 20
Buckley, Nadja, 114, 135
Bulgari, 192
Burr-McIntosh Monthly, 39
Bursalino, 148
Burton, Robert, 234
BVD Underwear, 104

Cagney, James, 115
Calet-Hirsch, 211
Calet, Neil, 211
Caligula, 12
Camarino, Roberta, 156
Campbell, Mrs. Patrick, 77
Canovas, Isabel, 212, 213, 224, 225, 226, 227, 228, 229
Capone, Al, 94
Cardin, Pierre, 163, 187, 201, 203
Cardinal Parfums, 99
Carnegie, Hattie, 110, 114, 154
Cartier, 114, 135, 201, 211
Castle, Vernon and Irene, 50, 52
Castlecliff, 161
Centennial Exposition, 85
Cerio, Keith, 190
Chanel, "Coco", 7, 67, 85, 89, 90, 93, 98, 109, 114, 199, 139, 141, 161, 173, 176, 179,

187, 201, 203, 210, 211, 213, 221
Charlemagne, The Emperor, 13
Charles II, 16, 17
Chen Yu, 116
Chow, Tina, 240
Christy, Howard Chandler, 106
Churchill, Alan, 26, 52
Ciner, 144
Ciro of Bond Street, 135
Clark, Dick, 160
Claudius, The Emperor, 12
Clausen, Susan, 221
Cleopatra, 173
Cne, Ora, 62
Cole of California, 135
College Humor, 71
Colombo, Michael, 233
Comm de Garcons, 211
Confucius, 191
Coro, 103, 114, 128
Corocraft, 103
Coty Award, The, 167, 212
Council of Fashion Design of America, 214
Courreges, Andre, 163, 173, 176, 178
Country Life, 95
Crawford, Joan, 111, 115
Cutex, 117

Dana Perfume, 135
Daniel, 149
de la Renta, Oscar, 179, 210
Delineator, The, 32, 85
DeLiso Debs, 161
Del'Olio, Louis, 214
de Pompadour, Madame, 18
Designer, The
Dior, Christian, 118, 119, 135, 139, 161, 185, 210, 213
Disraeli, Benjamin, 21
Dorset, 149
DuBarry Cosmetics, 112
Dubbs, John F., 106
Dufy, Raoul, 47
Duncan, Isadora, 71
Durbin, Deanna, 111

Echo, 178
Edward III, 13
Edward VII, 50
Eisenberg, 91, 100, 114
Elizabeth, The Empress, 21
Ellis, Perry, 240
Erte, 48, 49, 70, 181, 185, 201, 233
Esquire, 115
Eugenie, The Empress, 109, 119
Evans Compacts, 102, 129
Exquisite Form, 161

Fairchild, John, 214
Ferragamo, 193
Ferre, Gianfranco, 203
Fiorucci, 182
Fisher, Harrison, 32

Flato, Paul, 94
Florenza, 153
Forbes & Wallace, 38, 56, 65
Fortuny, Mariano, 30
Francis, Kay, 100
Fraser, Kennedy, 163, 167, 175
Frazier, Brenda, 94
Frederick II, 18
Frederics, John, 161
Frenchie, 118
Frowick, Roy, 169
Fuller, Arthur, 79

Gage, Elizabeth, 208
Galliano, John, 189
George IV, 19
Gernreich, Rudi, 163
Gherardi, Gai, 191
Gibson, Charles Dana, 77
Gigli, Romeo, 203
Ginza Art Space Gallery, 191
Glamour, 137
Glass, Leo, 158
Glentex, 109
Grable, Betty, 210
Gray, Dorothy, 115, 149
Greenwich Village, 50
Gualtier, Jean Paul, 188, 189, 191, 193, 203
Gucci, 185, 187

Halsey, Edwin, 62
Halston, 179, 201, 240
Hamilton, Andrew, 30
Hamilton Watch Co., The, 30, 88, 166
Harlow, Jean, 93, 214
Haring, Keith, 240
Harpers Bazaar, 48, 49, 56, 85, 70, 90, 93, 94, 104, 112, 113, 119, 135, 161, 175
Haskell, Miriam, 114, 128, 138, 144, 145, 152
Held, John, Jr., 77
Hendrix, Jimi, 172
Henriette, 113
Henry III, 14
Henry VIII, 14
Hepburn, Katharine, 111
Hermes, 90, 92, 187, 194, 204, 205
Hobe, 114
Homer, 163
Hudnut, Richard, 52, 63
Huston, Virginia, 126
Hutton, Barbara, 94

Icing, The, 232, 233
Illinois Watch Case Co., 149
Ingersoll Watch Co., 21
International Silver Co., 30

Joseff of Hollywood (Eugene Joseff), 100, 114, 126, 190
Josef, 161
Joseph, Franz, 21

Josephine, The Empress, 19
Jourdan, Charles, 173
Junot, Laure, 19
Justinian, The Emperor, 12
Juvenal, 12

K & K, 149
Karan, Donna, 233
Katz, Adolph, 114
Kazo, 210
Kelly, Grace, 204
Kelly, Patrick, 240
Kemp, Harry, 50
Kennedy, Jacqueline, 166
Kieselstein-Cord, Barry, 202, 212
Kieselstein-Cord, CeCe, 202
Klein, Anne, 214
Klein, Calvin, 186
Klensch, Elsa, 214
Knapp Hats, 104
Knickerbocker, Cholly, 71
Kramer, 161

l.a. Eyeworks, 142, 143, 165, 191
Lackawanna Underwear, 104
LaCroix, Christian, 210, 211
Ladies Home Journal, 20, 30, 45, 49, 62, 85
Lagerfeld, Karl, 114, 176, 203, 211, 212, 214, 216, 218, 219, 220, 223, 233
Landrigan, E.J., Inc./Verdura, 211
Lane, Kenneth Jay, 94, 146, 153, 170, 173, 180, 187, 190
Langtry, Lily, 20
Lauren, Ralph, 178, 187, 195
Laver, James, 13, 16, 175
La Vie Parisienne, 48
Lalique, 59, 85
Lanvin, 203
Leiber, Judith, 167, 198, 217
Leighton, Fred, 232
Lelong, Lucien, 109
Lepape, George, 48
Lesage, 127
Liberty, Arthur, 30
Liberty of London, 30, 71, 178
Life Magazine, 204
Limoges, 102
Lombard, Carole, 93
Lord & Taylor, 39, 105, 135
Louis XIV, 17
Ludot, Didier, 29, 141

Macaronis, 17, 19
Mackie, Bob, 190, 203
Macy, R. H. & Co., 85, 109
Mademoiselle Shoes, 165
Magli, Bruno, 212
Mandalian, 78
Marvella, 173
Matisse, 155
Mauboussin, 107
McLaren, Malcolm, 214
McMein, Neysa, 46
McReynolds, Barbara, 191
Mel and Me, 233
Menjou, Adolf, 93
Menichetti, Lee, 181
Mercier, Jean, 69, 78
Mikimoto, 109
Miller, Nicole, 213, 214, 215
Miller, Nolan, 190
Mirabella, 210
Miranda, Carmen, 114
Mix, Tom, 71
Miyake, Issey, 211
Molyneaux, 93
Monroe, Marilyn, 201

Montana, Claude, 203
Montgomery Ward & Co., 90
Mori, Hanae, 211
Morris, Robert Lee, 186, 188, 212, 213, 231
Morris, William, 20
Morton, Frederic, 21
Moschino, 213, 214
Motion Picture Magazine, 135
Muuntox, 181

Napier Co., The, 211
Nelson, Lord, 19
New Yorker, The, 175
New York Times, The, 175, 190

Olsen, Elida, 232, 233
Onyx Hosiery, 104
Orlane, 145
Ovid, 12

Panetta, 114
Paretti, Elsa, 208
Paris Vogue, 176
Parker, Dorothy, 77, 87
Patou, Jean, 85
Penn, William, 30
Pepys, Samuel, 16
Pershing, General Jack, 30
Phillipe Model Shoes, 213
Philippe, Alfred, 114
Picasso, Paloma, 188, 195, 200
Pictorial Review, 79
Picturesque Hosiery, 132
Plasir de France, 107
Plato, 10
Plaza Hotel, The, 77
Poiret, Paul, 47, 66, 67, 70, 74, 88, 119, 139, 167
Poiret Perfume Co., 73
Prince Matchabelli, 98
Pucci, Emilio, 166, 170, 176
Punch, 50

Quant, Mary, 163

Rabanne, Paco, 110, 163, 164
Rambova, Natasha, 52
Reikawa of Kubo, 211
Reja, 161
Rex Fifth Avenue, 149
Richelieu, 190
Robert (Robert Levy), 138, 145, 170, 171
Rockwell, Norman, 114
Rogers, Ginger, 93
Rolex, 187
Rose, Robert, 211
Rosenstein, Nettie, 114, 115, 121
Roth, Christian Francis, 214
Rousseau, 18
Roz and Sherm, 232, 233
Rufus, Aurelius, 208
Russian Ballet, The, 47

Saint Laurent, Yves, 139, 166, 168, 175, 179, 187, 188, 195, 211
Saks Fifth Avenue, 109
Samuels, Laura, 62
Sandor, 170, 171
Sarasola, Lisandro, 179
Sary, Anne, 148
Savoy Hotel, The, 48
Scarisbrick, Diana, 95
Scassi, Arnold, 210
Schiaparelli, Elsa, 7, 87, 89, 90, 98, 109, 114, 132, 149, 157

Schreiner, 153
Sears, Roebuck & Co., 45, 90
Selro, 155, 180
Shiseido Corporation, The, 191
Siegel, Bugsy, 94
Sik, Kai, 181
Silberstein, Nina, 138
Silberstein, Stanley, 232
Simpson, Wallis Warfield, 93
Smith, Willi, 240
Standard Spats, 56, 85
Stein, Catherine, 11
Strauss, Levi, 21
Stetson Hats, 117
Stratton Compacts, 149
Style, 70, 71
Sui, Ana, 214
Suzy, 93

Temple, Shirley, 94
Textile Color Card of America, 50
Theodora, The Empress, 12, 13, 163
Tiffany & Co., 114, 137, 208
Tre-Jur, 104
Trifari, 114, 130, 161
Turner, Lana, 111
Tuttankhamen, 70
Twain, Mark, 31, 203
Twiggy, 170

Ungaro, Emanuel, 203, 210
Uozumi, Sachiko, 197

Valentino, 203, 211
Valentino, Rudolph, 52, 71
Valle, A., 48
Vallee, Rudy, 71
Van Cleef & Arpels, 137, 161
Venida Hair Nets, 104
Vera, 146
Verdura, (The Duke di Verdura - Fulco Santostefano della Cerda), 93, 94, 95, 136, 211
Versace, Gianni, 210
Vertes, Marcel, 7, 9, 17, 18, 20, 29, 47, 67, 89, 175
Victoria, Queen, 20
Vionnet, Madeleine, 85, 87
Vogue, 49, 87, 90, 94, 109, 111, 114, 173, 185
Vogue European Ready-to-Wear, 176
Voltaire, 18
Volupte, 149
Vreeland, Diana, 94
Vuitton, Louis, 178, 194, 212, 213

"W", 114, 176, 214
Wadsworth, 161
Warhol, Andy, 240
Webb, David, 138, 169, 232
Webb, Wilfred Mark, 9, 14
Wellington, The Duke of, 21
Westwood, Vivienne, 6, 66, 214, 222, 223, 232
Whiting and Davis, 78, 84
Wilde, Oscar, 137
Windsor, The Duchess of, 187
Windsor, The Duke of, 93
Winston, Harry, 137, 199, 206, 209, 217
Woman's Home Companion, The, 29
Women's Wear Daily, 214
Woodbury Co., 103
"World's End," 214
Worth, Charles Frederick, 22

Yamamoto, Johji, 211